Child and Adolescent: Mental Health and Psychiatry

Child and Adolescent: Mental Health and Psychiatry

Edited by Laurel Harper

hayle
medical

New York

Hayle Medical,
750 Third Avenue, 9th Floor,
New York, NY 10017, USA

Visit us on the World Wide Web at:
www.haylemedical.com

ISBN: 978-1-63241-741-1

Cataloging-in-Publication Data

Child and adolescent : mental health and psychiatry / edited by Laurel Harper.
    p. cm.
Includes bibliographical references and index.
ISBN 978-1-63241-741-1
1. Child mental health. 2. Teenagers--Mental health. 3. Child psychiatry.
4. Young adults--Psychology. 5. Psychiatry. I. Harper, Laurel.
RJ499 .C45 2019
618.928 9--dc23

Table of Contents

Preface

This book has been a concerted effort by a group of academicians, researchers and scientists, who have contributed their research works for the realization of the book. This book has materialized in the wake of emerging advancements and innovations in this field. Therefore, the need of the hour was to compile all the required researches and disseminate the knowledge to a broad spectrum of people comprising of students, researchers and specialists of the field.

Psychiatry is a medical specialty dealing with the diagnosis and treatment of mental illnesses. The diagnosis usually begins with a review of the case history of the patient. Other diagnostic methods include mental status examination, physical examinations, psychological tests and neuroimaging. Child and adolescent psychiatry, also known as pediatric psychiatry, is an important sub-field of psychiatry. It is concerned with the diagnosis and treatment of mental illnesses in children and adolescents. Some of the common disorders related to child and adolescent psychiatry include learning disorders, attention deficit hyperactivity disorder, panic disorder, bipolar disorder, depression, obsessive compulsive disorder, anorexia nervosa, bulimia nervosa and childhood onset schizophrenia. This book elucidates the concepts and innovative models around prospective developments with respect to child and adolescent psychiatry. It strives to provide a fair idea about this discipline and to help develop a better understanding of the latest advances within this field. The extensive content of this book provides the readers with a thorough understanding of the subject.

At the end of the preface, I would like to thank the authors for their brilliant chapters and the publisher for guiding us all-through the making of the book till its final stage. Also, I would like to thank my family for providing the support and encouragement throughout my academic career and research projects.

Editor

Child maltreatment in Germany: prevalence rates in the general population

Andreas Witt[1*†], Rebecca C. Brown[1†], Paul L. Plener[1], Elmar Brähler[2,3] and Jörg M. Fegert[1]

Abstract

Background: Child maltreatment and its consequences are considered a major public health problem. So far, there is only one study from Germany reporting prevalence rates on different types of maltreatment.

Methods: A representative sample of the German general population was examined for experiences of child maltreatment using the Childhood Trauma Questionnaire (CTQ) between September and November 2016. A total of 2510 (53.3% female) participants between 14 and 94 years (M = 48.8 years) were enrolled. Besides the CTQ, a range of sociodemographic information was collected. The interrelatedness of different types of maltreatment was examined using configuration analysis and predictors for maltreatment were identified by performing binary logistic regression analyses.

Results: Overall, 2.6% (f: 3.9%, m: 1.2%) of all participants reported severe emotional abuse, 3.3% (f: 3.4%, m: 3.3%) severe physical abuse, 2.3% (f: 3.7%, m: 0.7%) severe sexual abuse, 7.1% (f: 8.1%, m: 5.9%) severe emotional neglect and 9% (f: 9.2%, m: 8.9%) severe physical neglect. Women were more likely to report at least moderate sexual and emotional abuse than men. The largest difference between age groups was reported for physical neglect, with participants aged over 70 years reporting the highest rates. Participants who reported childhood maltreatment were more likely to be unemployed or have lower educational outcomes. The most common combination of maltreatment types were physical and emotional neglect, all five types of maltreatment combined and physical and emotional neglect and physical abuse combined.

Conclusions: Child maltreatment, especially physical neglect is common in the German population. Women seem to be at greater risk for sexual and emotional abuse than men. Knowledge about different types of maltreatment based on the Childhood Trauma Questionnaire (CTQ) can help to put findings of future studies into an epidemiological and societal context.

Keywords: Prevalence, Child maltreatment, Child abuse and neglect, Representative study

Background

Child maltreatment is considered a major public health problem [1–3]. The consequences of maltreatment are diverse and may affect victims throughout their whole lifespan via psychological and behavioral problems, as well as somatic disorders [1, 4–11]. As a consequence, in addition to these individual consequences, maltreatment causes high financial burden for society. Previous studies estimated annual expenses caused by maltreatment between 11 to 30 billion Euros for Germany [7] and up to 124 billion US Dollars per year in the US [8].

Results from international studies show that child maltreatment is highly prevalent. This is also true in high income countries where prevalence rates are comparable to those of widespread diseases [9, 10]. Meta-analyses on the prevalence of different types of maltreatment exist, and especially child sexual abuse having been reviewed repeatedly [10–13]. One meta-analyses showed varying prevalence rates mostly due to varying definitions, but also due to methodological factors, like small sample sizes, geographical regions or non-random designs

*Correspondence: Andreas.Witt@uniklinik-ulm.de
†Andreas Witt and Rebecca C. Brown contributed equally to this work
[1] Department of Child and Adolescent Psychiatry/Psychotherapy, University of Ulm, Steinhövelstr. 5, 89073 Ulm, Germany
Full list of author information is available at the end of the article

[11, 13]. One review by Stoltenborgh and colleagues [11] focused on the assessment of child sexual abuse in adult populations and included 331 independent samples with a total of almost 10 million participants. The overall prevalence for self-reported child sexual abuse was reported at around 12.7% (95% confidence interval (CI) 10.7–15.0%), 18% for women and 7.6% for men. These rates are comparable to those found in other meta-analyses [10, 12] and also in a meta-analysis focusing on prevalence rates of sexual abuse in adolescent populations [13]. Overall, females seem to be more often affected by sexual abuse than men.

For other types of maltreatment like neglect, the data base is less comprehensive. The so-called "neglect of neglect" is still evident in research [3, 14, 15]. Meta-analyses on physical and emotional abuse, as well as neglect show a high variation in prevalence rates [15–17]. Regarding physical abuse, prevalence rates of 22.6% (95% CI 19.6–26.1%) were reported by Stoltenborgh and colleagues [16], similar to 22.9% by Sethi and colleagues for the European Region [10]. Larger differences were reported for emotional abuse with a rate of 36.3% worldwide [17] and 29.1% reported from the European Union [10]. With regard to child neglect, Stoltenborgh and colleagues identified 19 independent samples, underlining the need for further studies on neglect. Prevalence rates were reported at 16.3% (95% CI 12.1–21.5) for physical and 18.4% (95% CI 13.0–25.4) for emotional neglect. In contrast to findings on sexual abuse, there does not seem to be a gender preponderance for the other types of maltreatment [3, 15–17].

For Germany, data on the prevalence of child maltreatment in the general population is limited to three data sets: two studies, which were conducted almost 20 years apart from each other, focused on the assessment of child sexual abuse [18–20]. They reported a marked decline of sexual abuse over a period of almost 20 years. Only one study reported on the prevalence of different types of maltreatment in the general population. The study was conducted in 2010 using the Childhood Trauma Questionnaire (CTQ) [21, 22] and reported a prevalence of 1.6% for severe emotional, 2.8% for severe physical, 1.9% for severe sexual abuse, and 6.6% for severe emotional and 10.8% for severe physical neglect [22].

In summary, data on the prevalence of different types of child maltreatment exist, however usually only general prevalence rates for different types of maltreatment and males and females are reported. On closer examination, prevalence rates vary considerably across different subgroups (e.g. age cohorts or gender) [18, 22]. As the CTQ has been used in a range of brain imaging studies as a covariate [23, 24] and it is a widely used screening instrument for the assessment of child maltreatment [22, 25, 26] recent data need to be made available to set new scientific findings into context and inform the debate of societal burden by childhood maltreatment.

The aim of the present study is to provide recent and detailed prevalence rates for all types of maltreatment as assessed by the CTQ (emotional, physical, and sexual abuse, as well as physical and emotional neglect) in a representative sample of the general population in Germany.

Methods
Procedure
Data collection took place between September and November 2016. Using a random route procedure, a representative sample of the German population was obtained by a demographic consulting company (USUMA, Berlin, Germany). The sample was representative in regard to age, gender, and geographic region. Households of every third residence in a randomly chosen street were invited to participate in the study. In multi-person households, participants were randomly selected using a Kish-Selection-Grid. For inclusion, participants had to be at least 14 years of age and have sufficient German language skills. Of 4902 designated addresses, 2510 households participated in the study. The main reason for non-participation was failure to contact anyone in the residence after four attempts (14.9%), refusal by the individual who answered the door to have anyone in the household participate in the study (15.3%), failure to contact the randomly selected household member after four attempts (2.3%) and refusal by the selected member to participate (14.7%).

Individuals who agreed to participate were given information about the study and provided informed consent. Participants were told that the study was about psychological health and well-being. Responses were anonymous. In a first step, socio-demographic information was obtained in an interview-format by the research staff. Then, the researcher handed out a copy of the questionnaire and a sealable envelope. The researcher remained nearby in case the participants needed further information. The completed questionnaires were linked to the respondent's demographic data, but did not contain name, address, or any other identifying information.

The study was conducted in accordance with the Declaration of Helsinki, and fulfilled the ethical guidelines of the International Code of Marketing and Social Research Practice of the International Chamber of Commerce and of the European Society of Opinion and Marketing Research. The study was approved by the Ethics Committee of the Medical Department of the University of Leipzig.

Measures

The sociodemographic section contained information on age, gender, citizenship, geographical area (East vs. West Germany, rural vs. urban area), educational and occupational status and partnership status. Additionally, an estimation of the equivalence income (household income divided by the square root of household size), according to OECD [27] was calculated.

The prevalence of five types of child maltreatment was assessed using the 28 item brief version of the Childhood Trauma Questionnaire (CTQ) [21, 28, 29]. The CTQ is a screening measure for the assessment of child maltreatment. The CTQ contains five subscales each assessed by 5 items, including sexual, emotional and physical abuse as well as emotional and physical neglect. Additionally, three items assess whether participants tend to minimize problematic experiences within their family. The psychometric properties of the German version of the CTQ have been demonstrated by Klinitzke and colleagues [21]. The internal consistency ranged between 0.62 and 0.96 for the subscales. The intra-class coefficient for an interval of 6 weeks was 0.77 for the overall scale and for subscales between 0.58 and 0.81. Based on norm data by Häuser and colleagues [22] severity scores for each subscale can be calculated, ranging from "none–minimal", "minimal–moderate", "moderate–severe", to "severe–extreme". For the prevalence analysis of the different types of maltreatment, a cut-off of at least "moderate–severe" was chosen.

Participants

A total of 2510 participants were included in the sample. Participants were on average 48.4 years old (SD = 18.2) and 53.3% were female. 3.2% reported a place of birth outside Germany. The sample was representative for the German population in regard to age and gender. The sociodemographic characteristics are presented in Table 1.

Statistical analyses

All analyses were conducted using SPSS version 21. Descriptive analyses were conducted for prevalence rates. Comparisons were conducted using χ^2 tests. To

Table 1 Demographic data

	Total (N = 2510)	Female (N = 1339)	Male (N = 1171)
Age			
Mean (standard deviation)	48.4 (18.2)	48.9 (18.1)	47.8 (18.4)
Range	14–94	14–94	14–93
Living with partner			
Yes	1370 (55%)	719 (54%)	651 (56.2%)
No	1119 (45%)	612 (46%)	507 (43.8%)
Citizenship			
German	2429 (96.8%)	1303 (97.3%)	1126 (96.2%)
Not German	81 (3.2%)	36 (2.7%)	45 (3.8%)
Geographical area			
Eastern Germany	505 (20.1%)	255 (19%)	921 (78.7%)
Western Germany	2005 (79.9%)	1084 (81%)	250 (21.3%)
Rural	1026 (40.9%)	548 (40.9)	478 (40.8%)
Urban	1484 (59.1%)	791 (59.1%)	693 (59.2%)
Occupational status			
Full-time	1074 (42.8%)	407 (30.4%)	667 (57%)
Part-time	281 (11.2%)	246 (18.4%)	35 (3%)
Hourly	60 (2.4%)	54 (4%)	6 (0.5%)
Federal volunteer service/parental leave	25 (1%)	22 (1.6%)	3 (0.3%)
Unemployed	131 (5.2%)	64 (4.8%)	67 (5.7%)
Retiree	638 (25.4%)	368 (27.5%)	270 (23.1%)
Homemaker	79 (3.1%)	77 (5.8%)	2 (0.2%)
In training	42 (1.7%)	21 (1.6%)	21 (1.8%)
Student	161 (6.4%)	70 (5.2%)	91 (7.8%)
Employment status			
Unemployed	131 (5.3%)	64 (4.8%)	67 (5.8%)
Employed	2360 (94.7%)	1265 (95.2%)	1095 (94.2%)

assess the co-occurrence of different types of child maltreatment a configuration analysis was conducted. Binary logistic regression analyses were conducted to identify predictors of childhood maltreatment. Age and gender were entered in the analyses as potential predictors.

Results

Of the N = 2487 participants who completed the CTQ, 31.0% (n = 772) reported at least one type of child maltreatment. Of all participants, 6.5% reported at least moderate emotional abuse, 6.7% reported physical abuse, 7.6% sexual abuse, 13.3% emotional neglect, and 22.5% reported physical neglect (for details see Table 2).

Co-morbidity of types of child maltreatment

Overall, 58.10% (N = 416) of those reporting any form of child maltreatment reported only one type of maltreatment. In detail, 47.15% (N = 265) of those reporting physical neglect (N = 562) 31.58% (N = 60 out of N = 190) of those reporting sexual abuse, 14.76% (N = 49 out of N = 332) of those reporting emotional neglect, 13.17% (N = 22 out of N = 167) of those reporting physical abuse, and 12.27% (N = 20 out of 163) of those reporting emotional abuse did not report another type of maltreatment. The most common combination of types of child maltreatment were physical and emotional neglect (13.99%), all five types of maltreatment combined

(3.89%) and physical and emotional neglect and physical abuse combined (3.50%) (for details see Table 3).

Predictors of moderate to severe types of maltreatment

Gender was shown to be a predictor for emotional and sexual abuse, with women reporting higher rates of both types of abuse (see Table 4; details on gender differences by severity of maltreatment are also presented in Table 2). Furthermore, age was identified as a predictor for physical neglect, with higher age being associated with higher prevalence rates (see Table 4; Fig. 1 for details).

Age differences concerning the prevalence of child maltreatment

The experience of at least one type of child maltreatment was reported most frequently in the oldest age group of 70+ (50.4%) and least often in the youngest age group of 14–19 years olds (13.4%). Participants aged between 20 and 69 years reported rather consistent rates of 24.3–33.8% (for details see Fig. 1). The largest difference between age groups was reported for physical neglect, with participants aged over 70 years reported much higher rates (46%) than participants of other age groups (for details see Fig. 1).

Regarding child abuse, highest rates of emotional and sexual abuse were reported in the age group of 40–49 year olds. Rates of childhood physical abuse were

Table 2 Prevalence of child maltreatment by severity

	N	None–minimal N (%)	Low–moderate N (%)	Moderate–severe N (%)	Severe–extreme N (%)
Emotional abuse					
Total	2492	2027 (80.8)	302 (12.0)	98 (3.9)	65 (2.6)
Female	1324	1053 (79.5)	156 (11.8)	64 (4.8)	51 (3.9)
Male	1168	974 (83.4)	146 (12.5)	34 (2.9)	14 (1.2)
Physical abuse					
Total	2497	2185 (87.1)	145 (5.8)	83 (3.3)	84 (3.3)
Female	1330	1165 (87.6)	79 (5.9)	41 (3.1)	45 (3.4)
Male	1167	1020 (87.4)	66 (5.7)	42 (3.6)	39 (3.3)
Sexual abuse					
Total	2496	2148 (85.6)	158 (6.3)	133 (5.3)	57 (2.3)
Female	1329	1090 (82.0)	89 (6.7)	101 (7.6)	49 (3.7)
Male	1167	1058 (90.7)	69 (5.9)	32 (2.7)	8 (0.7)
Emotional neglect					
Total	2496	1486 (59.2)	678 (27.0)	155 (6.2)	177 (7.1)
Female	1329	809 (60.9)	334 (25.1)	78 (5.9)	108 (8.1)
Male	1167	677 (58.0)	344 (29.5)	77 (6.6)	69 (5.9)
Physical neglect					
Total	2496	1452 (57.8)	482 (19.2)	336 (13.4)	226 (9.0)
Female	1329	786 (59.1)	251 (18.9)	170 (12.8)	122 (9.2)
Male	1167	666 (57.1)	231 (19.8)	166 (14.2)	104 (8.9)

Table 3 Prevalence of different types and combinations of maltreatment

Type/combination of maltreatment	N	Percent in relation to participants with at least one type of maltreatment (N = 772)
Emotional abuse (EA) only	20	2.59
Physical abuse (PA) only	22	2.85
Sexual abuse (SA) only	60	7.77
Emotional neglect (EN) only	49	6.35
Physical neglect (PN) only	265	34.33
EA + PA	4	0.52
EA + SA	12	1.55
EA + EN	13	1.68
EA + PN	5	0.65
PA + SA	1	0.13
PA + EN	3	0.39
PA + PN	11	1.42
SA + EN	3	0.39
SA + PN	13	1.68
EN + PN	108	13.99
EA + PA + SA	3	0.39
EA + PA + EN	18	2.33
EA + PA + PN	4	0.52
EA + SA + EN	4	0.52
EA + SA + PN	3	0.39
EA + EN + PN	7	0.91
PA + SA + EN	1	0.13
PA + SA + PN	4	0.52
PA + EN + PN	27	3.50
SA + EN + PN	20	2.59
EA + PA + SA + EN	2	0.26
EA + PA + SA + PN	10	1.30
EA + PA + EN + PN	21	2.72
EA + SA + EN + PN	6	0.78
PA + SA + EN + PN	14	1.81
EA + PA + SA + EN + PN	30	3.89

EA emotional abuse, *PA* physical abuse, *SA* sexual abuse, *EN* emotional neglect, *PN* physical neglect

higher in older age groups than in younger participants (see Fig. 2).

Socio-demographic variables and childhood maltreatment

All five types of child maltreatment were analyzed separately regarding different socio-demographic variables (being employed or unemployed, level of education and equivalence income). Participants who were unemployed, had a lower level of education and a lower equivalence income reported highest rates of emotional abuse, physical abuse, and physical and emotional neglect. Sexual abuse was reported more often by unemployed participants (for details see Table 5).

Discussion
Prevalence rates

The aim of the present study was to provide recent prevalence data on five types of child maltreatment, assessed with the CTQ in the general population in Germany. Detailed prevalence rates are presented separately for 10 age cohorts, gender, different demographic variables and severity. Additionally, co-occurrences of and predictors for different types of maltreatment analysed. The methodology of the present study was identical to the study of Häuser and colleagues [22], who assessed child maltreatment using the CTQ in the general population of Germany. In general, prevalence rates found in the present study again underline that child maltreatment, especially physical neglect, is rather common in the general population of Germany. Overall, rates found by Häuser and colleagues, were replicated [22]. In the current sample 2.6% reported severe emotional, 3.3% severe physical and 2.3% severe sexual abuse. Additionally 7.1% reported severe emotional and 9% severe physical neglect. Compared to Häuser and colleagues [22], the rates for all types of maltreatment (except physical neglect, with 10.7), were higher: For severe emotional abuse, they reported a rate of 1.6, 2.8% for physical abuse, 1.9% for sexual abuse and 6.6% for emotional neglect. However, those higher

Table 4 Binary logistic regressions for predictors of different types of maltreatment

Dependent variable	Independent variable	Odds ratio (OR)	95% confidence interval (CI)	β	p
Emotional abuse	Gender	0.444	0.313–0.629	−0.812	<.001
	Age	0.997	0.988–1.006	−0.003	.547
Physical abuse	Gender	1.114	0.81–1.530	0.108	.504
	Age	1.008	0.999–1.017	0.008	.065
Sexual abuse	Gender	0.281	0.196–0.403	−1.269	<.001
	Age	1.004	0.995–1.012	0.004	.406
Emotional neglect	Gender	0.871	0.688–1.102	−0.139	.249
	Age	1.005	0.998–1.011	0.005	.148
Physical neglect	Gender	1.103	0.908–1.340	0.098	.325
	Age	1.027	1.021–1.032	0.026	<.001

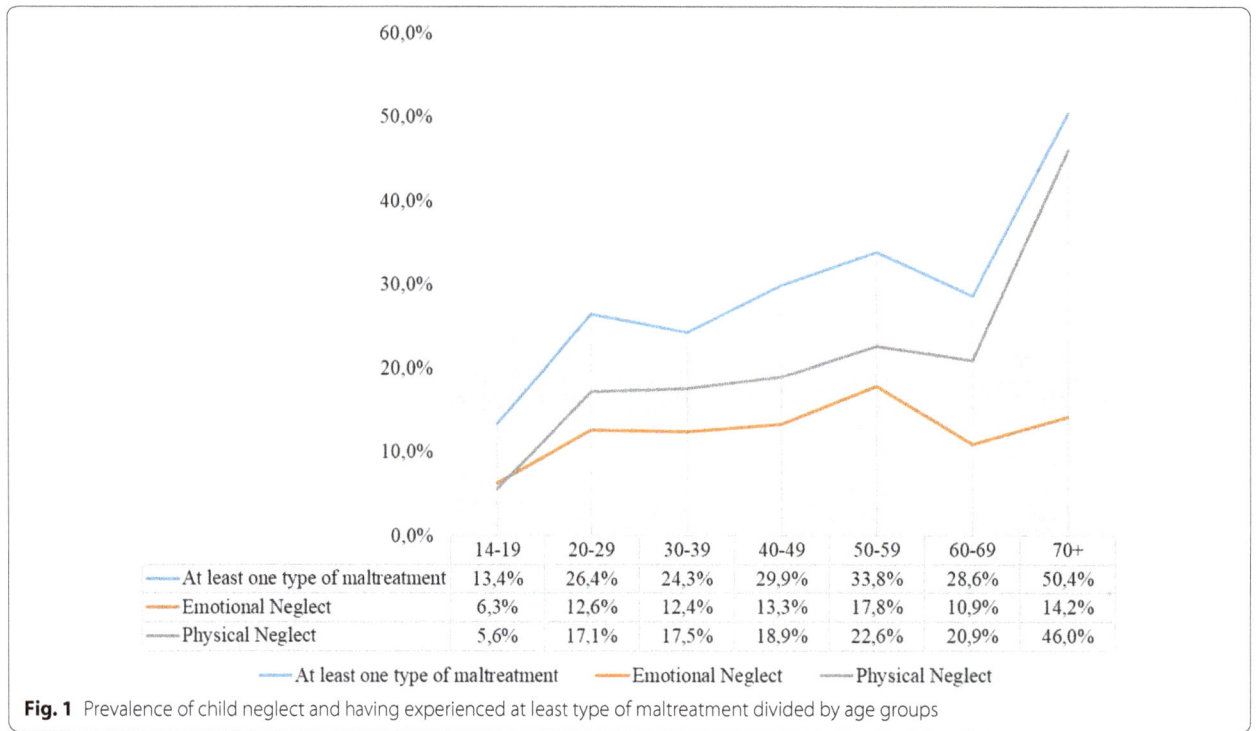

	14-19	20-29	30-39	40-49	50-59	60-69	70+
At least one type of maltreatment	13,4%	26,4%	24,3%	29,9%	33,8%	28,6%	50,4%
Emotional Neglect	6,3%	12,6%	12,4%	13,3%	17,8%	10,9%	14,2%
Physical Neglect	5,6%	17,1%	17,5%	18,9%	22,6%	20,9%	46,0%

Fig. 1 Prevalence of child neglect and having experienced at least type of maltreatment divided by age groups

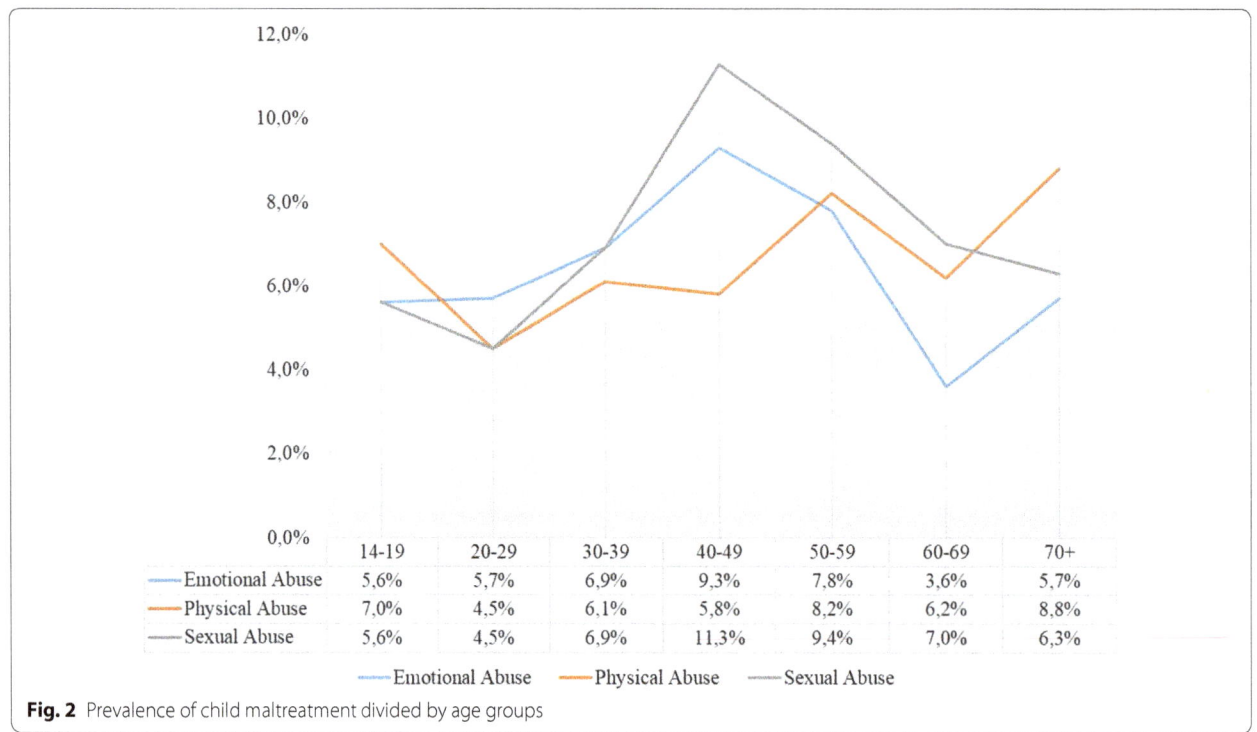

	14-19	20-29	30-39	40-49	50-59	60-69	70+
Emotional Abuse	5,6%	5,7%	6,9%	9,3%	7,8%	3,6%	5,7%
Physical Abuse	7,0%	4,5%	6,1%	5,8%	8,2%	6,2%	8,8%
Sexual Abuse	5,6%	4,5%	6,9%	11,3%	9,4%	7,0%	6,3%

Fig. 2 Prevalence of child maltreatment divided by age groups

rates might represent statistical variation and have to be examined for statistical significance. An explanation for the rise in prevalence rates may be due to an increased awareness in the general population. In 2010, right at the time, when the data collection of the study of Häuser and colleagues [22] took place, the so called abuse scandals in the Roman Catholic Church and in educational institutions with high reputations [30] came aware to the public. In its aftermath a public and political discussion about sexual abuse, but also other types of maltreatment started and a range of measures for intervention and better prevention were taken. This broad discussion might have led to a higher awareness about sexual abuse and child maltreatment in general and might have given rise to reported rates of childhood maltreatment in our study. In contrast the prevalence for physical neglect is smaller in the present study compared to Häuser and colleagues [22].

In comparison to prevalence rates for sexual abuse reported in meta-analyses, the rate of the present study for at least having experienced moderate sexual abuse is rather low [10–12]. The prevalence rate for physical neglect was higher compared to those found by Stoltenborgh and colleagues [15]. Emotional and physical neglect also have been found to be most common type of maltreatment in the US [31].

Comparison of age cohorts

Older age was a significant predictor of physical neglect. The rates for physical neglect were the highest among those of 70 years and older with about 46%. This generation was born in, or before 1946 and therefore survived World War II and the period after the war. This period was marked by hardship for the population, thus making high rates of physical neglect not astonishing among this particular group. This age group is no longer as strongly represented in the present study as compared to Häuser and colleagues [22] due to demographic changes in the population therefore explaining lower rates of physical neglect in our sample in comparison to this former study.

Although not significantly, rates for physical abuse seemed to be declining from the oldest age cohorts towards the youngest, albeit an increase among the youngest age cohort. This general decrease from the oldest age cohorts towards those between 20 and 29 years might be due to change in norms in the society and the legal ban on physical punishment in Germany in the year 2000 [32, 33], with the higher rates in the youngest age cohort maybe explained by a clearer recall of physical abuse. For emotional and sexual abuse the pattern was quite different. For both types of maltreatment, highest prevalence rates were observed in the age group of 40–49 year olds. Quite interestingly, the present study found a steep increase in prevalence rates for sexual abuse among the age cohorts of 40–49 year olds and 50–59 year olds. However, it remains unclear whether this result represents an actual increase in rates or represents an increase in reporting due to an increased perception of the problem because of changes in social norms. The rates for emotional neglect seemed to be relatively stable across age groups. In general repeated surveys in student populations would be necessary to identify changes over time.

Maltreatment and sociodemographic variables

Concerning other socio-demographic variables, the results generally show a higher prevalence of different types of maltreatment among those with a lower sociodemographic status. This becomes apparent in education and employment status and consequently in the monthly equivalence income, thus pointing towards the lifelong consequences of maltreatment also on the societal level that have been described in the literature [1, 5, 7, 8].

Table 5 Prevalence of child maltreatment by socio-demographic variables

	N total	Emotional abuse N (%)	Physical abuse N (%)	Sexual abuse N (%)	Emotional neglect N (%)	Physical neglect N (%)
Employed/unemployed						
Employed	2332	144 (6.1)	150 (6.4)	172 (7.3)	304 (13.0)	520 (22.1)
Unemployed	127	19 (14.6)	17 (13.2)	17 (13.1)	26 (20.0)	38 (29.7)
Chi²		14.35**	8.98*	5.78*	5.30*	3.97*
Education						
Did not graduate school	55	10 (18.2)	11 (20.0)	8 (14.5)	14 (25.5)	17 (30.9)
Graduated school	2103	136 (6.5)	148 (7.0)	164 (7.8)	299 (14.2)	507 (24.1)
University degree	247	15 (6.1)	4 (1.6)	15 (6.0)	16 (6.5)	34 (13.8)
Chi²		11.95*	25.87**	4.55	17.80**	14.85*
Equivalence income						
<1250€/month	544	47 (8.6)	43 (7.9)	46 (8.5)	91 (16.7)	152 (27.9)
1250–2500€/month	1469	75 (5.1)	80 (5.4)	94 (6.4)	168 (11.4)	311 (21.2)
>2500€/month	392	17 (4.3)	16 (4.1)	26 (6.6)	47 (12)	62 (15.8)
Chi²		10.94**	6.94*	2.7	10.2**	20.7***

* p<.05, ** p<.001

Female gender was found to be a significant predictor for sexual and emotional abuse. Especially the finding on sexual abuse is in line with findings from meta-analyses that report a preponderance for female gender [3, 10–12], and do not report a skewed distribution for the other types of maltreatment [15–17].

Co-occurrence of different types of maltreatment
As literature demonstrates, different types of child maltreatment are interrelated and the co-occurrence of different types of maltreatment is rather the rule than the exception [34]. Due to observing a population based sample, the rates of co-occurrences of different types of maltreatment were lower than reported from clinical samples [35]. Additionally, the present study included a high number of participants reporting physical neglect without having experienced any other type of maltreatment. However, results show that both types of neglect (physical and emotional) often co-occur, as well as combinations with other types of abuse, such as emotional and physical abuse.

Limitations
The retrospective assessment of child maltreatment may always be affected by different biases e.g. recollection biases. The random rout approach systematically excludes people that are currently residing in institutions. Therefore certain high risk-samples such as residents of child welfare institutions with a high prevalence of sexual abuse [36] may have been underrepresented in the current sample.

Conclusions
Child maltreatment, especially physical neglect, is common among the general population of Germany. Physical neglect is highly prevalent in the (post) World War II generation and steadily declines towards the youngest age group. In general, experiences of child maltreatment are associated with a lower sociodemographic status. Women are more likely to report at least moderate levels of emotional and sexual abuse than men. Different types of maltreatment, especially physical and emotional neglect, seem to co-occur frequently.

Authors' contributions
AW and RB analyzed and interpreted the data. RB carefully read the manuscript and provided a language editing. PLP, JMF and EB were involved in planning the study, drafting the manuscript and language editing. All authors read and approved the final manuscript.

Author details
[1] Department of Child and Adolescent Psychiatry/Psychotherapy, University of Ulm, Steinhövelstr. 5, 89073 Ulm, Germany. [2] Department of Psychosomatic Medicine and Psychotherapy, University Medical Center of Johannes Gutenberg University Mainz, Mainz, Germany. [3] Department of Medical Psychology and Medical Sociology, University of Leipzig, Leipzig, Germany.

Competing interests
AW, RB, EB state that they have no competing interests.

JMF has received research funding from the EU, DFG (German Research Foundation), BMG (Federal Ministry of Health), BMBF (Federal Ministry of Education and Research), BMFSFJ (Federal Ministry of Family, Senior Citizens, Women and Youth), German armed forces, several state ministries of social affairs, State Foundation Baden-Württemberg, Volkswagen Foundation, European Academy, Pontifical Gregorian University, RAZ, CJD, Caritas, Diocese of Rottenburg-Stuttgart. Moreover, he received travel grants, honoraria and sponsoring for conferences and medical educational purposes from DFG, AACAP, NIMH/NIH, EU, Pro Helvetia, Janssen-Cilag (J&J), Shire, several universities, professional associations, political foundations, and German federal and state ministries during the last 5 years. Every grant and every honorarium has to be declared to the law office of the University Hospital Ulm. Professor Fegert holds no stocks of pharmaceutical companies.

PLP has received research funding from the Bundesinstitut für Arzneimittel und Medizinprodukte, BMBF (Federal Ministry of Education and Research), VW-Foundation, Baden-Württemberg Stiftung, Lundbeck, Servier. Professor Plener holds no stocks of pharmaceutical companies.

Funding
Not applicable.

References
1. Gilbert R, Widom CS, Browne K, Fergusson DM, Webb E, Janson S. Burden and consequences of child maltreatment in high-income countries. Lancet. 2009;373:68–81.
2. Fegert JM, Stotzel M. Child protection: a universal concern and a permanent challenge in the field of child and adolescent mental health. Child Adolesc Psychiatry Ment Health. 2016;10:18.
3. Jud A, Fegert JM, Finkelhor D. On the incidence and prevalence of child maltreatment: a research agenda. Child Adolesc Psychiatry Ment Health. 2016;10:17.
4. Weber S, Jud A, Landolt MA. Quality of life in maltreated children and adult survivors of child maltreatment: a systematic review. Qual Life Res. 2016;25(2):237–55. doi:10.1007/s11136-015-1085-5.
5. De Bellis MD. Developmental traumatology: the psychobiological development of maltreated children and its implications for research, treatment, and policy. Dev Psychopathol. 2001;13:539–64.
6. Norman RE, Byambaa M, De R, Butchart A, Scott J, Vos T. The long-term health consequences of child physical abuse, emotional abuse, and neglect: a systematic review and meta-analysis. PLoS Med. 2012;9:e1001349.
7. Habetha S, Bleich S, Weidenhammer J, Fegert JM. A prevalence-based approach to societal costs occurring in consequence of child abuse and neglect. Child Adolesc Psychiatry Ment Health. 2012;6:35.
8. Fang X, Brown DS, Florence CS, Mercy JA. The economic burden of child maltreatment in the United States and implications for prevention. Child Abuse Negl. 2012;36:156–65.
9. Gilbert R, Fluke J, O'Donnell M, Gonzalez-Izquierdo A, Brownell M, Gulliver P, et al. Child maltreatment: variation in trends and policies in six developed countries. Lancet. 2012;379:758–72.
10. Sethi D, Bellis M, Hughes K, Gilbert R, Mitis F, Galea G. European report on preventing child maltreatment. Copenhagen: World Health Organisation Regional Office for Europe; 2013.
11. Stoltenborgh M, van Ijzendoorn MH, Euser EM, Bakermans-Kranenburg MJ. A global perspective on child sexual abuse: meta-analysis of prevalence around the world. Child Maltreat. 2011;16:79–101.
12. Pereda N, Guilera G, Forns M, Gomez-Benito J. The international epidemiology of child sexual abuse: a continuation of Finkelhor (1994). Child Abuse Negl. 2009;33:331–42.
13. Barth J, Bermetz L, Heim E, Trelle S, Tonia T. The current prevalence of child sexual abuse worldwide: a systematic review and meta-analysis. Int J Public Health. 2013;58:469–83.

14. McSherry D. Understanding and addressing the "neglect of neglect": why are we making a mole-hill out of a mountain? Child Abuse Negl. 2007;31:607–14.

15. Stoltenborgh M, Bakermans-Kranenburg MJ, van Ijzendoorn MH. The neglect of child neglect: a meta-analytic review of the prevalence of neglect. Soc Psychiatry Psychiatr Epidemiol. 2013;48:345–55.

16. Stoltenborgh M, Bakermans-Kranenburg MJ, van Ijzendoorn MH, Alink LR. Cultural–geographical differences in the occurrence of child physical abuse? A meta-analysis of global prevalence. Int J Psychol. 2013;48:81–94.

17. Stoltenborgh M, Bakermans-Kranenburg MJ, Alink LR, van Ijzendoorn MH. The universality of childhood emotional abuse: a meta-analysis of worldwide prevalence. J Aggress Maltreat Trauma. 2012;21:870–90.

18. Stadler L, Bieneck S, Wetzels P. Viktimisierung durch sexuellen Kindesmissbrauch: befunde national-repräsentativer Dunkelfeldforschung zu Entwicklungstrends in Deutschland. Praxis der Rechtspsychologie. 2012;22:190–220.

19. Wetzels P. Zur Epidemiologie physischer und sexueller Gewalterfahrungen in der Kindheit: Ergebnisse einer repräsentativen retrospektiven Prävalenzstudie für die BRD. Hannover: Kriminilogisches Forschungsinstitut Niedersachsen; 1997.

20. Stadler L, Bieneck S, Pfeiffer C. Repräsentativbefragung Sexueller Missbrauch 2011: Forschungsbericht Nr. 118. Hanover: Kriminologisches Forschungsinstitut Niedersachsen; 2012.

21. Klinitzke G, Romppel M, Hauser W, Brahler E, Glaesmer H. The German Version of the Childhood Trauma Questionnaire (CTQ): psychometric characteristics in a representative sample of the general population. Psychother Psychosom Med Psychol. 2012;62:47–51.

22. Häuser W, Schmutzer G, Brähler E, Glaesmer H. Misshandlung in Kindheit und Jugend: ergebnisse einer Umfrage in einer repräsentativen Stichprobe der deutschen Bevölkerung. Deutsches Ärzteblatt. 2011;108:287–311.

23. Quidé Y, Ong XH, Mohnke S, Schnell K, Walter H, Carr VJ, Green MJ. Childhood trauma-related alterations in brain function during a Theory-of-Mind task in schizophrenia. Schizophr Res. 2017. doi:10.1016/j.schres.2017.02.012.

24. Dannlowski U, Stuhrmann A, Beutelmann V, Zwanzger P, Lenzen T, Grotegerd D, et al. Limbic scars: long-term consequences of childhood maltreatment revealed by functional and structural magnetic resonance imaging. Biol Psychiatry. 2012;71:286–93.

25. Glaesmer H. Assessing childhood maltreatment on the population level in Germany: findings and methodological challenges. Child Adolesc Psychiatry Ment Health. 2016;10:15.

26. Hovdestad W, Campeau A, Potter D, Tonmyr L. A systematic review of childhood maltreatment assessments in population-representative surveys since 1990. PLoS ONE. 2015;10:e0123366.

27. OECD. OECD framework for statistics on the distribution of household income, consumption and wealth. Paris: OECD publishing; 2013.

28. Wingenfeld K, Spitzer C, Mensebach C, Grabe HJ, Hill A, Gast U, et al. The German version of the Childhood Trauma Questionnaire (CTQ): preliminary psychometric properties. Psychother Psychosom Med Psychol. 2010;60:e13.

29. Bernstein DP, Stein JA, Newcomb MD, Walker E, Pogge D, Ahluvalia T, et al. Development and validation of a brief screening version of the Childhood Trauma Questionnaire. Child Abuse Negl. 2003;27:169–90.

30. Rassenhofer M, Zimmer A, Sprober N, Fegert JM. Child sexual abuse in the Roman Catholic Church in Germany: comparison of victim-impact data collected through church-sponsored and government-sponsored programs. Child Abuse Negl. 2015;40:60–7.

31. US Department of Health and Human Services. Child maltreatment 2014. Washington: US Government Printing Office; 2015.

32. Bussmann KD, Erthak C, Schroth A. Effects of banning corporal punishment in Europe. In: Durrant JE, Smith AB, editors. Global pathways to abolishing physical punishment. Abingdon: Routledge; 2011. p. 299–322.

33. Bussmann KD. Familiengewalt report. 2005.

34. Herrenkohl RC, Herrenkohl TI. Assessing a child's experience of multiple maltreatment types: some unfinished business. J Fam Violence. 2009;24:485.

35. Witt A, Munzer A, Ganser HG, Fegert JM, Goldbeck L, Plener PL. Experience by children and adolescents of more than one type of maltreatment: association of different classes of maltreatment profiles with clinical outcome variables. Child Abuse Negl. 2016;57:1–11.

36. Allroggen M, Rau T, Ohlert J, Fegert JM. Lifetime prevalence and incidence of sexual victimization of adolescents in institutional care. Child Abuse Negl. 2017;66:23–30. doi:10.1016/j.chiabu.2017.02.015.

2

Disruptive behavior scale for adolescents (DISBA): development and psychometric properties

Mahmood Karimy[1], Ahmad Fakhri[2], Esmaeel Vali[1], Farzaneh Vali[1], Feliciano H. Veiga[3], L. A. R. Stein[4,5,6] and Marzieh Araban[7,8*] ⬤

Abstract

Background: Growing evidence indicates that if disruptive behavior is left unidentified and untreated, a significant proportion of these problems will persist and may develop into problems linked with delinquency, substance abuse, and violence. Research is needed to develop valid and reliable measures of disruptive behavior to assist recognition and impact of treatments on disruptive behavior. The aim of this study was to develop and evaluate the psychometric properties of a scale for disruptive behavior in adolescents.

Methods: Six hundred high school students (50% girls), ages ranged 15–18 years old, selected through multi stage random sampling. Psychometrics of the disruptive behavior scale for adolescents (DISBA) (Persian version) was assessed through content validity, explanatory factor analysis (EFA) using Varimax rotation and confirmatory factor analysis (CFA). The reliability of this scale was assessed via internal consistency and test–retest reliability.

Results: EFA revealed four factors accounting for 59% of observed variance. The final 29-item scale contained four factors: (1) aggressive school behavior, (2) classroom defiant behavior, (3) unimportance of school, and (4) defiance to school authorities. Furthermore, CFA produced a sufficient Goodness of Fit Index > 0.90. Test–retest and internal consistency reliabilities were acceptable at 0.85 and 0.89, respectively.

Conclusions: The findings from this study suggest that the Iranian version of DISBA questionnaire has content validity. Further studies are needed to evaluate stronger psychometric properties for DISBA.

Keywords: Adolescence, Disruptive behavior, Validity, Reliability, Psycho-educational development scale

Background

Adolescence is considered one of the major periods in structuring and establishing the personality [1]. Further, it is a crucial time in which mental and behavioral disorders may manifest [2, 3]. Early diagnosis and timely intervention of adolescents with mental and behavioral disorders is very important [4], and since 1950 many studies have been carried out on the prevalence of behavior disorders and problems among student adolescents [5, 6]. It is likely that the behavior problems which arise in this period appear later on in life as stable characteristics; therefore, detection of such behavior among students, and dealing with them correctly is essential [7].

In particular, disruptive behavior disorders (DBDs), including conduct disorder (CD), oppositional defiant disorder (ODD) and attention deficit hyperactivity disorder (ADHD), may manifest in children and adolescents and can be associated with a host of school difficulties and problems in later life. Common symptoms occurring in individuals with CD and ODD include: defiance of authority figures, angry outbursts, and other antisocial behaviors such as lying and stealing. It is felt that the difference between oppositional defiant disorder and conduct disorder is in the severity of symptoms and

*Correspondence: arabanm@ajums.ac.ir; araban62@gmail.com
[7] Social Determinants of Health Research Center, Department of Health Education and Promotion, Public Health School, Ahvaz Jundishapur University of Medical Sciences Campus, Golestan BLVD, Ahvaz 61375-15751, Iran
Full list of author information is available at the end of the article

that they may lie on a continuum often with a developmental progression from ODD to CD with increasing age [8]. Furthermore, ODD often includes problems of emotional dysregulation (i.e., angry and irritable mood) not included in definitions of CD (American Psychiatric Asso., 2013) [9].

Today, there is little doubt regarding the emergence of disruptive behavior in adolescence. According to surveys, two to six percent of adolescents from typical demographics of society have some level of disruptive behavior [10]. This behavior has caused concern for families, schools, and public health, constituting the most common reason for adolescents to visit psychiatric clinics [7]. Students with disruptive behavior are faced with educational problems such as academic failure, expulsion, dropping out, and low grades, as well as high-risk behavior such as drug and alcohol abuse, and high-risk sexual behavior [11].

Students with disruptive behavior interrupt the learning process for other students, and the teacher's ability to teach effectively; they also divert school resources and energy away from the main academic goals [12]. Adolescents with disruptive behavior have problems with their ability to understand and manage emotions [13] and higher risk of committing anti-social and criminal behavior [14]. Disruptive behavior is behavior which truly disrupts the learning and teaching processes in classroom or any other educational environment [15–17].

The cause of DBDs is not known. DBDs are more common among children aged 12 years and older; and child abuse or neglect and a traumatic life experience have been stated as risks for DBDs [18]. Additionally, It has been documented some socio-psychological and cultural factors may contribute to disruptive behavior [19]. For example, parent–child and school-child relationships may enhance the risk of developing DBD [20]; it has also been shown that life satisfaction and hope are negatively related to adolescent problem behaviour [21]. Disruptive behavior disorders are associated with psychological problems including anxiety, depression [22] and development of antisocial personality disorder later in life [19]. Psychosocial interventions that include parents, children, families and teachers, as well as behavioral support, can improve this disorder among adolescent [23].

DBD's are related to poor outcomes for youth including involvement in crime and numerous educational problems [16, 17]; therefore, timely screening, detection and management of DBDs are of critical importance [24]. A number of rating scales exist to assist in detecting DBDs including the Conner's Parent Rating Scale (CPRS), the disruptive behavior rating scale (DBRS), and the disruptive behavior scale-professed by students (DBS-PS). The CPRS focuses mainly on ADHD [8]; the DBRS consists of 45 questions, and has been validated among young children [25]; and the DBS-PS has only been validated among Portuguese students [15]. It is advantageous to develop screening that encompasses DBDs more generally, is brief, and is of relevance to older children. Furthermore, expanding validation of such screening tools to cultures other than Western cultures is important.

Because DBDs are association with important and potentially life-long impairment, and because DBDs are associated with significant societal costs, the current study aimed to design a suitable scale for screening DBDs. We therefore, designed a 29-item disruptive behavior screening scale among Iranian high school students and analyzed its psychometric properties.

Methods

The research population consisted of all the high school students aged fifteen to eighteen of Saveh city in the academic year 2015–2016. The sample size was determined four hundred people, considering the number of items in the scale (initially, 39 items) and following Munro [26] who recommended ten people for each item. To increase the accuracy of the study, six hundred students (300 girls and 300 boys) were selected for the study.

Sampling

A multi stage sampling was applied. Firstly, Saveh-a city located in the center of Iran, was divided into two parts: north and south. Among all high schools located in each region, four high schools (2 girls high schools and 2 boys high schools) were randomly selected from each district, which constituted a total of eight high schools. Then, among all students attending a high school, a random sample was selected using random numbers. It is worth mentioning that the required sample ratio for participation in the study was determined for each high school according to the number of students in each high school. In the last stage, the ratio of samples participating in the study from each class was determined for each of first and fourth grades according to the number of students in each grade.

The students were 15 to 18 years old and were the tenth, eleventh and twelfth grade students.

The students answered the anonymous scale without the presence of teachers, and without any compulsion, in a self-administered manner.

The scale

A student's disruptive behavior scale was developed for this study. The disruptive behavior scale for adolescents (DISBA) was designed in reference to literature review and semi-structured interviews with students and high school authorities. Disruptive behavior in this study was considered as any type of behavior, which truly disrupts the learning and teaching processes in classroom or educational environment.

To develop the item-pool, we considered previous scales on disruptive behavior and conducted semistructured interviews. The initial item pool consisted of 39 items, including the 16-item DBS-PS [15] along with 23 items derived from literature review [8, 24, 25] and interviews.

To develop the 23 items, focus groups were conducted with thirty students who were similar to the target population in terms of demographic properties, as well as with ten teachers and school staff Focus group data were analyzed for thematic content and then a panel of experts developed 23 items based on focus group themes and the literature. Finally, the research team then decided to utilize a 4-point Likert scale response option consisting of never (0), rarely (1), usually (2) and always (3) for each item.

Statistical analysis
Face validity
Both qualitative and quantitative methods were used to determine face validity. For quantitative face validity, 20 students were asked about the importance of each item in helping to identify disruptive classroom behavior. For the qualitative approach, students were asked to assess each item for ambiguity and difficulty. Overall, no problems in reading or understanding the items were expressed by the students. The quantitative face validity was evaluated through item impact score. Participants were asked to rate the importance of each item on a five-point Likert type scale form strongly important to not at all important. The scores ranged from 1 to 5 for each item. The item impact score for each item was calculated by multiplying the mean score of importance of an item with its frequency by relative frequency (percentage). The item impact scores of greater than 1.5 were considered suitable.

Content validity
A panel of experts (15 specialists in health education, psychiatry, health psychology, and educational psychology) rated items according to relevance. Each item was rated according to the following: (1) irrelevant, (2) important, but not essential, (3) essential. For each item a Content Validity Ratio (CVR) was computed as $(n_e - N/2)/(N/2)$, where n_e is the number of experts rating the item as essential and N is the number of experts. The overall CVR index of the scale is computed as a mean of the items' CVR values. The Content Validity Index (CVI) was also calculated Experts rated items on a four-point rating scale: (1) not relevant, (2) somewhat relevant, (3) quite

relevant, and (4) very relevant. CVI is the percentage of experts rating an item as quite or very relevant. The recommended value for CVR is 0.59, for CVR scale index it is determined using Lawshe's table, and for CVI the minimum recommended value is 0.79 [27, 28].

Construct validity
Exploratory factor analysis (EFA) was carried out to identify the underlying relationships between items. To determine the adequacy of the sample size, a Kaiser–Meyer–Olkin test was applied. A threshold of > 0.5 for corrected item–total–correlation was chosen as sufficient. SPSS 15 (SPSS, Inc., Chicago, IL, USA) was utilized for analyses, and items with factor loadings over 0.50 were retained. Confirmatory Factor Analysis (CFA) was carried out to test whether the data fit the hypothesized measurement model. The following cut-offs were considered appropriate [29]: 0.90 for the Comparative Fit Index (CFI), Goodness of Fit Index (GFI) and Normed Fit Index (NFI), 0.08 for the root mean square error approximation (RMSEA). Lisrel 8.8 (Scientific Software International, Inc., 2007) was used in this study for confirmatory factor analysis.

Reliability
Two methods were used to assess reliability: internal consistency and stability as described below:

1. Internal consistency: this was assessed using Cronbach's alpha coefficient. The value of 0.7 or above was considered satisfactory [30].
2. Test–retest analysis. N = 25 students from the study sample completed the scale twice with an interval of 2 weeks. The intraclass correlation coefficient (ICC) was calculated and a value of 0.4 or above was considered acceptable [30, 31].

Ethics statement
The study was approved by the Ethics Committee of Saveh University of Medical Sciences. All the participants had signed the informed written consent form, where the confidentiality of the information received and the anonymity of responses to the scales was stressed.

Results
The average age and its standard deviation was 16.83 ± 0.86 for the male students and 16.62 ± 0.85 for the female students. The grade point average (GPA) of students was 15.8 ± 2.3 in the year before, on a scale from 12 to 20, where 20 indicates better performance. One hundred fifty-nine students (26.5%) had a history of smoking cigarettes or hookah within the 7 days before

completing the study. One hundred fifty-three students (25.5%) were not happy with their lives.

Seven questions were omitted through examination of CVR, while three questions were omitted through examination of CVI. Twenty-nine out of thirty-nine questions, which had proper content validity, entered the stage of construct validity assessment using exploratory factor analysis. The Kaiser–Meyer–Olkin test for sampling adequacy and Bartlett's sphericity test both indicated the data were suitable for EFA.

In the next stage, the Exploratory Factor Analysis found four factors with Eigen values greater than one: (1) aggressive school behavior, (twelve questions), (2) classroom defiant behavior (six questions), (3) unimportance of school, (six questions), and (4) defiance to school

authorities (five questions). The factor loading matrix in Table 1 shows that all the extracted factor loadings are greater than 0.50, and these factors explain a total of fifty-nine percent of the cumulative variance.

Confirmatory factor analysis was carried out to assess the results from the Exploratory Factor Analysis. The results showed that the structural model provided a good fit to the data. The Chi square value was significant $\chi^2 = 17.16$, df $= 7.4$, p $= 0.02$). The Goodness-of-Fit Index was 0.91, the adjusted goodness-of-fit index was 0.90, the Normed Fit Index was 0.92, the Comparative Fit Index was 0.96, and the root mean square error of approximation as 0.05. These figures indicate that the four-factor model of disruptive behavior has satisfactory goodness-of-fit (Table 2).

Table 1 The result obtained from exploratory factor analysis with varimax rotation among adolescents aged 15–17 (n = 600)

Item	Factor 1	Factor 2	Factor 3	Factor 4
I hit the school trees and break their branches	0.722[a]			
I stick gum on the seats	0.668			
I love to carve on the school benches	0.611			
I tuck the back of my shoes like villains when I walk	0.610			
I sometimes come to school after taking drugs	0.606			
I bring explosives to school	0.600			
I deliberately break or damage school equipment	0.589			
I get expelled from class due to inappropriate and disruptive behavior	0.562			
I like to drag my feet when I walk	0.558			
I text messages in class while the teacher is teaching	0.549			
I kick the classroom door open	0.536			
I clash with teachers	0.503			
I make noise and disrupt the class		0.622		
I eat refreshments in class without permission		0.621		
I like to disrupt the class and the school		0.611		
I speak without permission and disrupt the class		0.594		
I argue with my classmates		0.570		
I sing out loud at school		0.543		
I don't turn up on time for school			0.711	
I turn up late for class			0.655	
I forget to bring the things I need to school			0.560	
I don't pay attention to the lessons in the classroom			0.532	
I skipping classes			0.530	
I can't relate well with my friends			0.511	
I don't care about school's teachers and authorities				0.650
I argue with teachers				0.640
I leave my seat without teacher's permission				0.607
I argue with the school's authorities				0.543
I don't stand up when the teacher enters the class				0.541
Total variance explained	59%			

[a] Factor loadings less than 0.3 were omitted

Table 2 The results obtained from confirmatory factor analysis

RMSEA	GF	NF	CFI	d	χ^2
0.05	0.91	0.92	0.9	7.4	17.16

RMSEA root mean square error of approximation; *GFI* goodness-of-fit index; *NFI* Normed Fit Index; *CFI* Comparative Fit Index

Table 3 Cronbach's α coefficient and ICC for the disruptive behavior scale and its subscales

Domain	Number of items	Cronbach's α coefficient	ICC
Aggressive school behavior	12	0.82	0.79
Classroom defiant behavior	6	0.91	0.87
Unimportance of school	6	0.77	0.71
Defiance to school authorities	5	0.86	0.88
Total scale	29	0.89	0.85

ICC intraclass correlation coefficient

The reliability of the scale was assessed in terms of internal consistency and temporal stability. The Cronbach's alpha coefficient ranged from 0.77 to 0.91, ICC's ranged from 0.71 to 0.88 indicating satisfactory stability (Table 3).

Discussion

It is critical to detect students who may have disruptive behavior disorder, given that such behavior may lead to high-risk behavior such as delinquency, violence, drug abuse and anti-social personality if left untreated [28, 30]. This study presents a brief, valid and reliable scale with sub-parts that may aid in screening for DBDs in youth. Furthermore, many such scales are primarily created and validated in Westernized cultures, and it is important to expand validation and use in other countries.

To study construct validity, factor analysis was used and showed a 4-factor construct that explained 59% of variance, which is consistent with other similar studies [32]. Results of confirmatory factor analysis show that the data with the four presented constructs have sufficient goodness-of-fit.

The four-factor structure is not consistent with results obtained for the DBS-PS which yielded a three-factor structure consisting of distraction-transgression, schoolmate aggression and aggression to school authorities [15]. The four-factor structure found in this study included (1) aggressive school behavior, (2) classroom defiant behavior, (3) unimportance of School, and (4) defiance to school authorities. One possible explanation for such a difference at factor-level may be due to the fact that these scales have different number of items and have been validated among different populations with different age ranges and cultural backgrounds.

Based on DSM-5 disruptive behavior and ADHD are two distinct disorders although they may present similarly and may be co-exist. Behavior of children with ADHD may be disruptive, but this behavior by itself does not violate social norms or others' rights and so does not usually meet criteria for CD [9]. As such, there are similarities between DISBA and scales that screen for ADHD symptoms including: losing things, making mistakes, arguing, damaging things or equipment, failing to do tasks, having problem with relationship and skipping schools. While screening can alert professionals to a potential behavioral problem, further assessment and diagnosis will help in determining how to target and tailor interventions for specific disorders.

The results of the study show that the students' disruptive behavior scale has good internal consistency ranging from 0.77 to 0.91. This is consistent with a similar study on Portuguese students that also showed the reliability ranged from 0.67 to 0.88 [15]. Test–retest results indicate a high degree of reliability in the DISBA, which is again consistent with the aforementioned study on Portuguese students that found test–retest reliability to be 0.85 [15].

Limitation

Future studies may wish to examine the correlations between scales and other phenomena associated with DBD, such as observations of stealing, fighting, etc. In addition, future studies may wish to examine how well scales distinguish between youth with and without a diagnosis of DBD (ODD, CD, or ADHD), and sensitivity to detect change in behavior over time (e.g., following intervention).

Conclusion

According to the results of this study, this brief 29-item scale evidences good validity and reliability. School authorities and teachers might use DISBA to screen students in order to identify problematic students in need of further evaluation for diagnosis and intervention. Although based in part on the DBS-PS, the DISBA evidences good psychometrics in a non-Westernized culture, allows for screening based on four relevant scales for the school setting as compared to only three, and can be used with youth ages 15–18 years old.

Abbreviations

CVR: content validity ratio; CVI: Content Validity Index; CFA: confirmatory factor analysis; RMSEA: root mean square error of approximation; NFI: Normed Fit Index; GFI: Goodness of Fit Index; CFI: Comparative Fit Index.

Authors' contributions

All author contributed in design, data gathering and analysis. All authors contributed to drafting the manuscript. All authors read and approved the final manuscript.

Author details

[1] Social Determinants of Health Research Center, Saveh University of Medical Sciences, Saveh, Iran. [2] Department of Psychiatry, Ahvaz Jundishapur University of Medical Sciences, Ahvaz, Iran. [3] Institute of Education, University of Lisbon, Lisbon, Portugal. [4] Psychology Dept., University of RI, Kingston, RI, USA. [5] Behavioral & Social Sciences Dept., Brown University School of Public Health, Providence, RI, USA. [6] RI Training School, Cranston, RI, USA. [7] Social Determinants of Health Research Center, Department of Health Education and Promotion, Public Health School, Ahvaz Jundishapur University of Medical Sciences Campus, Golestan BLVD, Ahvaz 61375-15751, Iran. [8] Department of Health Education and Promotion, Public Health School, Ahvaz Jundishapur University of Medical Sciences Campus, Golestan BLVD, Ahvaz 61375-15751, Iran.

Acknowledgements

The number S556 is associated with this research project. Financial support associated with this project and its home institution is recognized and appreciated. We sincerely acknowledge our gratitude to the Chairman of Saveh Education Office, the teachers and participating students in this study and all those who helped us to conduct this study. We are grateful to Professor Ali Montazeri for his valuable comments on the earlier version of the manuscript.

Competing interests

The authors declare that they have no competing interests.

Funding

Financial support was received from Saveh University of Medical Sciences.

References

1. Karimy M, Niknami S, Heidarnia AR, Hajizadeh I, Montazeri A. Prevalence and determinants of male adolescents' smoking in Iran: an explanation based on the theory of planned behavior. Iran Red Crescent Med J. 2013;15(3):187–93.
2. Stringaris A, Maughan B, Copeland WS, Costello EJ, Angold A. Irritable mood as a symptom of depression in youth: prevalence, developmental, and clinical correlates in the Great Smoky Mountains Study. J Am Acad Child Adolesc Psychiatry. 2013;52:831–40.
3. Dray J, Bowman J, Freund M, Campbell E, Hodder RK, Lecathelinais C, Wiggers J. Mental health problems in a regional population of Australian adolescents: association with socio-demographic characteristics. Child Adolesc Psychiatry Ment Health. 2016;10(1):32.
4. Undheim AM, Lydersen S, Kayed NS. Do school teachers and primary contacts in residential youth care institutions recognize mental health problems in adolescents? Child Adolesc Psychiatry Ment Health. 2016;10(1):19.
5. Manninen M, Pankakoski M, Gissler M, Suvisaari J. Adolescents in a residential school for behavior disorders have an elevated mortality risk in young adulthood. Child Adolesc Psychiatry Ment Health. 2015;9(1):46.
6. Buchanan T. Internet-based questionnaire assessment: appropriate use in clinical contexts. Cogn Behav Ther. 2003;32:100–9.
7. Moreland AD, Dumas JE. Categorical and dimensional approaches to the measurement of disruptive behavior in the preschool years: a meta-analysis. Clin Psychol Rev. 2008;28(6):1059–70.
8. Sadock BJ, Sadock VA. Kaplan and Sadock's synopsis of psychiatry. Behavioral sciences/clinical psychiatry. Philadelphia, US: Lippincott Williams and Wilkins and Wolter Kluwer Health; 2011.
9. Association AP. Diagnostic and statistical manual of mental disorders (DSM-5®). USA: American Psychiatric Pub; 2013.
10. Semke CA, Garbacz SA, Kwon K, Sheridan SM, Woods KE. Family involvement for children with disruptive behaviors: the role of parenting stress and motivational beliefs. J Sch Psychol. 2010;48(4):293–312.
11. Nock MK, Kazdin AE, Hiripi E, Kessler R. Prevalence, subtypes, and correlates of DSM-IV conduct disorder in the National Comorbidity Survey Replication. Psychol Med. 2006;36:699–710.
12. Amada G, Smith MC. Coping with misconduct in the college classroom: a practical model. Asheville: College Administration Publications; 1999.
13. Ciarrochi J, Chan AY, Bajgar J. Measuring emotional intelligence in adolescents. Personal Individ Differ. 2001;31(7):1105–19.
14. Motamedi M, Amini Z, Siavash M, Attari A, Shakibaei F, Azhar MM, Harandi RJ, Hassanzadeh A. Effects of parent training on salivary cortisol in children and adolescents with disruptive behavior disorder. J Res Med Sci. 2008;13(2):69–74.
15. Veiga F. Disruptive behavior scale professed by students (DBS-PS): development and validation. Int J Psychol Psychol Ther. 2008;8:203–16.
16. Lannie AL, McCurdy BL. Preventing disruptive behavior in the urban classroom: effects of the good behavior game on student and teacher behavior. Educ Treat Child. 2007;30(1):85–98.
17. Walker HM, Ramsey E, Gresham FM. Heading off disruptive behavior: how early intervention can reduce defiant behavior—and win back teaching time. Am Educ. 2003;26(4):6–45.
18. John M. Eisenberg Center for Clinical Decisions and Communications Science, AHRQ Comparative Effectiveness Reviews Treating Disruptive Behavior Disorders in Children and Teens. A review of the research for parents and caregivers, in comparative effectiveness review summary guides for consumers. Rockville: Agency for Healthcare Research and Quality; 2005.
19. Rijlaarsdam J, Tiemeier H, Ringoot AP, Ivanova MY, Jaddoe VWV, Verhulst FC, Roza SJ. Early family regularity protects against later disruptive behavior. Eur Child Adolesc Psychiatry. 2016;25(7):781–9.
20. Johnston C, Mash EJ. Families of children with attention-deficit/hyperactivity disorder: review and recommendations for future research. Clin Child Fam Psychol Rev. 2001;4(3):183–207.
21. Salami SO. Moderating effects of resilience, self-esteem and social support on adolescents' reactions to violence. Asian Soc Sci. 2010;6(1):101.
22. Butler AM, Titus C. Systematic review of engagement in culturally adapted parent training for disruptive behavior. J Early Interv. 2015;37(4):300–18.
23. Wolf NJ, Hopko DR. Psychosocial and pharmacological interventions for depressed adults in primary care: a critical review. Clin Psychol Rev. 2008;28(1):131–61.
24. Masi G, Milone A, Brovedani P, Pisano S, Muratori P. Psychiatric evaluation of youths with disruptive behavior disorders and psychopathic traits: a critical review of assessment measures. Neurosci Biobehav Rev. 2016. https://doi.org/10.1016/j.neubiorev.2016.09.023.
25. Friedman-Weieneth JL, Doctoroff GL, Harvey EA, Goldstein LH. The disruptive behavior rating scale—parent version (DBRS-PV) factor analytic

structure and validity among young preschool children. J Atten Disord. 2009;13(1):42–55.

26. Munro BH. Statistical methods for health care research. 1st ed. Philadelphia: Lippincott Williams & Wilkins; 2005.

27. Lawshe CH. A quantitative approach to content validity. Pers Psychol. 1975;28(4):563–75.

28. Waltz C, Bausell BR. Nursing research: design statistics and computer analysis. Philadelphia: Davis FA; 1981.

29. Hu LT, Bentler PM. Cut-off criteria for fit indexes in covariance structure analysis: conventional criteria versus new alternatives. Struct Equ Model. 1999;6:1–55.

30. Patterson P. Reliability, validity, and methodological response to the assessment of physical activity via self-report. Res Q Exerc Sport. 2000;71(sup2):15–20.

31. Polit DF, Beck CT. The content validity index: are you sure you know what's being reported? Critique and recommendations. Res Nurs Health. 2006;29(5):489–97.

32. Zuddas A, Marzocchi GM, Oosterlaan J, Cavolina P, Ancilletta B, Sergeant J. Factor structure and cultural factors of disruptive behaviour disorders symptoms in Italian children. Eur Psychiatry. 2006;21(6):410–8.

3

Responding to safety concerns and chronic needs: trends over time

Barbara Fallon[1*], Nico Trocmé[2], Joanne Filippelli[1], Tara Black[1] and Nicolette Joh-Carnella[1]

Abstract

Background: For the past 20 years, the Ontario child welfare sector has made significant legislative and policy changes. Changes to legislation and policy can impact the public and sector's response to child maltreatment and inform identified trends. Using an investigative taxonomy of urgent protection and chronic need this paper examines the shift in the nature of investigated maltreatment over time.

Methods: Data from five cycles of the Ontario Incidence Studies of Reported Child Abuse and Neglect (1993, 1998, 2003, 2008 and 2013) were used. Provincial incidence rates were calculated by dividing the weighted estimates by the child population 15 years of age and under and then multiplying by 1000 in order to produce an annual incidence rate per 1000 children. Investigations were divided into urgent (severe physical harm, sexual abuse, neglect and physical abuse of children under 4) and chronic (risk only, exposure to intimate partner violence, emotional maltreatment, neglect and physical abuse of children four or over). Tests of statistical significance were calculated to assess changes in subtypes between cycles.

Results: Between 1993 and 2013, the rate of child maltreatment related investigations completed in Ontario has increased from 20.48 per 1000 children to 53.27 per 1000 children. Overall there has been a decline in the incidence of urgent investigations from 9.31 per 1000 child maltreatment investigations in 1993 to 5.94 per 1000 maltreatment investigations in 2013. There has been a fourfold increase in the incidence of chronic investigations from 11.18 per 1000 child maltreatment investigations in 1993 to 47.33 per 1000 maltreatment investigations in 2013.

Conclusion: The nature of child protection work using the urgent-chronic taxonomy shows a dramatic shift in the types of concerns identified without a corresponding shift in the way families are assessed for need. The provision of a forensic investigation to all families does not distinguish between urgent safety concerns and needs that may require prolonged engagement. Effective service provision requires more precision in our response to these diverse concerns.

Background

Three children, ages 7, 9 and 11 are observed alone on public transit by a concerned citizen and a child welfare authority is contacted with an allegation that the children are not being provided with appropriate supervision. The next day, the same child welfare authority is contacted by a cousin of a woman who has been assaulted by her husband, worried that their teenager has witnessed the assault. The following day a teacher calls with a concern that a 2 year old sibling of one of her students is being left home alone when the mother walks her pupil to school in the morning. Each of these referrals to the child protection agency is judged to meet the threshold for investigation and while the number of "collaterals" interviewed may vary in each case, each family will receive a visit and an interview, the worker will complete a risk assessment and assess the child's safety. There will be a determination about whether a child has been maltreated and whether the family needs ongoing child welfare services. The assessment of maltreatment varies across provinces and is determined by the clinical judgement of the investigating worker based on the balance of probabilities of whether the child has been maltreated.

*Correspondence: barbara.fallon@utoronto.ca
[1] Factor-Inwentash Faculty of Social Work, University of Toronto, 246 Bloor Street West, Toronto, ON M6S 3W6, Canada
Full list of author information is available at the end of the article

Similar to other Canadian Provincial and Territorial statutes, safety and well-being are central and equal considerations within Ontario child welfare legislation [1]. Typically, a maltreatment-related concern for a child is reported to a child welfare authority. If the concern is deemed to be appropriate for an investigative response (i.e. screened-in), a series of decisions are made: whether or not to substantiate the concern, if ongoing child welfare services are required, and in rare cases, whether the child needs to be placed in out of home care. Investigative trends in Canada suggest a shift from urgent protection concerns to a greater focus on the consequences of family dysfunction on the development and well-being of children, or more chronic need [1]. For over 20 years, the Ontario child welfare sector has been undergoing significant legislative and policy changes. The approach to investigating a concern of abuse or neglect from the community about a child has largely remained unchanged. Using the investigative taxonomy of urgent protection and chronic need proposed by Trocmé and colleagues [1] and data from the five cycles of the Ontario Incidence Studies of Reported Child Abuse and Neglect [2–6], the purpose of this paper is to examine whether there has been a change in the type of maltreatment reported and investigated in Ontario from 1993 to 2013.

The Ontario practice and policy context

The Ontario Incidence Study of Reported Child Abuse and Neglect (OIS) is the only source of aggregated provincial data on reported child maltreatment and provides an opportunity to explore possible changes in the incidence of reported child abuse and neglect over time. Reported child abuse and neglect in the province of Ontario doubled between 1998 and 2003; from a rate of an estimated 27.42 investigations per 1000 children to a rate of 53.56 per 1000 children in 2003. Since 2003, the rate of investigated maltreatment has remained consistent with the latest estimate in 2013 indicating that 53.27 investigations per 1000 children were conducted [5]. In 2008 a study examining the incidence of reported maltreatment in five provinces revealed that Ontario had the highest rate of maltreatment-related investigations (54.05 per 1000 children) and Quebec had the lowest rate of 13.19 per 1000 children [7].

Changes to legislation and policy can impact the public and sector's response to alleged child maltreatment and inform identified trends. The increase in the incidence of investigations in Ontario is believed to be driven by the broadening of the child welfare mandate and the inclusion of children's exposure to intimate partner violence, as well as those who were at future risk of maltreatment [8, 9]. Greater awareness of the adverse consequences of child maltreatment such as the increased likelihood of

poor adult physical, mental health academic outcomes and economic hardship [10] may also be contributing to an increase in investigated reports [1].Child welfare practice and policy has been likened to a pendulum that swings between family-centred and more intrusive, child-centred service approaches [11]. Tragic events such as the death of a child can influence the orientation of the child welfare system. In Ontario, there were several high profile child deaths and coroner's inquests in the 1990s that led to legislative changes and policy directives [8, 11] because there were concerns about the capacity of the child welfare sector to adequately protect children [8]. This pressure to improve the capacity of the child welfare system to respond led to a series of policy and legislative changes, which resulted in a shift to a more child-centred approach and a greater focus on immediate protection and safety of the child [9]. A new risk assessment model, comprised of three standardized decision-making tools (Ontario Eligibility Spectrum, Ontario Safety Assessment, and Ontario Risk Assessment) for all child welfare authorities was implemented in the province of Ontario in 1998 [12]. Risk assessment tools are designed to assist workers with the assessment of the future risk of maltreatment. The Ontario Child and Family Services Act (CFSA) was amended in March of 2000 and the definition of a child in need of protection was expanded [8]. Changes to the Act included clarifying its paramount purpose to promote the safety, well-being and best interests of children, lowering the thresholds for risk of harm and intervention, recognizing cases of neglect, clarifying the duty to report [8]. All of these factors are believed to have contributed to the increase in investigations in Ontario between 1998 and 2003 [1].

In 2006, further policy reform was initiated through the Ontario Child Welfare Transformation Agenda (Transformation Agenda), which included a more balanced approach to practice that protected children while also promoting their well-being and supporting families [13]. The Transformation Agenda promoted early intervention and permanency in child welfare [5, 13]. Several changes were made to Ontario child welfare as a result of the 2006 Transformation Agenda. In keeping with the increased focus on accountability, the Eligibility Spectrum was revised and new practice standards were introduced for child welfare across the service provision continuum, commencing from the receipt of the report and ending at the completion of the case. These standards further promoted customized responses and offering supports to families [5].

In 2009, the Commission to Promote Sustainable Child Welfare (the Commission) was established to better understand the impact of the Transformation Agenda, and to develop and implement further changes to improve the child welfare sector [14, 15]. A sustainable child welfare system was conceptualized as one that is adaptable to change, uses resources effectively, and has the ability to manage both short and long term demands [5, 14, 15]. Several changes emerged as a result of the commission, including the implementation of Child Protection Information Network (CPIN), a province-wide information system. CPIN has yet to be fully implemented across the province due to challenges associated with integrating different and independent information systems used by organizations to document case and financial management. In addition, there have been further revisions to Ontario's Eligibility Spectrum and Standards in 2016 [16, 17]. Ontario will proclaim the Child, Youth and Family Services Act in 2018 in order to strengthen child welfare and improve outcomes for youth. It will raise the age of protection from 16 to 18 years, which is consistent with the United Nations Convention on the Rights of the Child [18]. The policy directions from the Transformation Agenda and the Commission have acted to highlight the importance of early intervention and support for at-risk children and families [9].

Despite significant policy and legislative changes that have occurred in Ontario over the last 20 years, there are concerns with traditional child welfare service models that emphasize child safety, and the ability of the sector to meet the complex, chronic needs of children and families served [1, 8, 11, 19]. Investigative trends in Canada have emphasized that differential or alternate response models are indicated [1, 11, 19]. There are a growing number of jurisdictions across North America that have implemented differential response models in child protection systems after several locations piloted this approach in the 1990s [20]. Differential response models typically assume a less adversarial approach with discrete pathways available to the family and the focus on the assessment of need traditional child welfare models emphasize more intrusive, forensic approaches [1]. Although several jurisdictions have implemented differential models to address the misalignment between client need and system response, there is no province-wide implementation of differential response models despite policy orientations that would support it. Child welfare systems need to refine their responses to meet the varied needs of children and families, and mobilize community resources [11].

The objective of this research is to determine rates at which child welfare authorities investigate maltreatment using the urgent-chronic taxonomy in Ontario to identify trends over time. A detailed analysis of investigative trends in Ontario by applying the urgent-chronic taxonomy can help to increase our understanding of how the child welfare system has been responding to population, policy and practice changes, and to its dual mandate of promoting safety and well-being.

Methods

Data from the five OIS cycles were analyzed to explore trends in the investigative taxonomy of urgent-chronic need. Each of the five cycles of the Ontario Incidence Study of Reported Child Abuse and Neglect (OIS) utilized a multi-stage sampling design [9]. The first stage of sampling included the selection of a representative sample of child welfare sites from a sampling frame that includes all mandated child welfare organizations in Ontario. Secondly cases that were opened in the study sites during the 3-month period from October 1 to December 31 in the year the study took place were selected. A 3-month sampling period is considered optimal for high participation rates and good compliance with study procedures [5]. Investigations were evaluated by study staff to ensure that they met the OIS definitions of maltreatment. In 2008 and 2013 the definition of maltreatment was expanded to include risk of future maltreatment. The 1993, 1998 and 2003 OIS cycles did not track cases where there was no specific maltreatment concern alleged or suspected during the course of the investigation or "risk only cases". Risk only cases where included beginning in 2008 and collected information about investigations in which there was no specific allegation of an incident of maltreatment, but rather the future risk of maltreatment was assessed.

The final stage of sampling includes identifying children investigated as a result of maltreatment concerns. In each of the five OIS cycles, estimates of the provincial annual rates of maltreatment investigations in Ontario were derived by applying a regionalization and annualization weights. Estimates for each of the cycles do not include incidents not reported to Ontario child welfare authorities, cases that were screened out and were not fully investigated, new reports on cases that were opened, and cases that were only investigated by police [5]. For greater detail on the design and weighting procedures, see the methods chapters specific to each of the five study cycles [2–6]. Please see Table 1 for the number of agencies, investigations and estimates of child maltreatment investigations completed across the OIS cycles.

Data for each of the OIS cycles is collected directly from investigating child welfare workers in each of the sampled organizations using a three-page standardized data collection instrument, the maltreatment assessment form. This instrument is completed at the conclusion of the investigation and collects clinical information that is routinely gathered by child welfare workers during the course conducting the investigation, including caregiver, child, case, and short-term service dispositions. In

Table 1 Sites and sample sizes for the Ontario Incidence Study of Reported Child Abuse (OIS) Cycles

	OIS-1993	OIS-1998	OIS-2003	OIS-2008	OIS-2013
Site selection (sample/total)	15/51	13/53	16/53	23/53	17/46
Case selection	1898	2193	4175	4415	3118
Investigated children	2447	3053	7172	7471	5265
Estimate of child maltreatment investigations	46,683	64,658	128,108	128,748	125,281

2008, the maltreatment assessment form was amended to include investigations that were conducted which focused not on an event of maltreatment that alleged or suspected but rather assessed the risk to the investigated child of future maltreatment or *risk only* investigations.

Analysis plan

SPSS Statistic version 23 was used to conduct the analyses. Provincial incidence rates were calculated by dividing the weighted estimates by the child population 15 years of age and under and then multiplying by 1000 in order to produce an annual incidence rate per 1000 children.

The population for Ontario children is based upon the appropriate Census data for the study cycle. The Census is conducted by Statistics Canada every 5 years.

First, the overall investigation rate for investigations in Ontario in each of the five OIS cycles (1993, 1998, 2003, 2008, and 2013) was compared over time. Next, we examined the change in the rates of investigations using the urgent-chronic taxonomy across cycles of the OIS. Investigations were classified as urgent or other maltreatment-related investigations or assessments (i.e. chronic need) by using the taxonomy developed by Trocmé and colleagues [1]. Classifications were by the primary form of maltreatment, child age and the presence of severe harm requiring medical treatment. Investigations were assessed as urgent protection if the child was younger than 4 years of age and was investigated for neglect of physical abuse, if the primary concern was sexual abuse, or if the child had sustained physical harm and required subsequent medical treatment. Urgent protection investigations were compared to other investigations or assessments.

Statistical significance was calculated to examine whether there had been a change in the incidence from the previous OIS cycle. Tests of significance were produced using WesVar 5.1 software.

Results

Figure 1 presents the incidence of reported maltreatment investigations in Ontario for each of the five cycles, between 1993 and 2013 in Ontario. Between 1993 and 2013, the rate of child maltreatment related investigations completed in Ontario since 1993 has gone from

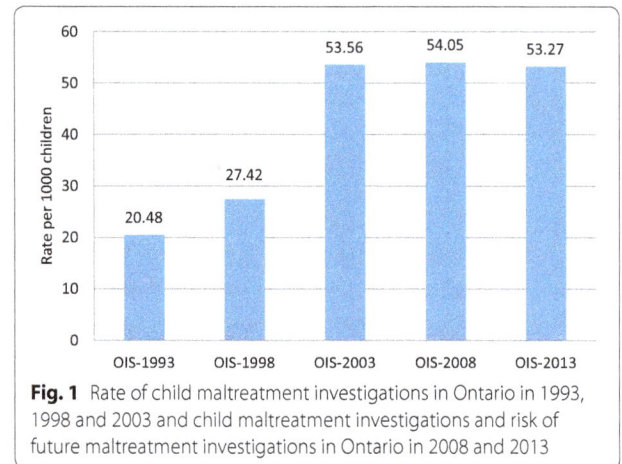

Fig. 1 Rate of child maltreatment investigations in Ontario in 1993, 1998 and 2003 and child maltreatment investigations and risk of future maltreatment investigations in Ontario in 2008 and 2013

20.48 per 1000 children to 53.27 per 1000 children. The incidence of investigations did not significantly change between 2003, 2008 and 2013.

Table 2 presents a classification of investigations by the urgent and chronic taxonomy from 1993, 1998, 2003, 2008 and 2013.

Urgent investigations

As shown in Table 2, the rate of severe physical harm is similar from 1993 to 2013. In 1998 the rate of severe physical harm rose to 1.02 per 1000 investigations from .41 per 1000 investigations in 1993; however, the proportion of cases with documented physical harm is consistently low, ranging from 1 to 4% of investigations. Similarly, the rate of investigated physical abuse for children under the age of 4 has remained consistent over time from a low of 0.96 per 1000 child maltreatment investigations in 2008 to a high of 1.79 in 2003. Reported sexual abuse investigations have declined with the largest reduction in investigations between 1993 and 1998: in 1993 the rate of investigated sexual abuse was 5.17 per 1000 child maltreatment investigations; in 1998 the incidence of reported sexual abuse was 2.58 per 1000 investigations (p < 0.01). For neglect investigations of children under the age of four, the rate of investigations nearly doubled between 1998 and 2003 from 2.57 per 1000 child maltreatment investigations in 1998 to 4.27 per 1000

Table 2 Incidence of urgent protection and chronic investigations and assessments in Ontario in 1993, 1998, 2003, 2008 and 2013

Type of investigation	OIS-1993			OIS-1998			OIS-2003			OIS-2008			OIS-2013		
	#	Rate per 1000	%	#	Rate per 1000	%	#	Rate per 1000	%	#	Rate per 1000	%	#	Rate per 1000	%
Urgent protection investigation															
Severe physical harm	890	0.41	2	2400	1.02*	4	1908	0.80	1	1729	0.73	1	1445	0.61	1
Physical abuse < 4	3472	1.59	8	3399	1.44	5	4283	1.79	4	2294	0.96	2	2704	1.15	2
Sexual abuse	11,315	5.17	25	6079	2.58*	9	6661	2.79	5	4557	1.91*	4	4212	1.79	3
Neglect < 4	4702	2.15	10	6059	2.57	9	10,197	4.27	8	7552	3.17	6	5603	2.38	4
Total urgent protection	20,379	9.31	45	17,937	7.61	28	23,049	9.64	18	16,132	6.77	13	13,964	5.94	11
Chronic investigations and assessments															
Physical abuse ≥4	14,930	6.82	33	19,207	8.15	30	31,777	13.29	25	20,142	8.46	16	21,804	9.28	17
Neglect ≥4	7546	3.45	17	15,795	6.70*	24	30,252	12.65*	24	20,493	8.60	16	20,291	8.64	16
Emotional maltreatment	1995	0.91	4	5076	2.15***	8	18,409	7.70***	14	8039	3.37*	6	10,566	4.50	8
Exposure to IPV	–	–	0	6607	2.80	10	24,564	10.27***	19	22,219	9.33	17	31,210	13.28	25
Overall risk	–	–	0	–	–	0	–	0	0	41,723	17.52	32	27,330	11.63	22
Total other investigations	24,471	11.18	55	46,685	19.81	72	105,002	43.94**	82	112,616	47.28	87	111,201	47.33	89
Total	44,850	20.48	100	64,622	27.42	100	128,051	53.56*	100	128,748	54.05	100	125,165	53.27	100

* $p < 0.05$, ** $p < 0.01$, *** $p < 0.001$

child maltreatment investigations in 2003, although this increase was not statistically significant.

Overall there has been a decline in the incidence of urgent investigations from 9.31 per 1000 child maltreatment investigations in 1993 to 5.94 per 1000 maltreatment investigations in 2013. As a proportion of all investigations, those of an urgent nature have declined from 45% of all investigations in the OIS-1993 to 11% of all investigations in the OIS-2013.

Chronic investigations

The nearly doubling of the rate of child maltreatment investigations in Ontario between 1998 and 2003 is reflected in some of the trends in the subtypes of chronic investigations. Physical abuse investigations for children 4 years of age and older went from a rate of 8.15 per 1000 investigations in 1998 to 13.29 per 1000 investigations in 2003, returning to 8.46 per 1000 investigations in 2008 and 9.28 per 1000 investigations in 2013. A very similar pattern is seen in the rate of neglect investigations for children 4 years of age and older.

In 1993, emotional maltreatment was investigated in only .91 per 1000 investigations. In 1998 there was a twofold increase to 2.15 per 1000 investigations and the rate of investigated emotional maltreatment continued to increase in 2003 to 7.70 per 1000 investigations. In 2008, there was a statistically significant decline in investigated emotional maltreatment to 3.37 per 1000 investigations. In 2008 one in three investigations focused on risk of future maltreatment (17.52 per 1000 investigations). In 2013 this proportion declined to one in five investigations (11.63 per 1000 investigations), although this decline was not statistically significant. Children exposed to intimate partner violence were not identified in 1993; in 2013 it had the highest incidence of investigations, 13.28 per 1000 investigations.

Overall there has been a fourfold increase in the incidence of chronic investigations from 11.18 per 1000 child maltreatment investigations in 1993 to 47.33 per 1000 maltreatment investigations in 2013. As a proportion of all investigations, those of a chronic nature have increased from 55% of all investigations to 89% of all investigations.

Discussion

The rate of child maltreatment related investigations completed in Ontario since 1993 has gone from 20.48 per 1000 children to 53.27 per 1000 children. Two decades of policy and legislative changes have resulted in a dramatic change in the type of situation that child protection workers are routinely faced with. The overall increase in child maltreatment investigations in Ontario is difficult to interpret; for instance, the rate of child homicides

has remained fairly consistent in Ontario for several decades [21]. Ontario's child population has varied little from 1993 to 2013. The child population increased by 8% between 1991 and 1996 but has remained stable from 1996 to present day [22–26]. The percentage of children in poverty has also remained consistent since the 1990s —approximately 15% of children in Ontario live below the poverty line [27], while unemployment rates have decreased from just over 8% in 2012 to 5.8% in January 2017 [28]. The incidence of reports to child welfare organizations for a child maltreatment related concern did not change after the 2008 Great Recession.

Urgent cases are investigations where the child has sustained harm serious enough to require medical treatment; there is an allegation of sexual abuse or there is a concern of physical abuse or neglect for a child under the age of four. The rate of urgent cases has both declined by nearly half (from 9.31 per 1000 investigations in 1993 to 5.94 investigations in 2013) and in proportion to the overall composition of investigations. The findings in this paper of a decline in reported sexual abuse investigations is consistent with a steady decline in sexual abuse since the 1990s in the United States [29, 30] and the Canadian incidence studies, although statistics from victimization surveys and police databases do not support the finding that child sexual abuse is in decline [31]. Severe physical harm is consistently noted in only a small proportion of investigations. In 1993 urgent investigations were almost half the work of an Ontario child protection worker, in 2013 a worker assessed an urgent investigation in one of every ten cases.

The Ontario child welfare legislation specifically includes situations where a child has been harmed or is at risk of being harmed, consistent with an emerging body of research that show chronic, unaddressed maltreatment results in behavioural, emotional, cognitive and health issues [1, 19, 32, 33]. This inclusion is reflected in some of the dramatic increases in the subtypes of chronic investigations. Strikingly, the assessment of future risk of maltreatment and investigations focusing on exposure to intimate partner violence was nearly half the investigative work of the child welfare system in Ontario in 2013. It is difficult to disentangle the complexity of issues by categorizing investigations through one subtype. In many investigations, intimate partner violence, mental health, substance use, poverty and few social supports co-occur but may not be the primary focus of the investigation [32, 34]. These families and children are at no less risk for dramatically poor outcomes than families and children involved in urgent investigations, but the nature of the concern requires less focus on the immediate physical safety of the child and more focus on the long term effects of family related problems. Standardized decision making tools have been helpful in assisting investigating workers in determining whether a child is at future risk of maltreatment. The results of this study demonstrate that one of the most important functions a child welfare worker can perform is the assessment of family functioning and need not only to mitigate the future risk of maltreatment but to align clinical and developmental concerns with the appropriate available services both within a child welfare agency but also in the broader community. The provision of effective child welfare services not only require the identification of the complex clinical needs of the children and families identified to the child welfare system but the ability to provide assistance and programs that are evidenced informed. Fundamentally, at present, there is a disconnect between the identified need and response.

Despite the changing nature of the type of maltreatment reported and investigated in Ontario, the response by the system is nearly identical to the investigation procedures. The concerns with a traditional or child protection response to maltreatment often considered adversarial and intrusive has led some jurisdictions in the United States and Canada to develop and implement a formal differential or alternative response to children and their families [20]. This response was aimed at aligning family needs to service through a detailed assessment. In Ontario, differential response has been implemented as the possibility that a worker can investigate the allegation in a more inclusive or customized manner. Nonetheless, the system still requires the use of the same tools and a determination about whether there is a protection concern. There is no discrete pathway in legislation, policy or practice to the provision of services without an investigation. If a child is determined to be in need of child welfare services, the case must be opened for protection services.

Limitations

The OIS collects information directly from the investigating worker and the data collected are not independently verified. The study only examines the case until the point of initial assessment—the data are not able to describe the longer term impact of the events described. The data do not include children who are only reported to the police, known to a community member or never disclose their abuse or neglect. There have been procedural and study definitional changes over time that reflect changes in legislation and procedures, in particular allowing workers to describe investigations as *risk only* in 2008 makes comparisons across cycles challenging. For example, the variation in reported emotional maltreatment investigations is likely to have been impacted by the inclusion of risk only investigations in 2008 as the chronic nature of these situations may be similar.

Conclusion

Data from the Ontario Incidence Studies of Reported Child Abuse and Neglect describe a child protection system that expanded rapidly between 1998 and 2003 and since then has consistently investigated five and a half percent of children 15 years of age and under for a child maltreatment-related concern. The nature of child protection work using the taxonomy developed by Trocmé and colleagues [1] shows a dramatic shift in the types of concerns identified without a corresponding shift in the way families are assessed for need. The provision of a forensic investigation to all families does not distinguish between urgent safety concerns and needs that may require prolonged engagement. Responding to the safety and longer term issues for the latency age children who are unsupervised on a bus, the toddler left alone in an apartment and the youth who witnesses his father assault his mother requires a system that can be attenuated to their distinct needs that aligns and advocates for services and supports within the child welfare system. Indeed, chronic conditions are ones that over-time will require the most extensive response not only from child welfare but from other related sectors. Effective service provision requires more precision in our response to these diverse concerns.

Abbreviation
OIS: Ontario Incidence Study of Reported Child Abuse and Neglect.

Authors' contributions
BF is the Principal Investigator of the OIS-2008 and OIS-2013. NT is the Principal Investigator of OIS-1993, OIS-1998, and OIS-2003. BF and NT provided the conceptual direction of the study. JF, BF and NJC synthesized the literature. BF, TB and JF conducted data analyses. All authors contributed to data interpretation and had input into the manuscript. All authors read and approved the final manuscript.

Author details
[1] Factor-Inwentash Faculty of Social Work, University of Toronto, 246 Bloor Street West, Toronto, ON M6S 3W6, Canada. [2] McGill University, 3506 University Street, Room#301, Montreal, QC H3A 2A7, Canada.

Acknowledgements
We acknowledge the support of the Social Sciences and Humanities Research Council Canada Research Chair in Child Welfare (#950-231186). Funding for the five cycles of the OIS was provided by the Ministry of Children and Youth Services.

Competing interests
The authors declare that they have no competing interests.

References

1. Trocmé N, Kyte A, Sinha V, Fallon B. Urgent protection versus chronic need: clarifying the dual mandate of child welfare services across Canada. Soc Sci. 2014;3:483–98.
2. Trocmé N, Fallon B, MacLaurin B, Daciuk J, Ortiz J. Ontario incidence study of reported child abuse and neglect 1998 (OIS-1998). Toronto: Centre of Excellence for Child Welfare, Faculty of Social Work, University of Toronto; 2002. http://cwrp.ca/publications/612. Accessed 24 July 2017.
3. Fallon B, Trocmé N, MacLaurin B, Knoke D, Black T, Daciuk J, et al. Ontario incidence study of reported child abuse and neglect 2003 (OIS 2003): major findings report. Toronto: Centre of Excellence for Child Welfare, Faculty of Social Work, University of Toronto. http://cwrp.ca/publications/613. Accessed 24 July 2017.
4. Fallon B, Trocmé N, MacLaurin B, Sinha V, Black T, Felstiner C, et al. Ontario incidence study of reported child abuse and neglect-2008 (OIS-2008). Toronto: Canadian Child Welfare Research Portal; 2010. http://cwrp.ca/publications/2293. Accessed 24 July 2017.
5. Fallon B, Van Wert M, Trocmé N, MacLaurin B, Sinha V, Lefebvre R, et al. Ontario incidence study of reported child abuse and neglect—2013 (OIS-2013). Toronto: Canadian Child Welfare Research Portal; 2015. http://cwrp.ca/publications/OIS-2013. Accessed 24 July 2017.
6. Trocmé N, McPhee D, Tam KK, Hay T. Ontario incidence study of reported child abuse or neglect 1993 (OIS-1993). Toronto: The Institute for the Prevention of Child Abuse; 1994.
7. Fallon B, Trocmé N, MacLaurin B, Sinha V, Hélie S. Provincial comparisons in the Canadian incidence study of reported child abuse and neglect-2008: context for variation in findings. Int J Child Youth Resil. 2015;3:125–42.
8. Trocmé N, Fallon B, MacLaurin B, Copp B. The changing face of child welfare investigations in Ontario: Ontario incidence study of reported child abuse and neglect (OIS 1993/1998). Toronto: Centre of Excellence for Child Welfare, Faculty of Social Work, University of Toronto; 2002.
9. Fallon B, Trocmé N, Sanders JE, Sewell KM, Houston EAL. Examining the impact of policy and legislation on the identification of neglect in Ontario: trends over-time. Int J Child Adolesc Resil. 2016;4:77–90.
10. Gilbert R, Kemp A, Thoburn J, Sidebotham P, Radford L, Glaser D, et al. Recognising and responding to child maltreatment. Lancet. 2009;373:167–80.
11. Trocmé N, Chamberland C. Re-involving the community: the need for a differential response to rising child welfare caseloads in Canada. In: Community collaboration and differential response: Canadian and international research and emerging models of practice. Ottawa: Child Welfare League of Canada; 2003. p. 45–56.
12. Trocmé N, Mertins-Kirkwood B, MacFadden R, Alaggia R, Goodman D. Ontario risk assessment model phase 1: implementation and training | Canadian Child Welfare Research Portal. Toronto: Centre for Applied Social Research, Bell Canada Child Welfare Research Unit, Faculty of Social Work, University of Toronto; 1999. http://cwrp.ca/publications/616. Accessed 21 Sept 2017.
13. Ministry of Children and Youth Services. Child welfare transformation 2005: a strategic plan for a flexible, sustainable and outcome-oriented service delivery model. Toronto: Government of Ontario; 2005.
14. Commission to Promote Sustainable Child Welfare. Towards sustainable child welfare in Ontario: First report. Ministry of Children and Youth Services, Government of Ontario; 2010. http://web.archive.org/web/20110601113748 http://www.sustainingchildwelfare.ca/assets/CPSCW-Towards-Sustainable-Child-Welfare-in-Ontario-201006.pdf. Accessed 19 Sept 2017.
15. Commission to Promote Sustainable Child Welfare. Realizing a sustainable child welfare system in Ontario. Final report. Toronto: Ministry of Children and Youth Services, Government of Ontario; 2012.
16. Ministry of Children and Youth Services. Ontario child protection tools manual: a companion to the child protection standards in Ontario. 2016.
17. Ontario Association of Children's Aid Societies. Ontario child welfare eligibility spectrum. 2016. http://www.oacas.org/publications-and-newsroom/professional-resources/eligibility-spectrum/. Accessed 19 Sep 2017.
18. United Nations Human Rights Office of the Commissioner. OHCHR Convention on the rights of the child. http://www.ohchr.org/EN/ProfessionalInterest/Pages/CRC.aspx. Accessed 30 Nov 2017.
19. Trocmé N, Fallon B, Sinha V, Van Wert M, Kozlowski A, Maclaurin B. Differentiating between child protection and family support in the Canadian child welfare system's response to intimate partner violence, corporal punishment, and child neglect. Int J Psychol J Int Psychol. 2013;48:128–40.
20. Fuller T. Beyond investigations: differential response in child protective services. In: Handbook of child maltreatment. New York: Springer; 2014. http://myaccess.library.utoronto.ca/login?url= http://books.scholarsportal.info/viewdoc.html?id=/ebooks/ebooks3/springer/2014-04-01/1/9789400772083. Accessed 31 May 2017.
21. Government of Canada SC. Family violence in Canada: a statistical profile 2010. 2012. https://www.statcan.gc.ca/pub/85-002-x/2012001/article/11643-eng.htm. Accessed 21 Sept 2017.
22. Trocmé N, McPhee D, Tam KK, Hay T. Chapter 3: Incidence of abuse and neglect. In: Ontario incidence study of reported child abuse or neglect 1993 (OIS-1993). Toronto: The Institute for the Prevention of Child Abuse; 1994.
23. Statistics Canada. Population by single years of age, showing sex, for Canada, provinces, territories, census divisions and census subdivisions. Ottawa: Statistics Canada; 1996.
24. Statistics Canada. Age and sex for population, for Canada, provinces, territories, census divisions and census subdivisions, 2001 census. Ottawa: Statistics Canada; 2001.
25. Statistics Canada. Census of Canada, 2006: age and sex for population, for Canada, provinces, territories, census divisions and census subdivisions. Ottawa: Statistics Canada; 2006.
26. Statistics Canada. Census of Canada, 2011: age and sex for population, for Canada, provinces, territories, census divisions and census subdivisions. Ottawa: Statistics Canada; 2011.
27. Khanna A, Friendly M, Guo L, Hilkewich M, Mulder E, Meisner A. Let's do this-let's end child poverty for good. Toronto: Campaign 2000; 2015. http://campaign2000.ca/wp-content/uploads/2016/03/C2000-National-Report-Card-Nov2015.pdf. Accessed 30 Nov 2017.
28. Government of Ontario. Labour market report, April 2017. https://www.ontario.ca/page/labour-market-report-April-2017. Accessed 30 Nov 2017.
29. Finkelhor D, Jones L, Shattuck A. Updated trends in child maltreatment, 2010. Durham: Crimes Against Children Research Centre; 2011.
30. Finkelhor D, Turner H, Ormrod R, Hamby SL. Trends in childhood violence and abuse exposure: evidence from 2 national surveys. Arch Pediatr Adolesc Med. 2010;164:238.
31. Collin-Vézina D, Hélie S, Trocmé N. Is child sexual abuse declining in Canada? An analysis of child welfare data. Child Abuse Negl. 2010;34:807–12.
32. Fallon R, Trocmé N, MacLaurin B. Should child protection services respond differently to maltreatment, risk of maltreatment, and risk of harm? Child Abuse Negl. 2011;35:236–9.
33. Gilbert R, Widom CS, Browne K, Fergusson D, Webb E, Janson S. Burden and consequences of child maltreatment in high-income countries. Lancet. 2009;373:68–81.
34. De Marco R, Tonmyr L, Fallon B, Trocmé N. The effect of maltreatment co-occurrence on emotional harm among sexually abused children. Vict Offenders. 2007;2:45–62.

4

Many, more, most: four risk profiles of adolescents in residential care with major psychiatric problems

Elisabeth A. W. Janssen-de Ruijter[1,2]* ⓘ, Eva A. Mulder[3,4], Jeroen K. Vermunt[5] and Chijs van Nieuwenhuizen[1,2]

Abstract

Background: The development of delinquent behaviour is largely determined by the presence of (multiple) risk factors. It is essential to focus on the patterns of co-occurring risk factors in different subgroups in order to better understand disruptive behaviour.

Aims and hypothesis: The aim of this study was to examine whether subgroups could be identified to obtain more insight into the patterns of co-occurring risk factors in a population of adolescents in residential care. Based on the results of prior studies, at least one subgroup with many risk factors in multiple domains and one subgroup with primarily risk factors in a single domain were expected.

Methods: The structured assessment of violence risk in youth and the juvenile forensic profile were used to operationalize eleven risk factors in four domains: individual, family, peer and school. Data from 270 male adolescents admitted to a hospital for youth forensic psychiatry and orthopsychiatry in the Netherlands were available. Latent class analysis was used to identify subgroups and significant differences between the subgroups were examined in more detail.

Results: Based on the fit statistics and the clinical interpretability, the four-class model was chosen. The four classes had different patterns of co-occurring risk factors, and differed in the included external variables such as psychopathology and criminal behaviour.

Conclusions: Two groups were found with many risk factors in multiple domains and two groups with fewer (but still several) risk factors in single domains. This study shed light on the complexity of disruptive behaviour, providing a better insight into the patterns of co-occurring risk factors in a heterogeneous population of adolescents with major psychiatric problems admitted to residential care.

Keywords: Disruptive behaviour, Risk factors, Latent class analysis, Forensic psychiatry

Background

The development and persistence of delinquent behaviour in youth is largely determined by the presence of (multiple) risk factors. Most research in youth forensic psychiatry has focused on which risk factors predict delinquency and how (persistent) delinquent behaviour in youth can be prevented [1–3]. These studies suggest that interventions that focus on delinquency must be aimed at reducing risk factors, in line with the risk-need-responsivity model (RNR-model) of Andrews and Bonta [4]. This model describes that the intensity of treatment should be adjusted to the nature, extent and severity of the problems. In addition to the nature, extent and severity of the risk factors, insight into the patterns of co-occurring risk factors is relevant to the treatment of this high-risk youth, because the interaction of multiple risk factors may influence treatment outcomes. Furthermore, studying the co-occurrence of risk factors in youth with major psychiatric problems manifesting behavioural

*Correspondence: Lisette.Janssen@ggze.nl
[1] GGzE Centre for Child & Adolescent Psychiatry, PO BOX 909 (DP 8001), 5600 AX Eindhoven, The Netherlands
Full list of author information is available at the end of the article

maladjustment, could gain more insight into the complexity of disruptive and delinquent behaviour.

In many studies on the development of delinquent behaviour, risk factors are divided into different domains: the individual, family, peer and school domains [2, 3, 5]. Examples of risk factors for delinquency are low IQ and prior history of substance use in the individual domain [3, 5, 6], exposure to violence in the home and parental criminality in the family domain [2, 3, 5, 7, 8], peer rejection and delinquent peers in the peer domain [3, 5, 6, 9] and low academic achievement and truancy in the school domain [2, 3, 5, 9]. Many adolescents with delinquent behaviour have multiple risk factors in numerous domains in their lives [9].

Possible consequences of being exposed to multiple risk factors have been described in the cumulative risk hypothesis [10, 11]. This hypothesis implies that the accumulation of risk factors, regardless of the presence or absence of particular risk factors, affects developmental outcomes: the greater the number of risk factors, the greater the prevalence of delinquent behaviour. Several studies have confirmed such a dose–response relationship between the number of risk factors and the likelihood of delinquent behaviour [2, 3, 5, 6, 9, 12]. Furthermore, exposure to an accumulation of risk factors in multiple domains, instead of risk factors in a single domain, increases the chance of later negative outcomes such as delinquent behaviour [12].

Despite the substantial number of studies on (multiple) risk factors for delinquent behaviour, little is known about the patterns of co-occurring risk factors among adolescents. To study the co-occurrence of risk factors, a person-centred approach instead of a variable-centred approach is needed. A person-centred approach examines how behaviours co-occur in groups of adolescents. In most research with a person-centred approach, subgroups are based on specific characteristics, such as committed offences, emotional and behavioural problems, or one single risk factor such as substance abuse [13–17]. In addition, the studies that used multiple risk factors to find subgroups have examined specific populations, such as childhood arrestees or first offenders [18–20]. However, studies on subgroups based on multiple risk factors in a broad population of adolescents in residential care are scarce.

Adolescents in residential care are a heterogeneous population, for example concerning psychiatric problems and exposure to risk factors [21, 22]. In addition, disruptive problem behaviour and delinquent behaviour are quite common in this population, although the frequency and severity of these behaviours may differ [23]. Insight into the patterns of co-occurring risk factors is a first step to better understanding the complexity of disruptive

behaviour. Therefore, the aim of this study was to examine whether subgroups could be identified to obtain more insight into the patterns of co-occurring risk factors in a heterogeneous population of adolescents in residential care with no, minor or serious delinquent behaviour and major psychiatric problems. Based on the results of prior studies on multiple risk factors, at least one subgroup with many risk factors in multiple domains and one subgroup with primarily risk factors in a single domain were expected [18, 19].

Methods

Setting

All participants were admitted to the Catamaran, a hospital for youth forensic psychiatry and orthopsychiatry in the Netherlands. This secure residential care setting offers intensive multidisciplinary treatment to male and female patients aged between 14 and 23 years. Patients admitted to this hospital are sentenced under juvenile criminal law or juvenile civil law, or are admitted voluntarily. Dutch juvenile criminal law comprises the treatment and rehabilitation of adolescents[1] who have committed serious offences. Measures under the Dutch juvenile civil law are applied to adolescents whose development is at risk and whose parents or caregivers are not able to provide the required care. Irrespective of the type of measure, all patients of this hospital display severe and multiple problems in different areas of their lives.

Participants

The total sample comprised all male patients admitted to the Catamaran with a minimal stay of 3 months between January 2005 and July 2014 (N = 275). Because 99% of the admitted adolescents are male, only male patients were included. Five patients who objected to the provision of the data for research purposes were excluded from the sample. Hence, the final sample comprised 270 patients. Of these patients, 129 were sentenced under Dutch juvenile criminal law (47.8%) and 118 under Dutch juvenile civil law (43.7%), while 23 patients were admitted voluntarily (8.5%). The majority of the patients (81.1%) were convicted of one or more offence(s) before their admission. Moderately violent offences (50.0%) and property offences without violence (45.2%) were the most common. As for psychopathology, most of the DSM-IV-TR disorders were in the category "disorders usually first diagnosed in infancy, childhood, or adolescence", in particular disruptive behaviour disorders (48.9%) and autism spectrum disorders (42.6%). Detailed demographic characteristics are displayed in Table 1.

---

[1] For reasons of brevity, the term 'adolescent' is used throughout the text to include young adults who were sentenced under the Dutch juvenile justice system.

Table 1 Demographic characteristics (N = 270)

	M (SD)	Range
Age at admission in years	16.9 (1.8)	14–23
IQ	93.9 (12.0)	63–127
	n	%
Judicial measure		
Criminal law	129	47.8
Civil law	118	43.7
Voluntary	23	8.5
Previous delinquent behaviour[a]		
No conviction	51	18.9
Drug offence	12	4.4
Vandalism (property)	83	30.7
Property offence without violence	122	45.2
Moderate violent offence	135	50.0
Violent property offence	53	19.6
Serious violent offence	21	7.8
Sex offence	36	13.3
Manslaughter	9	3.3
Arson	2	0.7
Murder	7	2.6
Axis-I classification of DSM-IV-TR[b,c]		
Disruptive behaviour disorder	132	48.9
Autism spectrum disorder	115	42.6
Attention deficit/hyperactivity disorder	63	23.3
Substance disorder	61	22.6
Reactive attachment disorder	34	12.6
Schizophrenia or other psychotic disorder	25	9.3
Mood disorder	23	8.5
Anxiety disorder	22	8.1
Other disorder usually first diagnosed in infancy, childhood, or adolescence	19	7.0
Other disorders[d]	18	6.7
Axis-II classification of DSM-IV-TR[b]		
Personality disorder	16	5.9
Mental retardation	16	5.9

[a] Classification of Van Kordelaar [28]

[b] Only DSM-IV-TR classifications with a prevalence of > 5% are displayed

[c] Due to comorbidity, percentages of DSM-IV-TR classifications do not sum up to 100

[d] Other disorders are sexual and gender identity disorders, sleep disorders, impulse control disorders not elsewhere classified, and adjustment disorders

Data collection

Data were collected through the structured assessment of violence risk in youth, the juvenile forensic profile and structured file analysis.

Structured assessment of violence risk in youth (SAVRY)

The SAVRY [24] is a risk assessment tool based on the structured professional judgement model. The SAVRY consists of 24 risk items and six protective items. The risk items have three coding possibilities (low, moderate and high), whereas the protective items are scored on a two-point scale (present or absent). The inter-rater reliability of the SAVRY risk total score is good and the predictive validity for physical violence against persons is excellent [24, 25].

Juvenile forensic profile (JFP)

The JFP [26] has been developed to measure risk factors in all life areas and for all types of offending behaviour using file data. The instrument contains seventy risk factors pertaining to seven domains: history of criminal behaviour, family and environment, offence-related risk factors and substance use, psychological factors, psychopathology, social behaviour/interpersonal relationships, and behaviour during stay at the institution. Each risk factor is measured on a three-point scale, where 0 = no problems, 1 = some problems, and 2 = severe problems. The inter-rater reliability of the JFP and the convergent validity, measured by SAVRY, were of satisfactory quality [26]. The predictive validity of the JFP was tested in a sample of 102 boys. A total score from nine risk factors of the JFP was found to be a good predictor of recidivism (AUC of 0.80; [27]).

Structured file analysis

Structured file analysis was used to register objective characteristics of the patients' lives. These characteristics included general background information (for example, ethnicity), life events, DSM-IV-TR classifications and committed offences. The committed offences were classified in accordance with the classification by Van Kordelaar ([28]; as used in [17]) and the life events were based on the 'Life Events' scoring list from a Dutch monitor system for youth health [29].

Data preparation

In this study, risk factors that were present at the moment of admission to the hospital were used to identify distinct subgroups. Therefore, eleven risk factors within the four domains (individual, family, peer and school), which were often described in the literature as prominent risk factors for disruptive problem behaviour or delinquency, were chosen. The best appropriate items of the SAVRY and JFP were used to operationalize these eleven risk factors.

The individual domain consisted of three risk factors: hyperactivity (item 43 of the JFP), cognitive impairment (item 39 of the JFP) and history of drug abuse (item 42 of the JFP). The family domain contained three risk factors: exposure to violence in the home (item 6 of the SAVRY), childhood history of maltreatment (item 7 of the SAVRY) and criminal behaviour of family members (item 14 of the JFP). The three risk factors in the peer domain were peer rejection (item 10 of the JFP), involvement in criminal environment (item 13 of the JFP) and lack of secondary network (item 55b of the JFP). The school domain comprised two risk factors: low academic achievement (item 25 of the JFP) and truancy (item 22 of the JFP).

After the identification of the different subgroups, possible differences between the subgroups were examined. For this, the objective characteristics from the file analysis and two age variables of the JFP (age of first criminal behaviour/violent behaviour) were used.

Procedure

Scoring of the SAVRY and JFP was done by officially trained and certified researchers and trainees under supervision. All instruments were completed by means of consensus scoring until an inter-rater reliability of at least 80% was achieved. After reaching an inter-rater reliability of at least 80%, the certified researchers scored individually. The trainees who were not officially trained remained under the supervision of a trained researcher, which means that each SAVRY and JFP they scored was checked by a trained researcher. The procedure scoring the structured file analysis was identical: after achieving an inter-rater reliability of at least 80%, the researchers scored individually and the trainees remained under the supervision of a researcher.

Scoring of the historical items of the SAVRY and JFP and the structured file analysis took place simultaneously 3 months after admission of the patient. At that time, all the required documents had been collected and the patient files were (mostly) complete. Risk factors, life events and other variables before admission were scored using information from all possible sources before admission, such as diagnostic reports from psychologists and psychiatrists, criminal records, treatment plans from previous settings and juridical documents. DSM-IV-TR classifications, demographic information and admission characteristics were collected from registration files and the first treatment plan of the Catamaran. All information was processed anonymously.

The Dutch Law on Medical Treatment Agreement Article 7: 458 states that scientific research is permitted without the consent of the patient if an active informed consent is not reasonably possible or, given the type and aim of the study, may not be required. The anonymity of the patient must be ensured using coded data. In addition, scientific research without the active consent of the patient is only permitted under three conditions: (1) the study is of general interest; (2) the study cannot be conducted without the requested information; and (3) the participant has not expressly objected to the provision of the data. This study fits within the conditions of this law, as the data were collected retrospectively. For an extra check, this type of study has been discussed thoroughly and approved by the science committee of the GGzE and by the Ethics Review Board of Tilburg University. In this study, patients' anonymity was guaranteed by using research numbers instead of names. Five patients in the initial sample (N = 275) explicitly objected to the provision of the data for research purposes and were therefore excluded. Hence, this study was conducted in accordance with the prevailing medical ethics in the Netherlands.

Statistical analyses

Latent class analysis (LCA) by means of Latent GOLD 5.0 [30, 31] was used to construct a clustering of latent classes based on a set of categorical latent variables [32]. In LCA, the following three steps were used: (1) a latent class model was built using the eleven risk factors as indicators; (2) subjects were assigned to latent classes based on their posterior class membership probabilities; and (3) the relationship between class membership and external variables was investigated [33].

In the first step, a latent class model was built with eleven ordinal risk factors as indicators. Of these factors, ten risk factors used a three-point scale: 0 (no risk), 1 (a small risk) and 2 (a high risk), and the eleventh risk factor (cognitive impairment) was recoded into a dichotomous variable (IQ less than or equal to 85 versus higher than 85). To identify the most suitable number of classes, several model fit indices were used. Firstly, the complexity of the latent class model was considered using three information criteria: the Bayesian information criterion (BIC), the Aikake information criterion (AIC) and the Aikake information criterion 3 (AIC3; [32, 34–37]). These criteria weight the fit and the parsimony of a model: the criteria are lowest for the best model. Secondly, a bootstrap likelihood ratio test (BLRT; [38]) was used to compare two models—for example, the three-class model with the four-class model. A significant p value ($p < .05$) rejects the null hypothesis that the three-class model, in this example, holds in the population.

In step two, the subjects were assigned to latent classes based on their posterior class membership probabilities. The classification method was a proportional assignment, which means that subjects were assigned to each class with a weight equal to the posterior membership probability for that class [32].

In the last step (step three), the association between class membership and external variables was investigated.

For this purpose, the BCH method for continuous data [39] and the maximum likelihood (ML) procedure for nominal data [40] were used. Wald tests were used to determine the significance ($p < .05$) of the encountered differences between classes in external variables (e.g. life events and committed offences). The significance tests are mainly used to eliminate the variables which are of less interest rather than to prove which effects really exist. Therefore, the alpha level is not adjusted for multiple testing (e.g. using a Bonferroni correction of a factor 53) since much stricter alpha levels would potentially hide possibly interesting correlates of the encountered classes.

Results

LCA

Table 2 shows the model fit statistics for models between one and eight latent classes. For the optimal modelling of the data, the information criteria suggest a range of a three-class model (BIC) to a seven-class model (AIC). The AIC3, which is the suitable criterion to use in small samples [34], is lowest for the four-class model. The p values of the BLRT were significant up to and including the four-class model. This means that the four-class model was preferred over the three-class model (BLRT = 44.44, $p < .000$). Therefore, the four-class solution was chosen, which was also in line with the clinical interpretability of the classes.

Class description

The means of the risk factors in the individual, family, peer and school domains for each of the four classes on a zero to one scale are shown in Fig. 1. Table 3 shows significant differences between the four classes on all risk factors except for hyperactivity, cognitive impairment and low academic achievement. Class 1 ($n = 119$, 44% of sample) represented adolescents with risk factors in the individual domain (drug abuse), peer domain (involvement in criminal environment) and school domain (truancy). In

addition, adolescents in Class 2 ($n = 70$, 26% of sample) had risk factors in all four domains, such as drug abuse, childhood history of maltreatment and lack of a secondary network. In contrast, adolescents in Class 3 ($n = 49$, 18% of sample) had the lowest risks overall. Notably, they had the highest risk for peer rejection compared to the adolescents in other classes. Finally, Class 4 ($n = 32$) represented the smallest group of adolescents (12% of sample). Risk factors that were common in this group were exposure to violence in the home and childhood history of maltreatment in the family domain.

Profiling the classes

To further describe the four classes, differences between the classes concerning the demographic and admission characteristics, psychopathology, drug use, criminal behaviour and life events were studied (see Additional file 1). The following variables were significantly different between the classes: judicial measure, age at admission, ethnicity and earliest age of (outpatient) care. More specifically, there were more first and second generation immigrants in Class 2 than in Classes 1 and 3 (Wald = 13.70, $p = .003$). The majority of adolescents in Class 2 were placed under the Dutch juvenile criminal law, whereas the majority of adolescents in Class 4 were placed under the Dutch civil law (Wald = 16.09, $p = .013$). In addition, adolescents in Class 4 had the earliest age of (outpatient) care (mean = 6.8; Wald = 8.33, $p = .040$) and were youngest at admission to the Catamaran (mean = 15.6; Wald = 24.44, $p = .000$).

As for psychopathology, the following disorders differed significantly between the classes: disruptive behaviour disorder, autism spectrum disorder, substance disorder, reactive attachment disorder and schizophrenia or other psychotic disorder. Adolescents in Classes 1 and 2 were, compared to adolescents in Classes 3 and 4, more often diagnosed with a disruptive behaviour disorder (Wald = 11.37, $p = .010$), a substance disorder (Wald = 194.67, $p = .000$), and schizophrenia or other

Table 2 Model fit statistics for latent classes

	LL	BIC	AIC	AIC3	No. of para-meters	p value BLRT	Entropy R^2
1-class	− 2444.22	5006.02	4930.45	4951.45	21		1.00
2-class	− 2396.34	4977.42	4858.67	4891.67	33	.000	.67
3-class	− 2359.75	4971.42	4809.49	4854.49	45	.000	.68
4-class	− 2337.52	4994.16	4789.05	4846.05	57	.000	.71
5-class	− 2322.49	5031.28	4782.99	4851.99	69	.064	.73
6-class	− 2308.20	5069.88	4778.41	4859.41	81	.168	.73
7-class	− 2294.16	5108.97	4774.32	4867.32	93	.116	.75
8-class	− 2282.86	5153.56	4775.72	4880.72	105	.296	.76

LL log likelihood, BIC Bayesian information criterion, AIC Aikake information criterion, AIC3 Aikake information criterion 3, BLRT bootstrap likelihood ratio test

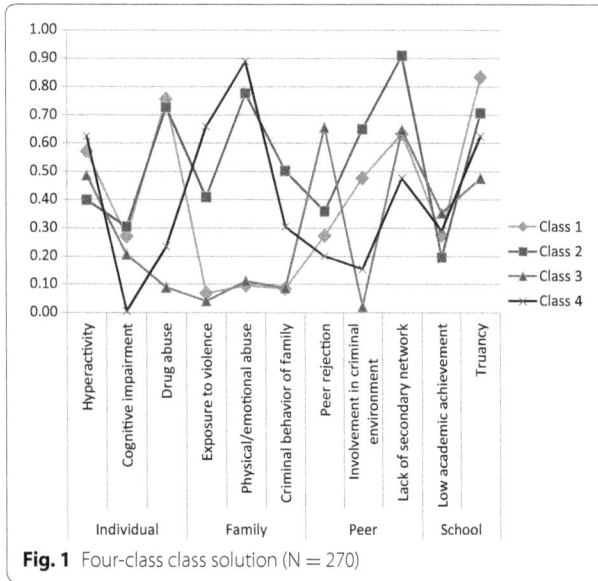

Fig. 1 Four-class class solution (N = 270)

psychotic disorder (Wald = 103.47, p = .000). Furthermore, autism spectrum disorders were more common in adolescents in Classes 1 and 3 (Wald = 28.64, p = .000), and reactive attachment disorders were more common in adolescents in Classes 2 and 4 (Wald = 15.83, p = .001). In addition, substance use differed significantly between the classes—soft drug use (Wald = 49.64, p = .000), hard drug use (Wald = 214.33, p = .000) and alcohol use (Wald = 41.83, p = .000)—and was more common in adolescents in Classes 1 and 2.

With regard to criminal behaviour, there were significant differences in no previous offences, vandalism, property offences without violence, moderate violent offences, violent property offences, serious violent offences, sex offences, arson and murder. Most types of offence—for example, property offences and violent offences—were

more common in adolescents in Classes 1 and 2 than in adolescents in Classes 3 and 4. Sex offences were, however, more common in adolescents in Class 3 (44.1%; Wald = 21.37, p = .000). Adolescents in Class 4 most often had no previous offences (53.1%; Wald = 18.03, p = .000).

Life events that differed significantly between the classes in the individual domain were victim of discrimination, financial problems, being a refugee from another country and out-of-home placement. For example, out-of-home placement before admission was more common in adolescents in Class 4 (82.4%; Wald = 11.42, p = .010). In addition, in the family domain, the following life events were significant: chronic illness or hospitalization of brother/sister, drug abuse parents, psychopathology parents, divorced parents, problems with new parent(s), financial problems parents and deceased brother/sister. Most of these life events in the family were more common in Classes 2 and 4 than in adolescents in Classes 1 and 3. Furthermore, two life events in the peer domain were significant: victim of bullying was most common in adolescents in Class 3 (86.1%; Wald = 18.10, p = .000), and impregnated a girl was more common in Classes 2 and 4 (respectively 2.2 and 10.2%; Wald = 19.03, p = .000).

Summary of the classes

Based on the risk factors of the first step of the LCA, two subgroups with many risk factors in multiple domains and two subgroups with fewer risk factors in single domains were found. Firstly, the adolescents in the classes with many risk factors (Classes 1 and 2), were mostly similar in respect of the types of offence they committed, except for the higher number of (attempted) murders in Class 2. In addition, the prevalence of psychopathology and substance use was also similar in both classes, except

Table 3 Means and comparison of LCA variables across four classes (N = 270)

Risk factors	Overall mean	Class 1 (n = 119)	Class 2 (n = 70)	Class 3 (n = 49)	Class 4 (n = 32)	Wald	p	Post hoc
Hyperactivity	1.03	1.14	.80	.97	1.25	5.59	.140	–
Cognitive impairment	.24	.27	.30	.21	.01	1.79	.620	–
History of drug abuse	1.12	1.51	1.46	.18	.47	26.88	.000	1,2 > 3,4
Exposure to violence in the home	.43	.14	.82	.08	1.32	26.01	.000	2,4 > 1; 4 > 3
Childhood history of maltreatment	.74	.19	1.55	.22	1.78	14.06	.003	2,4 > 1,3
Criminal behaviour of family members	.44	.17	1.00	.17	.61	21.47	.000	2,4 > 1; 2 > 3
Peer rejection	.72	.55	.72	1.31	.40	16.40	.001	3 > 1,2,4
Involvement in criminal environment	.78	.95	1.30	.04	.31	23.76	.000	1,2 > 3,4; 2 > 1
Lack of secondary network	1.38	1.27	1.82	1.30	.95	13.01	.005	2 > 1,3,4
Low academic achievement	.54	.55	.39	.71	.58	31.9	.36	–
Truancy	1.42	1.67	1.41	.95	1.25	15.81	.001	1,2 > 3; 1 > 4

for the higher prevalence of reactive attachment disorder in Class 2. Alternatively, the main difference between these two classes was the high family risk in Class 2. Other differences were ethnicity (more immigrants in Class 2) and financial problems (higher prevalence in Class 2).

The other two subgroups comprised adolescents with fewer, but still several, risk factors in single domains. The risk factors in these two subgroups were very different: adolescents in Class 3 experienced mainly risks in the peer domain, whereas adolescents in Class 4 experienced mainly family risks. Furthermore, adolescents in these two classes also differed in terms of psychopathology (highest prevalence of autism spectrum disorders in Class 3 versus highest prevalence of reactive attachment disorders in Class 4) and committed offences (the highest prevalence of sex offences in Class 3 versus the highest percentage of no previous conviction in Class 4).

Discussion

In this study, subgroups were investigated in a sample of adolescents in residential care with no, minor or serious delinquent behaviour and major psychiatric problems. The aim of this study was to obtain more insight into the patterns of co-occurring risk factors in order to better understand disruptive problem behaviour. Four subgroups were identified based on eleven risk factors in the individual, family, peer and school domains: Class 1 with many risk factors in the individual, peer and school domains; Class 2 with many risks in all four domains; Class 3 with mainly risks in the peer domain; and Class 4 with mainly risks in the family domain. These results were largely in line with the hypotheses, identifying not one but two subgroups with many risk factors and also not one but two subgroups with fewer risk factors in single domains.

As for the relationship between class membership and previous delinquent behaviour, this study, like many other studies, supports the cumulative risk hypothesis [10, 11]. Adolescents in the two groups with many risk factors had more often committed multiple offences than adolescents in the other two groups. Adolescents in the two groups with fewer, but still several, risk factors also had a history of delinquent behaviour. However, this behaviour was slightly less frequent than that of adolescents with more risk factors. This finding corresponds with a recent study by Wong et al. [9], who found a linear relationship between the accumulative risk level and delinquency: delinquent boys and girls turned out to have higher risk levels than boys and girls without delinquent behaviour.

Those adolescents in the two groups with many risk factors (Classes 1 and 2) have a similar history of criminal behaviour. The combination of committed offences and experienced risk factors in these two classes corresponds with the characteristics of the subgroup violent property offenders found by Mulder et al. [17]. This subgroup consisted of high-frequency offenders with violent and property offences, highest scores on alcohol abuse and high scores for conduct disorder, involvement with criminal peers, criminal behaviour in the family and truancy. Despite the similarities of the classes with this subgroup of violent property offenders, it is remarkable that the current study distinguished not one but two separate classes with one main difference.

The main difference between Classes 1 and 2 is the high number of family risk factors in Class 2, which is in line with the results of Geluk and colleagues [19]. They found an externalizing intermediate problem group that was characterized by externalizing problems in the individual and peer domains and relatively few parenting problems, and a pervasive high problem group with many problems across all domains. The results of this study on childhood arrestees who committed a first offence under the age of 12 imply that the classification of two separate groups based on the presence or absence of risks in the family domain can also be found in childhood.

Risk factors in the family domain were also seen in adolescents in Class 4 with childhood history of maltreatment as the highest family risk factor. In the literature, an association between maltreatment and later (violent) delinquency was found [41–43]. The pattern that abused children themselves commit violence or delinquent behaviour later in life is described as "the Cycle of Violence" [44, 45]. Bender [46] proposed an extension of this cycle with potential intervening risk factors in order to answer the question of why some maltreated youths become juvenile offenders. She found a potential intervention of two factors for males, namely running away from home and association with deviant peers. The association with deviant peers, which mainly occurred in adolescents in Class 2, could possibly explain why the adolescents in Class 2 were more often involved in criminal behaviour than those in Class 4.

Class 3 is a specific class with distinctive risk factors and characteristics different from the other classes. Adolescents in this class were most often diagnosed with an autism spectrum disorder, had the highest risk for peer rejection, and committed sexual offences more often compared to the other classes. The coincidence of an autism spectrum disorder and peer rejection is in line with the literature, which describes that children with autism spectrum disorders have an increased risk of being victims of bullying [47–49]. In addition, the highest prevalence of sexual offences in this class corresponds with a study by 't Hart-Kerkhoffs et al. [50] who found higher levels of symptoms of autism spectrum disorder in juvenile suspects of sex offences compared with the non-delinquent population. Furthermore, in a review by Van Wijk et al. [51], a relationship was mentioned between peer relationship problems and sexual offences, both of which were present in this group of adolescents.

Strengths of this study include the use of a reasonably large and complex clinical sample and a sophisticated approach to identifying heterogeneous clusters of youths. Nevertheless, there are also limitations to consider. Firstly, a limitation of this study is the use of file information to gather data. In most cases, the files were complete with corresponding information from various sources. However, in some cases, information from different sources was inconsistent. In these cases, additional information about the patient and/or his parents would have been very useful. Although the structured file analysis and scoring of the SAVRY and JFP was thoroughly conducted with all available information, only 4% of the files were double coded in order to achieve an inter-rater reliability of 80%. However, given the small differences between the raters in the training phase (range 68–88%), we concluded that the individually scored cases were reliable scored. Another limitation to consider is that of the generalizability of the findings. Our sample of male patients was admitted to one hospital for youth forensic psychiatry and orthopsychiatry in the Netherlands, which of course calls into question the generalizability of the findings. However, since the Catamaran offers treatment to a specific group of adolescents with major psychiatric problems from all over the country, this sample might well be representative of the population of adolescents with major psychiatric problems and behavioural problems in the Netherlands.

Despite these limitations, the findings of this study may have implications for practice. The risk, needs, and responsivity principles of the RNR-model [4] are important to take into account. First, according to the risk principle, more intensive treatment should be provided to persons with a risk profile with higher risks (adolescents in Classes 1 and 2) than to persons with a risk profile with lower risks (adolescents in Classes 3 and 4). Second, according to the needs principle, interventions should focus on the criminogenic needs of a person, which can be found in the described risk factors of each subgroup. For example, in adolescents in Classes 2 and 4 with high family risks interventions that strengthen protective factors in the family system could be valuable, because in past research protective factors were found to neutralize risk factors [2, 52]. Third, regarding responsivity, interventions must be adapted to the responsivity of the adolescents, which in this study is provided by information concerning cognitive functioning and low academic

achievement in the past. Hence, intervention decisions based on these three principles should finally lead to a reduction of recidivism [4].

In conclusion, this study underscores the importance of person-centred research using multiple risk factors and provides a better insight into the patterns of co-occurring risk factors in a heterogeneous population of adolescents in residential care with major psychiatric problems. Obviously, future research on these subgroups is needed, but this study is a first step towards a better understanding of the complexity of disruptive behaviour in this population of adolescents in residential care.

Authors' contributions
ChvN and EJ were responsible for the study concept and design. EJ was responsible for the acquisition and collection of the data. JV and EJ analysed and interpreted the data in collaboration with EM and ChvN. EJ was a major contributor in writing the manuscript. EM and ChvN were involved in critically revising the work. All authors read and approved the final manuscript.

Author details
[1] GGzE Centre for Child & Adolescent Psychiatry, PO BOX 909 (DP 8001), 5600 AX Eindhoven, The Netherlands. [2] Scientific Center for Care & Welfare (Tranzo), Tilburg University, Tilburg, The Netherlands. [3] Leiden University Medical Center, Leiden, The Netherlands. [4] Intermetzo-Pluryn, Nijmegen, The Netherlands. [5] Department of Methodology and Statistics, Tilburg University, Tilburg, The Netherlands.

Acknowledgements
We thank Marloes van Lierop, Meddy Weijmans and Marilyn Peeters for their help in the data collection. We also thank Ilja Bongers for her advice during the preparation of this manuscript.

Competing interests
The authors declare that they have no competing interests.

Funding
This study was facilitated by GGzE Centre for Child & Adolescent Psychiatry.

References

1. Farrington DP. Developmental and life-course criminology: key theoretical and empirical issues. The 2002 Sutherland Award Address. Criminology. 2003. https://doi.org/10.1111/j.1745-9125.2003.tb00987.x.
2. Van der Laan AM, Veenstra R, Bogaerts S, Verhulst FC, Ormel J. Serious, minor, and non-delinquents in early adolescence: the impact of cumulative risk and promotive factors. The TRAILS study. J Abnorm Child Psychol. 2010. https://doi.org/10.1007/s10802-009-9368-3.
3. Loeber R, Slot NW, Stouthamer-Loeber M. A cumulative developmental model of risk and promotive factors. In: Loeber R, Slot NW, Van der Laan AM, Hoeve M, editors. Tomorrow's criminals. The development of child delinquency and effective interventions. Farnham: Ashgate; 2008. p. 133–61.
4. Andrews DA, Bonta J. The psychology of criminal conduct. 5th ed. New Provence: Matthew Bender & Company, Inc., LexisNexis Group; 2010.
5. Murray J, Farrington DP. Risk factors for conduct disorder and delinquency: key findings from longitudinal studies. Can J Psychiatry. 2010;55(10):633–42.
6. Johansson P, Kempf-Leonard K. A gender-specific pathway to serious, violent, and chronic offending? Exploring Howell's risk factors for serious delinquency. Crime Delinquency. 2009. https://doi.org/10.1177//0011128708330652.
7. Hoeve M, Semon Dubas J, Eichelsheim VI, Van der Laan PH, Smeenk W, Gerris JRM. The relationship between parenting and delinquency: a meta-analysis. J Abnorm Child Psychol. 2009. https://doi.org/10.1007/s10802-009-9310-8.
8. Wong TML. Girls delinquency. A study on sex differences in (risk factors for) delinquency [Doctoral dissertation]. Vrije Universiteit Amsterdam; 2012.
9. Wong TML, Loeber R, Slotboom A, Bijleveld CCJH, Hipwell AE, Stepps SD, Koot HM. Sex and age differences in the risk threshold for delinquency. J Abnorm Child Psychol. 2013. https://doi.org/10.1007/s10802-012-9695-7.
10. Rutter M. Protective factors in children's responses to stress and disadvantage. In: Kent MW, Rolf JE, editors. Primary prevention of psychopathology, vol 3: social competence in children. Hanover: University of New England Press; 1979. p. 49–74.
11. Sameroff AJ. Dialectical processes in developmental psychopathology. In: Sameroff A, Lewis M, Miller S, editors. Handbook of developmental psychopathology. 2nd ed. New York: Kluwer Academic/Plenum Publishers; 2000. p. 23–40.
12. Loeber R, Burke JD, Pardini DA. Development and etiology of disruptive and delinquent behavior. Annu Rev Clin Psychol. 2009. https://doi.org/10.1146/annurev.clinpsy.032408.153631.
13. DeLisi M, Vaughn MG, Salas-Wright CP, Jennings WG. Drugged and dangerous: prevalence and variants of substance use comorbidity among seriously violent offenders in the United States. J Drug Issues. 2015;45(3):232–48.
14. Hasking PA, Scheier LM, Abdallah A. The three latent classes of adolescent delinquency and the risk factors for membership in each class. Aggress Behav. 2011;37:19–35.
15. Vaughn MG, DeLisi M, Gunter T, Fu Q, Beaver KM, Perron BE, Howard MO. The severe 5%: a latent class analysis of the externalizing behavior spectrum in the United States. J Crim Justice. 2011. https://doi.org/10.1016/j.crimjus2010.12.001.
16. Bianchi V, Brambilla P, Garzitto M, Colombo P, Fornasari L, Bellina M, Bonivento C. Latent classes of emotional and behavioural problems in epidemiological and referred samples and their relations to DSM-IV diagnoses. Eur Child Adolesc Psychiatry. 2017. https://doi.org/10.1007/s00787-016-0918-2.
17. Mulder EA, Vermunt JK, Brand EFJM, Bullens R, Van Marle H. Recidivism in subgroups of serious juvenile offenders: different profiles, different risks? Crim Behav Ment Health. 2012. https://doi.org/10.1002/cbm.1819.
18. Dembo R, Wareham J, Poythress N, Meyers K, Schmeidler J. Psychosocial functioning problems over time among high-risk youths. A latent class transition analysis. Crime Delinquency. 2008. https://doi.org/10.1177/0011128707306016.
19. Geluk CAML, Van Domburgh L, Doreleijers TAH, Jansen LMC, Bouwmeester S, Garre FG, Vermeiren R. Identifying children at risk of problematic development: latent clusters among childhood arrestees. J Abnorm Child Psychol. 2013. https://doi.org/10.1007/s10802-013-9811-3.
20. Schwalbe CS, Macy RJ, Day SH, Fraser MW. Classifying offenders: an application of latent class analysis to needs assessment in juvenile justice. Youth Violence Juv Justice. 2008. https://doi.org/10.1177/1541204007313383.
21. Yampolskaya S, Mowery D, Dollard N. Profile of children placed in residential psychiatric program: association with delinquency, involuntary mental health commitment, and reentry into care. Am J Orthopsychiatry. 2014. https://doi.org/10.1037/h0099808.
22. Yampolskaya S, Mowery D. Profiles of youth in therapeutic group care: associations with involuntary psychiatric examinations and readmissions. Am J Orthopsychiatry. 2017. https://doi.org/10.1037/ort0000156.
23. Dölitzsch C, Schmid M, Keller F, Besier T, Fegert JM, Schmeck K, Kölch M. Professional caregiver's knowledge of self-reported delinquency in an adolescent sample in Swiss youth welfare and juvenile justice institutions. Int J Law Psychiatry. 2016. https://doi.org/10.1016/j.ijlp.2016.02.026.
24. Lodewijks HPB, Doreleijers TAH, De Ruiter C, De Wit-Grouls HF. SAVRY. Handleiding voor de gestructureerde risicotaxatie van gewelddadig gedrag bij jongeren [SAVRY. Manual for the structured assessment of violence risk in youth]. Zutphen: Rentray; 2006.
25. Lodewijks HPB, Doreleijers TAH, De Ruiter C, Borum R. Predictive validity of the structured assessment of violence risk in youth (SAVRY) during residential treatment. Int J Law Psychiatry. 2008. https://doi.org/10.1016/j.ijlp.2008.04.2009.
26. Brand EFJM, Van Heerde WK, Handleiding FPJ. Forensisch profiel justitiële jeugdigen [Scoring manual JFP-list. Juvenile forensic profile]. The Hague: Department of Justice, National Agency of Correctional Institutions; 2010.
27. Brand EFJM. Onderzoeksrapport PIJ-dossiers 2003C: Predictieve validiteit van de FPJ-lijst [Research study PIJ-files 2003C: predictive validity of the JFP-list]. The Hague: Department of Justice, National Agency of Correctional Institutions; 2005.
28. Van Kordelaar WFJM. BOOG. Beslissingsondersteuning onderzoek geestvermogens in het strafrecht voor volwassenen. Een forensisch psychologische studie [Decision support in research on mental ability in criminal law. A forensic psychological study]. Deventer: Kluwer; 2002.
29. RIVM. Indicatoren voor de Monitor Jeugdgezondheid. Ingrijpende gebeurtenissen 1219 vragenlijst kind. [Indicators of the Monitor Youth Health. Life events 1219 questionnaire child]. 2005. http://www.monitorgezondheid.nl/jeugdindicatoren.aspx. Accessed 13 June 2011.
30. Vermunt JK, Magidson J. Latent GOLD 4.0 user's guide. Belmont: Statistical Innovations Inc; 2005.
31. Vermunt JK, Magidson J. Latent GOLD 5.0 upgrade manual. Belmont: Statistical Innovations Inc; 2013.
32. Vermunt JK, Magidson J. Technical guide for latent GOLD 5.0: basic, advanced, and syntax. Belmont: Statistical Innovations Inc; 2013.
33. Bakk Z, Tekle FB, Vermunt JK. Estimating the association between latent class membership and external variables using bias-adjusted three-step approaches. Sociol Methodol. 2013. https://doi.org/10.1177/0081175012470644.
34. Andrews RL, Currim IS. A comparison of segment retention criteria for finite mixture logit models. J Mark Res. 2003. https://doi.org/10.1509/jmkr.40.2.235.19225.
35. Bozdogan H. Choosing the number of component clusters in the mixture-model using a new informational complexity criterion of the inverse-Fisher information matrix. In: Opitz O, Lausen B, Klar R, editors. Information and classification, concepts, methods and applications. Berlin: Springer; 1993. p. 40–52.
36. Dias JG. Finite mixture models: review, applications, and computer intensive methods. Groningen: Rijksuniversiteit Groningen; 2004.
37. Lukociene O, Varriale R, Vermunt JK. The simultaneous decision(s) about the number of lower- and higher-level classes in multilevel latent class analysis. Sociol Methodol. 2010. https://doi.org/10.1111/j.1467-9531.2010.01231.x.
38. Langeheine R, Pannekoek J, Van De Pol F. Bootstrapping goodness-of-fit measures in categorical data analysis. Sociol Methods Res. 1996. https://doi.org/10.1177/0049124196024004004.
39. Bolck A, Croon MA, Hagenaars JA. Estimating latent structure models with categorical variables: one-step versus three-step estimators. Polit Anal. 2004;12:3–27.
40. Vermunt JK. Latent class modeling with covariates: two improved three-step approaches. Polit Anal. 2010;18:450–69.

41. Lansford JE, Miller-Johnson S, Berlin LJ, Dodge KA, Bates JE, Pettit GS. Early physical abuse and later violent delinquency: a prospective longitudinal study. Child Maltreat. 2007. https://doi.org/10.1177/1077559507301841.

42. Mersky JP, Reynolds AJ. Child matreatment and violent delinquency: disentangling main effects and subgroup effects. Child Maltreat. 2007. https://doi.org/10.1177/1077559507301842.

43. Salzinger S, Rosario M, Feldman RS. Physical child abuse and adolescent violent delinquency: the mediating and moderating roles of personal relationships. Child Maltreat. 2007. https://doi.org/10.1177/1077559507301839.

44. Widom CS. The cycle of violence. Science. 1989;244:160–6.

45. Widom CS, Maxfield MG. An update on the "cycle of violence". Washington DC: US Department of Justice, Office of Justice Programs 2001, National Institute of Justice; 2001.

46. Bender K. Why do some maltreated youth become juvenile offenders? A call for further investigation and adaptation of youth services. Child Youth Serv Rev. 2010. https://doi.org/10.1016/j.childyouth.2009.10.022.

47. Zablotsky B, Bradshaw CP, Anderson C, Law PA. The association between bullying and the psychological functioning of children with autism spectrum disorders. J Dev Behav Pediatr. 2013. https://doi.org/10.1097/DBP.0b013e31827a7c3a.

48. Zablotsky B, Bradshaw CP, Anderson CM, Law PA. Risk factors for bullying among children with autism spectrum disorders. Autism. 2014. https://doi.org/10.1177/1362361313477920

49. Zeedyk SM, Rodriguez G, Lipton LA, Baker BL, Blacher J. Bullying of youth with autism spectrum disorder, intellectual disability, or typical development: victim and parent perspectives. Res Autism Spectr Disord. 2014;8(9):1173–83.

50. 't Hart-Kerkhoffs LA, Jansen LM, Doreleijers TA, Vermeiren R, Minderaa RB, Hartman CA. Autism spectrum disorder symptoms in juvenile suspects of sex offenses. J Clin Psychiatry. 2009;70:266–72.

51. Van Wijk A, Vermeiren R, Loeber R, 't Hart-Kerkhoffs L, Doreleijers T, Bullens R. Juvenile sex offenders compared to non-sex offenders: a review of the literature 1995–2005. Trauma Violence Abuse. 2006. https://doi.org/10.1177/1524838006292519.

52. De Vries Robbé M, Geers MCK, Stapel M, Hilterman ELB, Vogel V. SAP-ROF—Youth Version Dutch. Richtlijnen voor het beoordelen van beschermende factoren voor gewelddadig gedrag bij jeugd. [Guidelines for the assessment of protective factors for violence risk in juveniles]. Utrecht: De Forensische Zorgspecialisten; 2014.

5

The role of self-esteem in the development of psychiatric problems: a three-year prospective study in a clinical sample of adolescents

Ingvild Oxås Henriksen[1], Ingunn Ranøyen[1,2], Marit Sæbø Indredavik[1,2] and Frode Stenseng[1,3]*

Abstract

Background: Self-esteem is fundamentally linked to mental health, but its' role in trajectories of psychiatric problems is unclear. In particular, few studies have addressed the role of self-esteem in the development of attention problems. Hence, we examined the role of global self-esteem in the development of symptoms of anxiety/depression and attention problems, simultaneously, in a clinical sample of adolescents while accounting for gender, therapy, and medication.

Methods: Longitudinal data were obtained from a sample of 201 adolescents—aged 13–18—referred to the Department of Child and Adolescent Psychiatry in Trondheim, Norway. In the baseline study, self-esteem, and symptoms of anxiety/depression and attention problems were measured by means of self-report. Participants were reassessed 3 years later, with a participation rate of 77% in the clinical sample.

Results: Analyses showed that high self-esteem at baseline predicted fewer symptoms of both anxiety/depression *and* attention problems 3 years later after controlling for prior symptom levels, gender, therapy (or not), and medication.

Conclusions: Results highlight the relevance of global self-esteem in the clinical practice, not only with regard to emotional problems, but also to attention problems. Implications for clinicians, parents, and others are discussed.

Keywords: Mental health, Identity, Resilience, Internalizing and externalizing problems, Structural equation modeling

Background

Self-esteem—in its broadest sense—is how much value a person place on his or herself [1]. Self-esteem is related to a person's ability to hold a favorable attitude towards one self [2], and to retain such positive beliefs in situations that are challenging, especially situations that include being evaluated by others [3, 4]. Adults possessing high global self-esteem are more likely to have e.g. higher well-being, better social relations, and experience more job satisfaction than their counterparts [5]. Low self-esteem is related to e.g. emotional problems, substance abuse, and eating disorders [6]. Although self-esteem is regarded as a rather stable part of personality, it also fluctuates dependent on recent fails or accomplishments [7, 8], and sublevels of self-esteem also exists in relation to particular domains of one's life, such as sports and spare time activities [9, 10].

Perhaps due to its idiosyncratic nature, the concept of self-esteem has been widely debated in the psychological literature [1, 11, 12]. Nevertheless, in spite of its unsettled definition, the concept of self-esteem has been extensively studied, and in particular in community samples. It has been widely studied in relation to subjective well-being and quality of life, and in domains such as schools, work, and sport activities [1, 13]. Meanwhile,

*Correspondence: frode.stenseng@ntnu.no
[1] Regional Centre for Child and Youth Mental Health and Child Welfare, Faculty of Medicine, NTNU, Trondheim, Norway
Full list of author information is available at the end of the article

few researchers have investigated the potential protective role of self-esteem in the development of psychiatric problems in adolescence. Hence, the role of self-esteem in the development of psychiatric conditions is largely unknown.

In the present study, then, based on 3-year longitudinal data on adolescents with psychiatric problems, we examined the potential protective role of self-esteem on later development of psychiatric problems. Before we turn to the empirical part of this report, we review studies relevant to this scope.

As mentioned above, several studies have explored the relationship between self-esteem and psychological outcomes in community samples. For example, Greenberg et al. [10] found that high self-esteem had an anxiety-buffering function among students in an experimental setting. Likewise, threats to self-esteem have been shown to induce anxiety [14, 15] and to activate strategies that defend or restore a person's self-esteem [16]. In a longitudinal study, including nearly 3000 participants from two samples aged 15–21 years, Orth, Robins and Roberts [17] showed that low self-esteem more strongly predicted depression, than depression predicted low self-esteem. Moreover, a large meta-analysis by Sowislo and Orth [18], comprising a total of 85 longitudinal studies, concluded that the effect of low self-esteem on negative affectivity is solid and holds across different samples and design characteristics of studies, but notably, mostly limited to community samples. This corresponds with a review by Orth and Robins [19], concluding that there is massive empirical evidence in support of the vulnerability hypothesis of the *self-esteem and depression link*, which suggests that low self-esteem contributes to depression, and not vice versa. In other words, high self-esteem seems to play a protective role in the development of poor mental health, perhaps through higher levels of self-efficacy and better coping mechanisms [20, 21] but studies on clinical samples are lacking.

The majority of research on self-esteem and mental health has focused on internalizing problems, but it is also plausible to suggest that self-esteem may be related to externalizing problems, such as attention-deficit/hyperactivity disorder (ADHD). Impulsivity, inattention, and hyperactivity are core symptoms of ADHD, and the disorder is associated with impairments in social, emotional, academic, and behavioral domains [22]. Although there is some controversy linked to the onset of ADHD [23], symptoms often becomes evident in early childhood and persist throughout adulthood [24, 25]. It has been shown that self-esteem is lower among children with ADHD than children without the diagnosis [26, 27], and untreated ADHD is associated with low global self-esteem [28]. In a clinical study, Slomkowski, Klein, and

Mannuzza [29] found that adolescents with ADHD who reported higher than average self-esteem reported fewer symptoms, indicating a protective role of self-esteem in the development of ADHD symptoms. Indeed, higher self-esteem and better social adjustment are considered important treatment targets for children with ADHD [28]. Nevertheless, the exact role of self-esteem in trajectories of longer-term attention problems is unclear.

In sum, self-esteem has been explored in a great number of studies conducted in community samples, and results indicate that low self-esteem may increase negative affectivity and anxiety. However, with regards to behavior problems, such as ADHD, results are inconclusive. To the best of our knowledge, virtually no studies have investigated the potential protective role of self-esteem on the development of attention problems and symptoms of anxiety/depression among adolescents in a clinical psychiatric setting. We approach this subject through a semi-reciprocal longitudinal model, with the aim of contributing to enhanced understanding of the relationship between self-esteem and mental health.

The following main hypotheses were stipulated in this study:

1. Self-esteem protects against the development of more anxiety/depression symptoms in a clinical psychiatric sample of adolescents.
2. Self-esteem protects against the development of more attention problems, but to a lesser extent than for internalizing problems (anxiety and depression symptoms).
3. Self-esteem is negatively correlated to both anxiety/depression symptoms and attention problems in a clinical psychiatric sample of adolescents.

Methods
Study design
The study is part of The Health Survey in the Department of Child and Adolescent Psychiatry (CAP), St. Olavs Hospital, Trondheim University Hospital, Norway. This clinic provides diagnostic assessment and treatment for all psychiatric conditions in referred children and adolescents, aged 0–18 years. This was a prospective study of a defined clinical population. Inclusion criteria in the baseline study were: referred adolescents, aged 13–18 years, who had at least one personal attendance at the clinic between February 2009 and February 2011. Exclusion criteria were: major difficulties in answering the questionnaire due to their psychiatric state, cognitive function, visual impairments, or lack of sufficient language skills. Emergency patients were invited to take part once they entered a stable phase. Follow-up of participants was conducted from 2012 to 2014, approximately 3 years

after their first assessment, depending on the time for their first visit at the clinic Participation in the follow-up study did not require attendance at the CAP clinic.

Study procedure
Newly referred patients as well as patients already enrolled at the CAP clinic received oral and written invitations at their first attendance after the project started. Written informed consent was obtained from adolescents and parents prior to inclusion, according to the CAP survey procedures. Relevant for this study: the participating adolescents responded to an electronic questionnaire about his or her mental and physical health in conjunction with an appointment at the clinic, without the presence of their parents. The questionnaire was accessed via a password-protected website. A project coordinator provided assistance if needed. Participants had a unique ID-code linked to their questionnaire. Once the questionnaire was submitted, it was not possible to resubmit a new questionnaire using the same code. In addition, data were collected from clinical charts. At follow-up, adolescents from baseline were invited to respond to an electronic questionnaire measuring physical and mental health status, using the same ID-code.

Study population
In the first study period, 2032 adolescent patients had at least one attendance at the CAP clinic. Of these, 289 were excluded on the basis of the exclusion criteria. Also, 95 were lost to registration (missing). Inclusion criteria were: adolescents aged 13–18 years, who had at least one personal attendance at the clinic over a 2-year period (February 15, 2009 to February 15, 2011). Exclusion criteria were: major difficulties in answering the questionnaire due to their psychiatric state, cognitive function, visual impairments or lack of sufficient language skills. Emergency patients were invited to take part once they entered a stable phase. Hence, 1648 patients (81.1%) were invited to participate. Of these, a total of 717 adolescents (43.5%), aged 13–18 years, participated in the baseline CAP survey; 393 girls (54.8%) and 324 boys (45.2%). All baseline participants, who had consented to being contacted for follow-up ($n = 685$), by then aged 16–21 years, were invited. Among the invited 570 participated (83%) at follow-up: 324 girls (57%) and 246 boys (43%). Mean birth year of participants was 1994. Mean age was 15.66 years ($SD = 1.65$). To explore the representativeness of the baseline study population, anonymous information about the reference population was collected from annual reports from St. Olav's University Hospital, 2009–2011. All adolescents in the study period ($N = 2032$) minus those excluded ($n = 289$) were defined as reference population ($n = 1743$). In accordance with

the permission given by the Norwegian Social Science Data Services, Data Protection Official for Research, we compared age, sex, and main reason for referral between participants ($n = 717$) and non-participants ($n = 1026$) of the reference population. Participants were 0.27 years older, 95% CI (.10, .45), than non-participants, $M = 15.66$, $SD = 1.65$ versus $M = 15.39$, $SD = 1.95$, $p = .002$. There were more girls in the study group than in the non-participating group, 393 girls (54.8%) versus 509 girls (49.6%), $p = .032$. Main reason for referral did not differ between participants and non-participants (Pearson exact Chi square test; $p = .11$). Five hundred and ninety-four of these participants (86.5%) received therapy at T1, and 278 participants (40.5%) received medication. Of the 570 participating at follow-up, 201 subjects (122 girls, 61%, and 79 boys, 39%), had been assessed for attention problems and/or emotional problems at baseline, and thus constitute the sample of the present study. Of these 201 eligible participants from T1, a total of 155 participants responded to all study variables in T2, 96 girls (62%) and 59 boys (38%), which corresponds to a participation rate of 77% (see Fig. 1) in the clinical sample.

Ethics
At both baseline and follow-up, written informed consent was obtained from the adolescents and parents prior to inclusion and from the parents of participants younger than 16 years of age, according to the study procedures in the CAP survey. Study approval was given by the Regional Committee for Medical and Health Research Ethics (reference numbers CAP survey T1: 4.2008.1393, T2: 2011/1435/REK Midt; present study: 2015/845/REK Midt), and by the Norwegian Social Science Data Services (reference number CAP survey: 19976).

Measures
Self-esteem
The Rosenberg Self-Esteem Scale [2] (RSES) is a Likert-type scale with items answered by self-report on a 4-point scale (1 = *strongly agree*, 4 = *strongly agree*). In the present study, self-esteem was scored on a scale ranging from 4 to 16 using a short version of the RSES, consisting of four statements: "I take a positive attitude towards myself"; "I feel I am a valuable person, at least on par with others"; "I really feel useless at times"; and "I feel I do not have much to be proud of". Scores on negative phrases were inverted. The RSES has exhibited high validity in several studies [30–32] and is widely used across nations in exploring self-esteem [33]. Cronbach's alpha was .85.

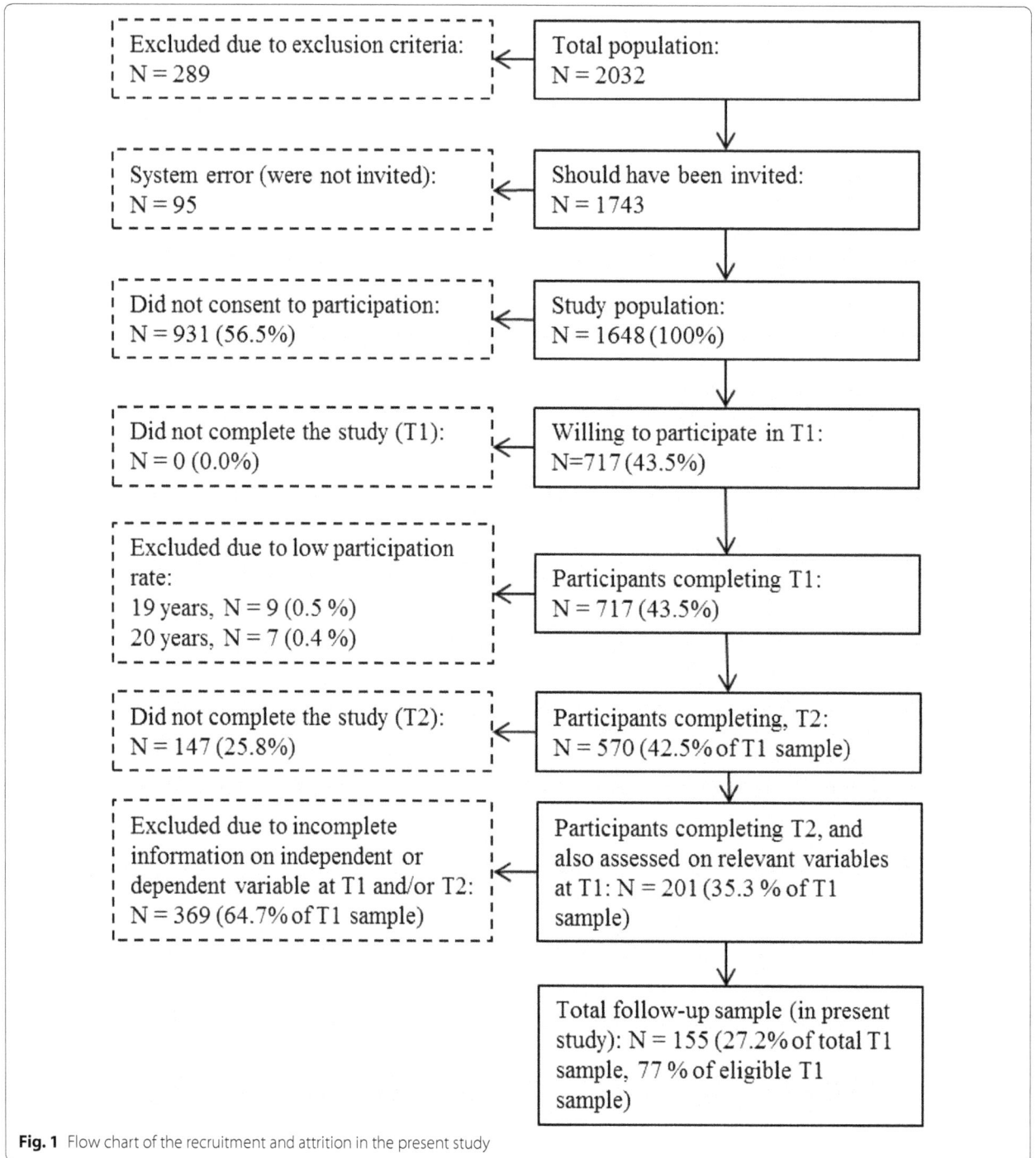

Fig. 1 Flow chart of the recruitment and attrition in the present study

Anxiety/depression and attention problems

The Youth Self-Report [34] (YSR) is a part of the Achenbach System of Empirically Based Assessment. It provides self-rating on 112 problem items. Each item is rated on a scale of 0–2 (0 = *not true*, 1 = *somewhat or sometimes true*, 2 = *very true or often true*). The problem checklist contains eight core syndrome scales [34].

In this study, the syndrome scales anxious/depressed and attention problems were used. Baseline YSR was collected from clinical charts of those participants who had responded to YSR as part of the clinicians' diagnostic evaluation. At follow-up the YSR was obtained directly by the Hel-BUP project as the YSR was incorporated in the questionnaire answered by all participants. The study population for this particular study consists of participants who answered YSR both at baseline and follow-up.

Results

Descriptive analyses
Descriptive analyses were performed in SPSS Version 21. Mean values and standard deviations for study variables are presented in Table 1. Mean level of self-esteem in the total sample was 9.41 ($SD = 3.08$) at baseline. Symptoms of anxiety/depression significantly decreased from 8.92 ($SD = 6.39$) at baseline to 7.44 ($SD = 5.95$) at follow-up. Additionally, mean levels of attention problems decreased from 7.83 ($SD = 3.87$) at baseline to 6.80 ($SD = 3.70$) at follow-up.

Correlation analysis
There were significant negative correlations between self-esteem and symptoms of anxiety/depression and attention problems (see Table 1) at baseline. There was a strong positive correlation between symptoms of anxiety/depression at baseline and at follow-up. Similarly, the correlation between attention problems at baseline and follow-up was moderately significant. Anxiety/depression at baseline was positively correlated with attention problems, both at baseline and at follow-up. The cross-time correlation between psychiatric problems at baseline and follow-up was significant for both categories of problems. There was a weak negative correlation between year of birth and anxiety/depression at follow-up, and a very weak positive correlation between birth year and gender, there were no significant correlations between birth year and other variables. Medication was associated with both anxiety/depression symptoms and attention problems at T1 and T2, but more strongly at T2. On the other hand, therapy was more strongly correlated with therapy at T1 compared to T2, and medication and therapy was positively correlated. Self-esteem was nonsignificantly associated with medication and therapy.

Structural equation modeling
Structural equation modeling was used to assess the effect of self-esteem on the stability of emotion problems and attention problems in the sample. In structural equation modeling, it is possible to combine latent factor analysis with standard regression analyses using sum scores, as well as many other modeling features [35]. In the present study, a semi cross-lagged model was defined, where each type of symptoms at follow-up were regressed on the other type of symptoms, as well as on their same type of symptoms at baseline. Also, to assess the effect of self-esteem on changes in symptoms from baseline to follow-up, a latent construct of the four self-esteem items at baseline was included as a predictor of symptoms at follow-up, and covariates were freed between self-esteem and the two symptoms-measures. A covariate was also freed between the two types of symptoms at baseline and the residuals at follow-up.

The path model was tested in AMOS Version 22 for potential correlations and cross-lagged paths (see Fig. 2), using maximum likelihood estimation Missing data was not imputed or estimated, only subjects with responses at baseline and follow up were included in the longitudinal analyses. The model had good fit with the data: χ^2 (16, N = 717) = 77.07, $p < .001$, CFI = .965, TLI = .920, RMSEA = .073. In the model, there was a high negative correlation between self-esteem and anxiety/depression at baseline ($\beta = -.58$, $p < .01$), as well as between self-esteem and symptoms of attention problems ($\beta = -.37$, $p < .01$). However, the correlation was stronger between self-esteem and symptoms of anxiety/depression. Furthermore, the stability over time of symptoms of both anxiety/depression ($\beta = .40$, $p < .01$) and attention problems ($\beta = .52$, $p < .01$) was relatively high, controlled for each other at identical measure points.

Our main hypothesis was related to the influence of self-esteem on change in levels of symptoms over time. Results showed that high self-esteem at baseline

Table 1 Correlations, mean values, and standard deviations among study variables at baseline (T1) and follow-up (T2)

	1	2	3	4	5	6	7	8	Mean	SD
1. Birth year	1								1994.2	1.572
2. Gender[a]	.188*	1							.38	0.487
3. Therapy[b]	− .275**	− .212**	1						.88	.32
4. Medication[c]	− .198*	.170*	.299**	1					.40	.49
5. Self-esteem T1	.106	.477**	− .116	.126	1				9.413	3.079
6. Anxious/depressed T1	− .151	− .451**	.201*	− .072	− .583**	1			8.916	6.393
7. Attention problems T1	− .136	− .184*	.169*	.165*	− .331**	.410**	1		7.832	3.871
8. Anxious/depressed T2	− .146	− .220**	− .334**	.298**	− .566**	.608**	.328**	1	7.439	5.954
9. Attention problems T2	− .148	− .229**	.143	.239**	− .332**	.300**	.564**	.540**	6.800	3.702

*p < .05, **p < .01

[a] Boy = 1, Girl = 2; [b] 1 = No, 2 = Yes; [c] 1 = No, 2 = Yes

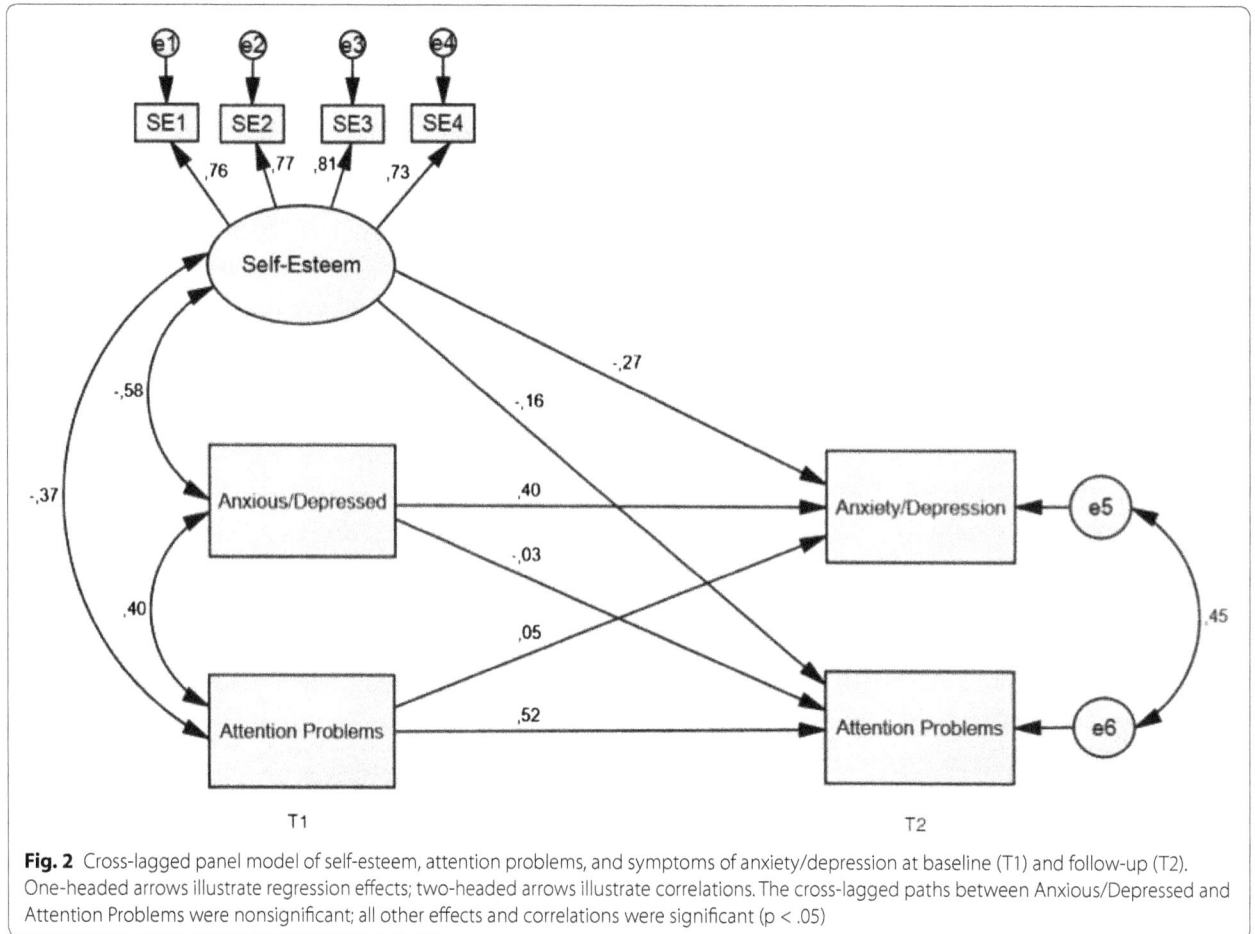

Fig. 2 Cross-lagged panel model of self-esteem, attention problems, and symptoms of anxiety/depression at baseline (T1) and follow-up (T2). One-headed arrows illustrate regression effects; two-headed arrows illustrate correlations. The cross-lagged paths between Anxious/Depressed and Attention Problems were nonsignificant; all other effects and correlations were significant (p < .05)

predicted a reduction in symptoms of both anxiety/depression ($\beta = -.27$, $p < .01$) and attention problems ($\beta = -.16$, $p < .01$) at follow-up. These results support the assumption self-esteem is protective towards the development of both emotional problems and attention problems. Moreover, the difference between these paths was not significant ($z = 1.72$, $p = .08$, two-tailed test).

Finally, when we controlled for gender, medication and therapy at T1 in the model, it did not affect the longitudinal findings in any substantial manner. The self-esteem → anxiety/depression path weakened from $\beta = -.27$ to $\beta = -.23$, whereas the self-esteem → attention problems path remained unchanged at $\beta = -.16$. Model fits were good: χ^2 (27, N = 717) = 85.26, $p < .001$, CFI = .972, TLI = .931, RMSEA = .055.

Discussion

In the present study, we assessed the longitudinal relationship of self-esteem and symptoms of anxiety/depression and attention problems among adolescents. In contrast to previous studies, we examined the role of self-esteem in the development of anxiety/depression

symptoms and attention problems in a clinical psychiatric sample of adolescents, with particular focus on the relationship between self-esteem and attention problems.

First, and cross-sectionally, results showed that self-esteem was negatively related to symptoms of depression/anxiety and attention problems in our clinical sample of adolescents. These findings are consistent with previous studies on depression/anxiety, attention problems, and self-esteem conducted in both clinical samples and community samples [17–20, 24, 36, 37]. Also, and as expected, symptoms of depression/anxiety were positively related to attention problems at both baseline and follow-up. Symptoms of anxiety/depression and attention problems were moderately stable over time, more so for attention problems than for anxiety/depression. Second, and in accordance with our main hypotheses, the path model showed that high self-esteem at baseline predicted a dampening in symptoms of *both* anxiety/depression and attention problems at follow-up. Notably, these effects remained highly significant after we controlled for gender, medication, and therapy.

The present results indicate that self-esteem protects against the development of attention problems and anxiety/depression among adolescents under treatment for mental health problems. Thus, self-esteem may be of clinical relevance, despite not being regarded as a clinical term. Self-esteem may tap into positive aspects of one's self, and as such constitute a source for resilience. When adolescents are under treatment, it may be fruitful for the clinician to focus on the strengths and qualities of the patient, in order to build a solid foundation for further treatment. A positive evaluation of the self may counteract symptoms of mental health problems in adolescence, although the actual mechanism for this is unclear. However, the protective effect of self-esteem found in the present study may in part be explained by how self-esteem affects stress coping, which is partly related to self-efficacy [21]. Studies have shown that high self-esteem acts as a buffer under stress, hence reducing harmful effects of stress on mental health [38]. When an individual is exposed to stress, he/she will utilize different strategies, or coping mechanisms. Lazarus and Folkman [39] described coping mechanisms as cognitive and behavioral efforts that individuals apply in order to tolerate, escape or minimize the effects of stress [40]. They described two main strategies: (a) the active problem-solving strategy, and (b) the avoidant strategy. Problem-solving strategies are considered functional because they allow confrontation of the problem, processing of the stress, and thus functional adaption. Avoidant strategies, on the other hand, are considered dysfunctional [41]. A possible explanation for this is that avoidant strategies disable processing of, and adaption to, the problem. It has been shown that individuals with low self-esteem often adopt passive-avoidant coping styles focused on emotions, whereas individuals with high self-esteem will adopt active problem focused coping strategies [38, 41]. Also, some studies have shown that high self-esteem is associated with persistence when facing adversities [1]. These are possible mechanisms/explanations for how high self-esteem can act as a resilience factor against long-term internalizing problems, such as depression and anxiety.

Furthermore, self-esteem was also negatively associated with attention problems. A study on adults with ADHD found that these subjects favored the use of maladaptive coping strategies [42]. Furthermore, attention problems were negatively associated with seeking advice and support from others. It is likely that maladaptive coping strategies and lack of social support in problem solving may lead to reduced self-esteem. Some researchers have suggested that children with attention problems may struggle to attend to social cues that allow them to engage in successful social interactions [43]. Tseng and Kawabata [44] suggested that problem with behaviors such as sharing and listening, could by others be perceived as inattentive or unsupportive behavior, which in turn may lead to poor peer liking. Negative peer feedback and rejection is likely to cause a negative sense of self, which in turn may lead to an increase in maladaptive behavior. Adolescents rejected by peers might also miss out on practicing reciprocal social interactions. Stenseng, Belsky, Skalicka, and Wichstrøm [45] found that lack of social belonging led to increased symptoms of hyperactivity-impulsivity and inattentiveness. It is possible that this manifests as a vicious cycle, where attention problems lead to peer rejection and low self-esteem, which in turn increases symptoms. If self-esteem is a protective factor against symptoms, appraising self-esteem may affect long-term outcome of ADHD in adolescents.

Symptoms of both anxiety/depression and attention problems were moderately stable over time. Stability of attention problems was higher than for anxiety/depression, as expected. This may be due to the neurobiological nature of attention problems [46]. Furthermore, whereas ADHD is mostly attributed to genetic makeup [47], symptoms of anxiety and depression are considered to be more dependent upon contextual factors and life circumstances. This may partly explain why attention problems were more stable over time than emotional problems. Although the stability of attention problems was relatively high, even greater stability of symptoms may have been expected within a clinical population. The decrease in symptoms shows that—despite a strong genetic disposition in the development of ADHD—self-esteem may act as a resilience factor against future symptoms of both attention problems and anxiety/depression. This emphasizes the gravity of self-esteem and indicates that self-esteem is of importance, also in a clinical setting. When self-esteem also inflicts on the development of attention problems, this indicates that clinicians should take a holistic view on their patients' challenges, and be carful to tie diagnoses to their patients' problems at an early stage in the treatment process. Symptoms are highly overlapping, so treatment of one category of mental health problems will often also reduce symptoms of another category of problems.

The present study has some limitations. First, analyses were based on symptoms of mental health problems, not diagnoses. Hence, findings cannot be directly transferred to adolescents with anxiety disorders, depressive disorders, or ADHD. However, within a clinical population, it is likely that a considerable part of the subjects with symptoms of attention problems will have a diagnosis of ADHD. Similarly, subjects with symptoms of anxiety and depression in a clinical sample are likely to be diagnosed with anxiety and/or depression. It is also possible that the prospective effects on the anxiety/depression scale found in the present study, may have turned out differently if we had measured anxiety and depression symptoms separately. Second, subjects diagnosed with ADHD, anxiety or depression may have received medical treatment during the study period, which may have reduced or altered symptoms. Third, a short version of the RSES was used in the present study. Although this may have affected self-esteem scores, the four-item version correlates highly with the original scale, and has demonstrated validity as a measure of self-esteem [48, 49]. Finally, as this study was performed in a clinical population, results are not representative for the general population.

Conclusions

The present study demonstrates that clinically assessed adolescents with high self-esteem suffer fewer symptoms of anxiety/depression and attention problems over time, indicating that self-esteem acts as a resilience factor against such symptoms. Hence, the present study highlights the importance of self-esteem in a clinical setting, and that addressing self-esteem in clinical practice may affect the long-term outcome of both anxiety/depression symptoms and attention problems among adolescents.

Abbreviations
ADHD: attention deficit/hyperactivity disorder; CAP: The Health Survey in the Department of Child and Adolescent Psychiatry; YSR: Youth Self-Report; RSES: Rosenberg Self-Esteem Scale; SPSS: Statistical Package for the Social Sciences; AMOS: analysis of moment structures.

Authors' contributions
All authors contributed to the design of the study. IR, IOH, and FS were responsible for the analyses and drafting of the manuscript. MSI was responsible for the data collection. All authors read and approved the final manuscript.

Author details
[1] Regional Centre for Child and Youth Mental Health and Child Welfare, Faculty of Medicine, NTNU, Trondheim, Norway. [2] Department of Child and Adolescent Psychiatry, St. Olavs Hospital, Trondheim University Hospital, Trondheim, Norway. [3] Queen Maud University College, Trondheim, Norway.

Acknowledgements
We thank the participants of the CAP survey.

Competing interests
The authors declare that they have no competing interests.

Funding
This study was financed by the Regional Centre for Child and Youth Mental Health and Child Welfare (RKBU), Faculty of Medicine, Norwegian University of Science and Technology, NTNU. The CAP survey is a product of the collaboration between St. Olavs Hospital/Trondheim University Hospital and the Regional Centre for Child and Youth Mental Health and Child Welfare (RKBU). It is also funded by Unimed Innovation at St. Olavs Hospital/Trondheim University Hospital and the Liaison Committee between the Central Norway Regional Health Authority and the NTNU.

References
1. Baumeister RF, Campbell JD, Krueger JI, Vohs KD. Does high self-esteem cause better performance, interpersonal success, happiness, or healthier lifestyles? Psychol Sci Public Interest. 2003;4(1):1–44.
2. Rosenberg M. Society and the adolescent self-image. Princeton: Princeton University Press; 1965.
3. Britt TW, Doherty K, Schlenker BR. Self-evaluation as a function of self-esteem, performance feedback, and self-presentational role. J Soc Clin Psychol. 1997;16(4):463–83.
4. Leary MR, Tambor ES, Terdal SK, Downs DL. Self-esteem as an interpersonal monitor: the sociometer hypothesis. J Pers Soc Psychol. 1995;68(3):518–30.
5. Orth U, Robins RW, Widaman KF. Life-span development of self-esteem and its effects on important life outcomes. J Pers Soc Psychol. 2012;102(6):1271–88.
6. Leary MR, Schreindorfer LS, Haupt AL. The role of low self-esteem in emotional and behavioral problems: why is low self-esteem dysfunctional? J Soc Clin Psychol. 1995;14(3):297–314.
7. Kernis MH, Grannemann BD, Mathis LC. Stability of self-esteem as a moderator of the relation between level of self-esteem and depression. J Pers Soc Psychol. 1991;61(1):80–4.
8. Telles S, Singh N, Bhardwaj AK, Kumar A, Balkrishna A. Effect of yoga or physical exercise on physical, cognitive and emotional measures in children: a randomized controlled trial. Child Adolesc Psychiatry Ment Health. 2013;7(1):37.
9. Rosenberg M, Schooler C, Schoenbach C, Rosenberg F. Global self-esteem and specific self-esteem: different concepts, different outcomes. Am Sociol Rev. 1995;60(1):141–56.
10. Stenseng F, Dalskau LH. Passion, self-esteem, and the role of comparative performance evaluation. J Sport Exerc Psychol. 2010;32(6):881–94.
11. Greenberg J, Solomon S, Pyszczynski T, Rosenblatt A, Burling J, Lyon D, Simon L, Pinel E. Why do people need self-esteem? Converging evidence that self-esteem serves an anxiety-buffering function. J Pers Soc Psychol. 1992;63(6):913–22.
12. Ryan RM, Brown KW. Why we don't need self-esteem: on fundamental needs, contingent love, and mindfulness. Psych Inq. 2003;14(1):71–6.
13. Gentile B, Grabe S, Dolan-Pascoe B, Twenge JM, Wells BE, Maitino A. Gender differences in domain-specific self-esteem: a meta-analysis. Rev Gen Psychol. 2009;13(1):34–45.
14. Bennett DH, Holmes DS. Influence of denial (situation redefinition) and projection on anxiety associated with threat to self-esteem. J Pers Soc Psychol. 1975;32(5):915–21.
15. Burish TG, Houston BK. Causal projection, similarity projection, and coping with threat to self-esteem. J Pers. 1979;47(1):57–70.
16. Greenberg J, Pyszczynski T, Solomon S. The causes and consequences of a need for self-esteem: a terror management theory. In: Baumeister RF, editor. Public self and private self. New York: Springer; 1986. p. 189–212.
17. Orth U, Robins RW, Roberts BW. Low self-esteem prospectively predicts depression in adolescence and young adulthood. J Pers Soc Psychol. 2008;95(3):695–708.
18. Sowislo JF, Orth U. Does low self-esteem predict depression and anxiety? A meta-analysis of longitudinal studies. Psychol Bull. 2013;139(1):213–40.
19. Orth U, Robins RW. Understanding the link between low self-esteem and depression. Curr Dir Psychol Sci. 2013;22(6):455–60.
20. Wehmeier PM, Schacht A, Barkley RA. Social and emotional impairment in children and adolescents with ADHD and the impact on quality of life. J Adolesc Health. 2010;46(3):209–17.

21. Bandura A. Self-efficacy: toward a unifying theory of behavioral change. Pscyhol Rev. 1977;84(2):191–215.

22. Schwarzer R, Bässler J, Kwiatek P, Schröder K. The assessment of optimistic self-beliefs: comparison of the German, Spanish, and Chinese versions of the General Self-efficacy Scale. Appl Psychol. 1997;46(1):69–88.

23. Caye A, Rocha TBM, Anselmi L, Murray J, Menezes AM, Barros FC, Swanson JM. Attention-deficit/hyperactivity disorder trajectories from childhood to young adulthood: evidence from a birth cohort supporting a late-onset syndrome. JAMA Psych. 2016;73(7):705–12.

24. Biederman J, Petty CR, Clarke A, Lomedico A, Faraone SV. Predictors of persistent ADHD: an 11-year follow-up study. J Psychiatr Res. 2011;45(2):150–5.

25. Faraone SV, Biederman J, Mick E. The age-dependent decline of attention deficit hyperactivity disorder: a meta-analysis of follow-up studies. Psychol Med. 2006;36(02):159–65.

26. Hechtman L, Weiss G, Perlman T. Hyperactives as young adults: self-esteem and social skills. Can J Psychiatry. 1980;25:478–83.

27. Mazzone L, Postorino V, Reale L, Guarnera M, Mannino V, Armando M, Fatta L, De Peppo L, Vicari S. Self-esteem evaluation in children and adolescents suffering from ADHD. Clin Pract Epidemiol Ment Health. 2013;9:96–102.

28. Harpin V, Mazzone L, Raynaud J-P, Kahle J, Hodgkins P. Long-term outcomes of ADHD a systematic review of self-esteem and social function. J Atten Disord. 2016;20(4):295–305.

29. Slomkowski C, Klein RG, Mannuzza S. Is self-esteem an important outcome in hyperactive children? J Abnorm Child Psychol. 1995;23(3):303–15.

30. Blascovich J, Tomaka J. Measures of self-esteem. In: Robinson JP, Shaver PR, Wrightsman LS, editors. Measures of personality and social psychological attitudes. New York: Elsevier; 1991. p. 115–60.

31. Robins RW, Hendin HM, Trzesniewski KH. Measuring global self-esteem: construct validation of a single-item measure and the rosenberg self-esteem scale. Personal Soc Psychol Bull. 2001;27(2):151–61.

32. von Soest T. Rosenbergs selvfølelsesskala: validering av en norsk oversettelse (rosenberg's self-esteem scale: validation of a Norwegian translation). Tidsskrift Norsk Psykologforening. 2005;42:226–8.

33. Schmitt DP, Allik J. Simultaneous administration of the rosenberg self-esteem scale in 53 nations: exploring the universal and culture-specific features of global self-esteem. J Pers Soc Psychol. 2005;89(4):623–42.

34. Achenbach TM, Rescorla LA. Manual for ASEBA school-age forms & profiles. Burlington: University of Vermont, Research Center for Children, Youth & Families; 2001.

35. Kline RB. Principles and practice of structural equation modeling. 3rd ed. New York City: Guilford Press; 2011.

36. Ranøyen I, Stenseng F, Klöckner CA, Wallander J, Jozefiak T. Familial aggregation of anxiety and depression in the community: the role of adolescents' self-esteem and physical activity level (the HUNT Study). BMC Public Health. 2015;15:78.

37. Schei J, Nøvik TS, Thomsen PH, Lydersen S, Indredavik MS, Jozefiak T. What predicts a good adolescent to adult transition in ADHD? The role of self-reported resilience. J Attent Disord. 2015. https://doi.org/10.1177/1087054715604362.

38. Dumont M, Provost MA. Resilience in adolescents: protective role of social support, coping strategies, self-esteem, and social activities on experience of stress and depression. J Youth Adolesc. 1999;28(3):343–63.

39. Lazarus RS, Folkman S. Stress, appraisal, and coping. New York: Springer; 1984.

40. Seiffge-Krenke I. Causal links between stressful events, coping style, and adolescent symptomatology. J Adolesc. 2000;23(6):675–91.

41. Thoits PA. Stress, coping, and social support processes: where are we? What next? J Health Soc Behav. 1995;35:53–79.

42. Young S. Coping strategies used by adults with ADHD. Personal Ind Diff. 2005;38(4):809–16.

43. Waschbusch DA, Andrade BF, King S. Attention-deficit/hyperactivity disorder. In: Essau CA, editor. Child and adolescent psychopathology: theoretical and clinical implications. New York: Routledge; 2006. p. 52–77.

44. Tseng W-L, Kawabata Y, Gau SSF, Crick NR. Symptoms of attention-deficit/hyperactivity disorder and peer functioning: a transactional model of development. J Abn Child Psychol. 2014;42(8):1353–65.

45. Stenseng F, Belsky J, Skalicka V, Wichstrøm L. Social exclusion predicts impaired self-regulation: a 2-year longitudinal panel study including the transition from preschool to school. J Pers. 2015;83(2):212–20.

46. Konrad K, Eickhoff SB. Is the ADHD brain wired differently? A review on structural and functional connectivity in attention deficit hyperactivity disorder. Hum Brain Mapp. 2010;31(6):904–16.

47. Larsson J-O, Larsson H, Lichtenstein P. Genetic and environmental contributions to stability and change of ADHD symptoms between 8 and 13 years of age: a longitudinal twin study. J Am Acad Child Adolesc Psych. 2004;43(10):1267–75.

48. Derdikman-Eiron R, Indredavik MS, Bratberg GH, Taraldsen G, Bakken IJ, Colton M. Gender differences in subjective well-being, self-esteem and psychosocial functioning in adolescents with symptoms of anxiety and depression: findings from the Nord-Trøndelag health study. Scand J Psychol. 2011;52(3):261–7.

49. Ranøyen I, Klöckner CA, Wallander J, Jozefiak T. Associations between internalizing problems in adolescent daughters versus sons and mental health problems in mothers versus fathers (The HUNT study). J Child Fam Stud. 2014;24:2008–20.

6

Predictors of adolescents' mental health problems in Saudi Arabia: findings from the Jeeluna® national study

Oraynab Abou Abbas[1] and Fadia AlBuhairan[1,2,3]*

Abstract

Background: Depression and anxiety among adolescents require further attention as they have profound harmful implications on several aspects of adolescents' wellbeing and can be associated with life threatening risk behaviors such as suicide.

Objective: To examine the underlying risk factors for feeling so sad or hopeless and for feeling worried among adolescents in Saudi Arabia.

Methods: Data from Jeeluna® national survey was used. A cross-sectional, multi-stage, stratified, cluster random sampling technique was applied among a sample of students aged 10–19 years attending intermediate and secondary schools in Saudi Arabia. A self-administered questionnaire assessing several domains, including feeling so sad or hopeless and worried, was used to collect data. Logistic regression models were fitted to determine the different factors associated with mental health.

Results: A sample of 12,121 students was included in this study. Feeling so sad or hopeless and feeling worried were significantly more prevalent among females and older adolescents ($p < 0.0001$). The results showed that poor relationship with parents, negative body image, and chronic illness to be significantly associated with feeling so sad or hopeless and worried.

Conclusions: Symptoms suggestive of mental health problems among adolescents in Saudi Arabia are prevalent and deserve special attention. Adopting effective strategies, including regular screening and intervention programs are highly needed to better address, detect, and control early signs of these problems.

Keywords: Adolescents, School, Mental health, Sadness, Hopelessness, Worrisome, Saudi Arabia

Background

Adolescents aged 10–24 years comprise nearly 25% (1.8 billion) of the world's 7.3 billion population. Out of the 1.8 billion, almost 9 out of 10 live in less developed countries [1]. In the Arab region, the majority of the population is below the age of 25 years [2]. Likewise, in the Kingdom of Saudi Arabia (KSA), 20% out of a 28 million population is between the ages 10–19 years [3].

Although it is believed that adolescence is a healthy time in an individual's life, around 15% of the global burden of disease accounted for by disability adjusted life years (DALYs) is in the 10–24 years old age group [4]. During adolescence, several biological, cognitive, physiological, psychological, emotional and social changes emerge, and certain risky behaviors arise and are linked to adolescents' health [4]. During this period, some mental health issues are also more likely to develop [5]. While mental disorders—in general—account for 45% of the burden of disease in 10–24 year olds [6], depression and anxiety are considered to be among its leading causes [7].

Mental health is an integral part of individuals' wellbeing that is influenced not only by individual attributes or

*Correspondence: buhairanfs@ngha.med.sa
[1] King Abdullah International Medical Research Center and King Saud Bin Abdulaziz University for Health Sciences, Riyadh, Kingdom of Saudi Arabia
Full list of author information is available at the end of the article

behaviors, but also by the overall social and economic circumstances and environmental factors [5]. A study by Collishaw and colleagues [8] showed a significant increase in the proportion of adolescents reporting frequent feelings of depression and anxiety where the figures had doubled between the 1980s and the 2000s.

Research on mental health problems including depression and anxiety among adolescents has found it to be associated with poor familial bonds [9], smoking [10, 11], substance use [12, 13], bullying and physical violence [14], suicide ideation and behavior [15–17], and other factors that have direct impact on adolescents' health and wellbeing. Moreover, mental health problems during adolescence tend to persist into adulthood. Adults who suffer from depression during adolescence are at higher risk of developing major depressive disorders [18].

Although a major public health issue, adolescents' mental health has not been granted much attention within the Arab region [19]. Gender disparities in mental health conditions are wider in the region and the burden of mental health disease is expected to continue to grow with the recent increases in regional crises over the years [19–21]. Results of the analysis of the Global School-based Student Health Survey (GSHS) that was conducted among 104,614 students from 19 low and middle income countries including Arab countries such as Jordan, United Arab Emirates, Lebanon and Morocco showed that around 35% of students reported having symptoms of depression [22]. In the KSA, individual studies have reported on the prevalence and risk factors of depression and/or anxiety [23–26] in subpopulations. The only nationally representative study addressing the prevalence of depression and anxiety among adolescents in the KSA is the Jeeluna® study, in which symptoms suggestive of depression and anxiety were found to be present among 14 and 6.7% of adolescents respectively [27]. With this current study, we aim to build on previous reports and identify the underlying correlates of symptoms of depression and anxiety among adolescents in the KSA, so as to better inform policy makers, plan suitable interventions, and find sustainable solutions.

Methods

Data for this study was taken from the 2012 Jeeluna® national cross-sectional study. Jeeluna® is the first national study to assess the health status and health needs of adolescents in the KSA. It was conducted during the 2011–2012 academic year using student population proportionate, stratified, multistage, cluster sampling method. The sampling occurred at the district level and the sample size per district was proportionate to the student population within that district. Male and female students aged 10–19 years, and attending intermediate and secondary schools in public and private schools throughout the 13 regions of Saudi Arabia were invited to participate in the study, yielding a school response rate of 92.5% and a student response rate of 32%. Evening schools and schools serving special needs students were excluded. Data was weighted to ensure that it was nationally representative. The detailed methodology of Jeeluna® study was published earlier [27, 28].

Mental health domain is one of many other domains that were addressed in the Jeeluna® questionnaire. The questions were self-reported, and most of them were guided by the GSHS as well as the Youth Risk Behavior Surveillance System (YRBSS). For the current study, different variables including socio-demographics, chronic illness, relationship with parents, and others were extracted and analyzed. Symptoms of depression, referred hereafter as "feeling so sad or hopeless" was measured with the question *"during the past 12 months, how often did you feel excessively sad or hopeless daily for 2 weeks or more to the extent that you stopped doing your usual activities?"*, whereas symptoms of anxiety, referred hereafter as "feeling worried", was measured with the question *"during the past 12 months, how often have you felt so worried about something to the extent that you stopped doing your usual activities?"*. These questions have been used in the past in adolescent health surveys [29] and are guided by the Diagnostic and Statistical Manual (DSM) of Mental Disorders criteria for identifying underlying mental health disease. Answers were categorized as most of the time/always; or never/rarely/sometimes. Those who answered always or most of the time to those questions were considered as feeling so sad or hopeless and worried.

Data were weighted to account for the probability of selection of students within each school, hence obtaining unbiased results. Statistical analysis was performed using STATA 14.

p values less than 0.05 were considered to be statistically significant. Descriptive statistics were obtained for the whole sample and results were reported in terms of percentages. Bivariate analysis was then performed to test for all possible associations between the dependent and independent variable. Adjusted and unadjusted odds ratios were then generated and presented.

Ethical approval for the study was obtained from the Institutional Review Board (IRB) at King Abdullah International Medical Research Center (KAIMRC), as well as the Ministry of Education. Consent and assent forms were obtained from parents and students respectively, prior to participation in the study.

Results

Sample characteristics

Table 1 shows participants' demographics. For the purpose of this paper, a secondary data analysis was

Table 1 Sample characteristics

Variable	N = 12,121 % (95% CI)
Age (years)	
≤15	46.83 (41.34–52.39)
>15	53.17 (47.61–58.66)
Gender	
Male	52.97 (43.82–61.93)
Female	47.03 (38.07–56.18)
Nationality	
Saudi	86.33 (83.09–89.03)
Non-Saudi	13.67 (10.97–16.91)
Grade	
Intermediate	53.44 (46.68–60.07)
Secondary	46.56 (39.93–53.32)
Region	
Central	25.90 (22.47–29.66)
Western	32.36 (27.85–37.22)
Eastern	14 (10.33–18.70)
Northern	10.42 (6.84–15.58)
Southern	17.32 (13.70–21.66)
Chronic illness	
No	91.61 (91.0–92.18)
Yes	8.39 (7.82–9.0)
Relationship with mother	
Good	93.12 (92.37–93.79)
Neither good nor bad	5.26 (4.69–5.89)
Poor	1.63 (1.37–1.93)
Relationship with father	
Good	84.75 (83.58–85.85)
Neither good nor bad	11.2 (10.33–12.12)
Poor	4.05 (3.56–4.62)
Body image	
Happy with my body	39.65 (38.18–41.14)
Need to lose weight	45.04 (43.31–46.78)
Need to gain weight	15.31 (14.44–16.23)
Exercise during last week	
None	44.28 (41.27–47.34)
≤3 times	33.93 (32.39–35.50)
>3 times	21.79 (19.84–23.86)
Feeling so sad or hopeless	
No	85.75 (84.42–86.98)
Yes	14.25 (13.02–13.02)
Feeling worried	
No	93.34 (92.51–94.09)
Yes	6.66 (5.91–7.49)

CI confidence interval

conducted and a total number of 12,121 observations were considered. Fifty-three percent were males, and 53% were above 15 years of age. The mean age was 15.7 ± 3.4 years. The majority of participants were Saudis (86%). Most of the students (53%) were in intermediate schools and (46%) were in secondary schools. The distribution of the students differed across the four regions in proportion to the student population per region. As for the relationship with father and mother, the majority reported having a good relationship with 84 and 93% respectively. Overall, 14% reported feeling so sad or hopeless and 6% reported feeling worried during the past 12 months prior the survey. More females (62%) and older adolescents (>15 years of age) (59%) reported feeling so sad or hopeless. The same thing applies to feeling worried that was found to be more common among females and older adolescents (63% and 66% respectively) (all p values <0.001). Feeling so sad or hopeless and feeling worried were more common among Saudis vs non-Saudis. On the other hand, region showed no significant association with feeling so sad or hopeless and feeling worried.

Association of feeling so sad or hopeless and feeling worried with the different variables

At the bivariate level, our results revealed that age, gender, relationship with father and mother, chronic illness, body image, and exercise to be significantly associated with feeling so sad or hopeless and feeling worried (all p values <0.005). Nationality was not significantly associated with symptoms of feeling so sad or hopeless, yet it was significantly associated with feeling worried ($p < 0.05$) (Table 2).

Feeling so sad or hopeless

At the multivariate level, the associations revealed that females and older adolescents are more likely to feel so sad or hopeless with (OR 1.94; 95% CI 1.69–2.23) and (OR 1.18; 95% CI 1.00–1.40) respectively. Moreover, adolescents who had "neither good nor bad" and "poor" relationship with father had higher odds of feeling so sad or hopeless as compared to those who had a good relationship with father (OR 1.77; 95% CI 1.44–2.16) and (OR 3.44; 95% CI 2.65–4.47) respectively. The same trend continues when it comes to the relationship with mother, the poorer the relationship was, the higher the odds of feeling so sad or hopeless as compared to those who had a good relationship with mother. Adolescents who believed they needed to lose weight were more likely to feel so sad or hopeless as compared to those who were happy with their bodies. Chronic illness was also positively associated with feeling so sad or hopeless. Adolescents who self-reported having chronic illness had more than twice

Table 2 Adjusted and un-adjusted odds ratios (OR) for feeling so sad or hopeless and feeling worried

	Feeling so sad or hopeless				Feeling worried			
	U-OR	95% CI	A-OR	95% CI	U-OR	95% CI	A-OR	95% CI
Age (years)								
≤15	1		1		1		1	
>15	1.35*	1.11–1.65	1.18*	1.00–1.40	1.75*	1.39–2.21	1.56*	1.25–1.94
Gender								
Male	1		1		1		1	
Female	2.08*	1.81–2.39	1.94*	1.69–2.23	2.02*	1.65–2.47	1.88*	1.56–2.28
Nationality								
Saudi	1		1		1		1	
Non-Saudi	1.07	0.90–1.29	1.11	0.93– 1.32	1.26*	1.00–1.60	1.30*	1.04–1.63
Region								
Central	1		1		1		1	
Western	0.79	0.60–1.0	0.77	0.64–0.93	0.82	0.57–1.16	0.82	0.62–1.08
Eastern	0.80	0.57–1.11	0.75	0.59–0.93	0.90	0.61–1.31	0.88	0.65–1.20
Northern	0.79	0.52–1.21	0.87	0.63–1.21	0.58	0.56–1.29	0.94	0.66–1.35
Southern	0.82	0.60–1.11	0.82	0.68–1.00	0.89	0.59–1.33	0.93	0.66–1.30
Chronic illness								
No	1		1		1		1	
Yes	2.14*	1.75–2.61	2.31*	1.86–2.87	2.74*	2.16–3.47	2.79*	2.15–3.62
Relationship with father								
Good	1		1		1		1	
Neither good nor poor	2.13*	1.77–2.56	1.77*	1.44–2.16	2.07*	1.62–2.64	1.74*	1.34–2.26
Poor	4.58*	3.65–5.72	3.44*	2.65–4.47	5.99*	4.51–7.95	4.30*	3.22–5.74
Relationship with mother								
Good	1		1		1		1	
Neither good nor poor	2.30*	1.86–2.85	1.47*	1.13–1.92	2.36*	1.76–3.15	1.47*	1.05–2.04
Poor	4.91*	3.57–6.77	2.72*	1.85–4.02	6.01*	3.95–9.17	2.64*	1.60–4.36
Body image								
Happy with my body	1		1		1		1	
Need to lose weight	1.48*	1.32–1.66	1.38*	1.22–1.56	1.45*	1.20–1.76	1.29	1.06–1.57
Need to gain weight	1.33*	1.13–1.58	1.23*	1.02–1.49	1.34*	1.07–1.69	1.13	0.89–1.44
Exercise during last week								
None	1		1		1		1	
≤3 times	0.63*	0.57–0.71	0.78	0.70–0.88	0.69*	0.58–0.83	0.88	0.72–1.08
>3 times	0.68*	0.57–0.80	0.93	0.77–1.12	0.70*	0.56–0.88	0.94	0.72–1.22

* p < 0.05

the odds of reporting feeling so sad or hopeless (OR 2.31; 95% CI 1.86–2.87).

Feeling worried

In terms of statistical significance, results for the correlates of anxiety symptoms did not differ much from those of feeling so sad or hopeless. In particular, females (OR 1.88; 95% CI 1.56–2.28) and older adolescents (OR 1.56; 95% CI 1.25–1.94) were at higher odds of feeling worried as compared to males and younger adolescents. Adolescents who had a poor relationship with father or mother

had respectively 4.3 and 2.64 times the risk of feeling worried as compared to those who had a good relationship with father or mother. As for nationality, our results showed that non-Saudis had higher odds of feeling worried as compared to Saudis (OR 1.3; 95% CI 1.04–1.63). Feeling of worrisome was also significantly associated with chronic illness, with adolescents with chronic illness having twice the risk of feeling worried as compared to those who were generally healthy. On the other hand, body image, exercise and region showed no statistical significance at the multivariate level.

Discussion

The prevalence rate of depression (14%) and anxiety (6%) symptoms previously reported by the Jeeluna® [27] fall within the wide range reported by different studies on depression and anxiety in the region [25, 30, 31] which made us realize the importance highlighting this issue and further investigating its underlying risk factors.

Our findings of feeling so sad or hopeless and feeling worried being more prevalent among females and older adolescents, was found to be consistent with others' findings [32–34]. This was also supported by results reported by the analysis of the GSHS data that was conducted across 19 low and middle income countries including Morocco, Lebanon, Jordan and United Arab Emirates [22]. The higher prevalence rates among females can be attributed to different factors including genetics, biological, psychological or behavioral factors [35].

Poor family relationships or conflictual interactions within a family environment, as well as the lack of affection and support are correlated with depressive symptoms [36], as it is with other risk behaviors, such as bullying and violence [14]. This was also shown in our study, where poor relationship with mother or father was found to be significant risk factors feeling so sad or hopeless and feeling worried among adolescents in the KSA. The poorer the relationship with parents was, the higher the odds of feeling so sad or hopeless and feeling worried. Those results are aligned with the literature on this issue [26, 36, 37]. A study conducted among female adolescents in Riyadh has shown depression to be more prevalent among those who had bad relationship with their family members [26]. Other studies have also documented the importance of family roles in protecting adolescents from risky behaviors. For example, a national study about suicide ideation among adolescents in Lebanon showed that parental understanding was a protective factor against suicide ideation [15]. A regional study about adolescent and family connectedness among eight Arab societies, including Saudi Arabia, found that Arab adolescents, despite the social and cultural disparities among these societies, scored high on the connectedness to their families with females showing more connectedness than males [38]. These findings highlight the opportunity to capitalize on family relationships and connectedness and work towards focusing on building positive, strong and effective parenting and communication skills through launching awareness and educational campaigns or programs that target parents. Such programs may aim at enhancing parenting matters through equipping parents with the necessary knowledge about adolescents' physical, emotional and mental development. After all, knowledge is a key variable in this equation; if parents are made aware of the protective impact of positive relationship with children, and their significant role in shaping their children's well-being, they might become more engaged and more willing to take a step forward and make a difference.

Similar to other reports from different parts of the world [39–41], body image has been found to be a significant predictor of feeling so sad or hopeless and feeling worried among adolescents; those who thought they need to gain weight or lose weight were more likely to be feel so sad or hopeless. Similarly, a longitudinal study among 2139 US adolescent boys conducted between 1996 and 2009 found that distorted body image to be a risk factor for elevated depressive symptoms and tend to persist to adulthood [39]. This result is not surprising in a time where people have become deeply immersed in social media and so influenced by the 'perfect-body' image that may eventually affect their satisfaction with their bodies.

As for adolescents with chronic illnesses, our findings showed it to be significantly associated with mental health; similarly, a huge body of literature have documented the serious effects that chronic illness has on adolescents' mental health [42, 43]. In their meta-analysis, Pinquart and colleagues [44] had shown that children and adolescents with chronic physical illnesses had higher levels of depressive symptoms as compared to their healthy peers. This was also documented in a study among a subpopulation of high school students in KSA, in which they found chronic illness to be a significant risk factor for depression [24].

Given the cross-sectional nature of this study, the causal inference between the dependent and independent variables cannot be established; however, our study reveals several underlying risk factors for feeling so sad or hopeless and feeling worried among adolescents in the KSA and sets the ground for more in-depth longitudinal studies that can better reflect on this situation. On the other hand, the strength of this study resides in the generalizability of the results being the first study to address mental health and associated risk factors among a nationally representative sample of adolescents in Saudi Arabia, which in turn sets a baseline for research on adolescents' mental health in the country. Adolescents' mental health is an important issue that is, unfortunately, being widely underestimated. A huge body of research unveils the deleterious effects that depression during adolescence has on their wellbeing, not only as adolescents but as future adults too. This can be avoided through early detection of symptoms when present and effective school and community-based interventions that are tailored to the Saudi cultural context where, as in many other Middles Eastern countries, mental health problems are still stigmatized [45]. Accordingly, mental health interventions in the Middle East should take into account the fundamental role of families, adolescent-family connectedness and stigma associated with mental health [38, 46].

Ministry of Health and School Health Programs should work hand in hand in planning public awareness campaigns and training programs that target adolescents, parents and teachers. Parents should be well educated about the importance of positive communications with adolescents and this should not be difficult for an Arab country like Saudi Arabia, where family ties are highly cherished and families are considered to be the first line of support and protection.

Annual screening for depression, as recommended by the United States Preventive Services Task Force [47] should be implemented in schools. Effective professional counseling services should be implemented at all schools to help support students better cope with their problems, be it social, emotional or behavioral. Attention to capacity building in adolescent health, including adolescent mental health, is much needed [48] and will provide healthcare providers with the necessary knowledge, awareness, and skills for addressing adolescents' health needs. Though some attention to this has begun with the first Adolescent Health and Medicine Capacity Building Workshop in the Region in 2016 (AlBuhairan, unpublished), much more is needed. Lastly, the civil society should also be held accountable for planning prevention programs that promote positive mental health and creating a supporting environment so as to overcome shame and stigma linked to mental health.

Conclusions

Mental health issues are a major public health concern that have serious implications on adolescents' wellbeing. This study reveals the underlying risk factors of symptoms of depression and anxiety among adolescents in Saudi Arabia and highlights the importance of taking the necessary actions and planning suitable interventions that can lessen its harmful impact if not preventing it. Further in-depth research studies that assess adolescents' mental health using diagnostic tools for depression and anxiety are needed. Also, parents–adolescents research in Saudi Arabia is missing and requires closer investigation.

Abbreviations
CI: confidence interval; KSA: Kingdom of Saudi Arabia; OR: odds ratio; PV: physical violence; GSHS: Global School-based Student Health Survey; YRBSS: Youth Risk Behavior Surveillance System.

Authors' contributions
OA participated in analytic plan, data analysis and interpretation, and drafting of article. FA conceived of the study, acquired the funding, participated in its design, analytic plan, data management, and drafting of article. Both authors read and approved the final manuscript.

Author details
[1] King Abdullah International Medical Research Center and King Saud Bin Abdulaziz University for Health Sciences, Riyadh, Kingdom of Saudi Arabia. [2] Department of Pediatrics, King Abdullah Specialized Children's Hospital, King Abdulaziz Medical City, Riyadh, Kingdom of Saudi Arabia. [3] Bloomberg School of Public Health, Johns Hopkins University, Baltimore, MD, USA.

Acknowledgements
The authors would like to thank King Abdullah International Medical Research Center for supporting and funding the Jeeluna® project.

Competing interests
The authors declare that they have no competing interests.

Funding
This study was supported and funded by King Abdullah International Medical Research Center (Protocol Number RC08-092).

References
1. United Nations Population Funds. The power of 1.8 billion adolescents, youth and the transformation of the future. United Nations Population Funds; 2014. http://www.unfpa.org/sites/default/files/pub-pdf/EN-SWOP14-Report_FINAL-web.pdf. Accessed 23 Feb 2017.
2. UNPY. Regional overview: youth in the Arab region. New York: United Nations Economic and Social Commission for Western Asia and the United Nations Programme on Youth (UNPY).
3. US Census Bureau. International Programs. International Data Base. 2016. Accessed 23 Feb 2017.
4. Sawyer SM, Afifi RA, Bearinger LH, Blakemore S-J, Dick B, Ezeh AC, et al. Adolescence: a foundation for future health. Lancet. 2012;379:1630–40.
5. World Health Organization. Risks to mental health: an overview of vulnerabilities and risk factors. Geneva: WHO; 2012.
6. Gore FM, Bloem PJ, Patton GC, Ferguson J, Joseph V, Coffey C, et al. Global burden of disease in young people aged 10–24 years: a systematic analysis. Lancet. 2011;377:2093–102.
7. Patel V. Why adolescent depression is a global health priority and what we should do about it. J Adolesc Health. 2013;52:511.
8. Collishaw S, Maughan B, Natarajan L, Pickles A. Trends in adolescent emotional problems in England: a comparison of two national cohorts twenty years apart. J Child Psychol Psychiatry. 2010;51:885–94.
9. Séguin M, Manion I, Cloutier P, Mcevoy L, et al. Adolescent depression, family psychopathology and parent/child relations: a case control study. Can Child Adolesc Psychiatr Rev. 2003;12:2–9.
10. Fergusson DM, Goodwin RD, Horwood LJ. Major depression and cigarette smoking: results of a 21-year longitudinal study. Psychol Med. 2003;33:1357–67.
11. Johnson JG, Cohen P, Pine DS, Klein DF, Kasen S, Brook JS. Association between cigarette smoking and anxiety disorders during adolescence and early adulthood. JAMA. 2000;284:2348–51.
12. Skogen JC, Sivertsen B, Lundervold AJ, Stormark KM, Jakobsen R, Hysing M. Alcohol and drug use among adolescents : and the co-occurrence of mental health problems. Ung@hordaland, a population-based study. BMJ Open. 2014;4:e005357.
13. Wu P, Goodwin RD, Fuller C, Liu X, Comer JS, Cohen P, et al. The relationship between anxiety disorders and substance use among adolescents in the community: specificity and gender differences. J Youth Adolesc. 2010;39:177–88.
14. AlBuhairan F, Abbas OA, El Sayed D, Badri M, Alshahri S, de Vries N. The relationship of bullying and physical violence to mental health and aca-

demic performance: a cross-sectional study among adolescents in Saudi Arabia. Int J Pediatr Adolesc Med. 2017;4:61–5.

15. Mahfoud ZR, Afifi RA, Haddad PH, Dejong J. Prevalence and determinants of suicide ideation among Lebanese adolescents: results of the GSHS Lebanon 2005. J Adolesc. 2011;34:379–84.

16. Fotti SA, Katz LY, Afifi TO, Cox BJ. The associations between peer and parental relationships and suicidal behaviours in early adolescents. Can J Psychiatry. 2006;51:698–703.

17. Thompson EA, Mazza JJ, Herting JR, Randell BP, Eggert LL. The mediating roles of anxiety, depression, and hopelessness on adolescent suicidal behaviors. Suicide Life Threat Behav. 2005;35:14–34.

18. Pine DS, Cohen P, Gurley D, Brook J, Ma Y. The risk for early-adulthood anxiety and depressive disorders in adolescents with anxiety and depressive disorders. Arch Gen Psychiatry. 1998;55:56–64.

19. Obermeyer CM. Adolescents in Arab countries: health statistics and social context. DIFI Fam Res Proc. 2015;1.

20. AlBuhairan FS. Adolescent and young adult health in the Arab region: where we are and what we must do. J Adolesc Health. 2015;57:249–51. doi:10.1016/j.jadohealth.2015.06.010.

21. World Health Organization. Health for the world's adolescents: a second chance in the second decade. Geneva: World Health Organization; 2014.

22. Fleming LC, Jacobsen KH. Bullying among middle-school students in low and middle income countries. Health Promot Int. 2010;25:73–84. doi:10.1093/heapro/dap046.

23. Al Gelban K. Prevalence of psychological symptoms in Saudi secondary school girls in Abha, Saudi Arabia. Ann Saudi Med. 2009;29:275.

24. Abdel-Fattah MM, Asal ARA. Prevalence, symptomatology, and risk factors for depression among high school students in Saudi Arabia. Neurosciences. 2007;12:8–16.

25. Mahfouz AA, Al-Gelban KS, Al Amri H, Khan MY, Abdelmoneim I, Daffalla AA, et al. Adolescents' mental health in Abha city, southwestern Saudi Arabia. Int J Psychiatry Med. 2009;39:169–77.

26. Raheel H. Depression and associated factors among adolescent females in Riyadh, Kingdom of Saudi Arabia, a cross-sectional study. Int J Prev Med. 2015;6:90.

27. AlBuhairan FS, Tamim H, Al Dubayee M, AlDhukair S, Al Shehri S, Tamimi W, et al. Time for an adolescent health surveillance system in Saudi Arabia: findings from "Jeeluna". J Adolesc Health. 2015;57:263–9. doi:10.1016/j.jadohealth.2015.06.009.

28. AlBuhairan FS. Jeeluna study: national assessment of the health needs of adolescents in Saudi Arabia. Riyadh: King Adbullah International Medical Research Center; 2016.

29. Centers for Disease Control and Prevention. YRBSS|Youth Risk Behavior Surveillance System|Data|Adolescent and School Health|CDC. https://www.cdc.gov/healthyyouth/data/yrbs/index.htm. Accessed 13 June 2017.

30. Ismayilova L, Hmoud O, Alkhasawneh E, Shaw S, El-Bassel N. Depressive symptoms among Jordanian youth: results of a national survey. Community Ment Health J. 2013;49:133–40.

31. World Health Organization. Maternal, child and adolescent mental health : challenges and strategic directions 2010–2015. Geneva: World Health Organization; 2010.

32. Hankin BL, Mermelstein R, Roesch L. Sex differences in adolescent depression: stress exposure and reactivity models. Child Dev. 2007;78:279–95.

33. Bennett DS, Ambrosini PJ, Kudes D, Metz C, Rabinovich H. Gender differences in adolescent depression: do symptoms differ for boys and girls? J Affect Disord. 2005;89:35–44.

34. Lewinsohn PM, Gotlib IH, Lewinsohn M, Seeley JR, Allen NB. Gender differences in anxiety disorders and anxiety symptoms in adolescents. J Abnorm Psychol. 1998;107:109–17.

35. Piccinelli M, Wilkinson G. Gender differences in depression. Br J Psychiatry. 2000;177:486–92.

36. Sheeber L, Hops H, Davis B. Family processes in adolescent depression. Clin Child Fam Psychol Rev. 2001;4:19–35.

37. Sheeber LB, Davis B, Leve C, Hops H, Tildesley E. NIH public access. J Abnorm Psychol. 2007;116:144–54.

38. Dwairy M, Achoui M, Abouserie R, Farah A. Adolescent-family connectedness among Arabs: a second cross-regional research study. J Cross Cult Psychol. 2006;37:248–61. doi:10.1177/0022022106286923.

39. Blashill AJ, Wilhelm S. Body image distortions, weight, and depression in adolescent boys: longitudinal trajectories into adulthood. Psychol Men Masc. 2014;15:445–51.

40. Ozmen D, Ozmen E, Ergin D, Cetinkaya AC, Sen N, Dundar PE, et al. The association of self-esteem, depression and body satisfaction with obesity among Turkish adolescents. BMC Public Health. 2007;7:80.

41. Marcotte D, Fortin L, Potvin P, Papillon M. Gender differences in depressive symptoms during adolescence: role of gender-typed characteristics, self-esteem, body image, stressful life events, and pubertal status. J Emot Behav Disord. 2002;10:29–42.

42. Greydanus D, Patel D, Pratt H. Suicide risk in adolescents with chronic illness: implications for primary care and specialty pediatric practice: a review. Dev Med Child Neurol. 2010;52:1083–7.

43. Haarasilta L, Marttunen M, Kaprio J, Aro H. Major depressive episode and physical health in adolescents and young adults: results from a population-based interview survey. Eur J Public Health. 2005;15:489–93.

44. Pinquart M, Shen Y. Depressive symptoms in children and adolescents with chronic physical illness: an updated meta-analysis. J Pediatr Psychol. 2011;36:375–84.

45. Sewilam AM, Watson AMM, Kassem AM, Clifton S, McDonald MC, Lipski R, et al. Roadmap to reduce the stigma of mental illness in the Middle East. Int J Soc Psychiatry. 2015;61:111–20. doi:10.1177/0020764014537234.

46. Almakhamreh S, Hundt GL. An examination of models of social work intervention for use with displaced Iraqi households in Jordan. Eur J Soc Work. 2012;15:377–91.

47. US Preventive Services Task Force (USPSTF). Final recommendation statement: depression in children and adolescents: screening. 2016. https://www.uspreventiveservicestaskforce.org/Page/Document/RecommendationStatementFinal/depression-in-children-and-adolescents-screening1. Accessed 14 Mar 2017.

48. AlBuhairan FS, Olsson TM. Advancing adolescent health and health services in Saudi Arabia: exploring health-care providers' training, interest, and perceptions of the health-care needs of young people. Adv Med Educ Pract. 2014;5:281–7. doi:10.2147/AMEP.S66272.

7

Treatment expectancy, working alliance, and outcome of Trauma-Focused Cognitive Behavioral Therapy with children and adolescents

Veronica Kirsch* 🆔, Ferdinand Keller, Dunja Tutus and Lutz Goldbeck^

Abstract

Background: It has been shown that positive treatment expectancy (TE) and good working alliance increase psychotherapeutic success in adult patients, either directly or mediated by other common treatment factors like collaboration. However, the effects of TE in psychotherapy with children, adolescents and their caregivers are mostly unknown. Due to characteristics of the disorder such as avoidant behavior, common factors may be especially important in evidence-based treatment of posttraumatic stress symptoms (PTSS), e.g. for the initiation of exposure based techniques.

Methods: TE, collaboration, working alliance and PTSS were assessed in 65 children and adolescents (age $M = 12.5$; $SD = 2.9$) and their caregivers. Patients' and caregivers' TE were assessed before initiation of Trauma-Focused Cognitive Behavioral Therapy (TF-CBT). Patients' and caregivers' working alliance, as well as patients' collaboration were assessed at mid-treatment, patients' PTSS at pre- and post-treatment. Path analysis tested both direct and indirect effects (by collaboration and working alliance) of pre-treatment TE on post-treatment PTSS, and on PTSS difference scores.

Results: Patients' or caregivers' TE did not directly predict PTSS after TF-CBT. Post-treatment PTSS was not predicted by patients' or caregivers' TE via patients' collaboration or patients' or caregivers' working alliance. Caregivers' working alliance with therapists significantly contributed to the reduction of PTSS in children and adolescents (post-treatment PTSS: $\beta = -0.553$; $p < 0.001$; PTSS difference score: $\beta = 0.335$; $p = 0.031$).

Conclusions: TE seems less important than caregivers' working alliance in TF-CBT for decreasing PTSS. Future studies should assess TE and working alliance repeatedly during treatment and from different perspectives to understand their effects on outcome. The inclusion of a supportive caregiver and the formation of a good relationship between therapists and caregivers can be regarded as essential for treatment success in children and adolescents with PTSS.

Keywords: Caregiver, Children and adolescents, Collaboration, Posttraumatic stress symptoms, TF-CBT, Treatment expectancy, Working alliance

Background

For decades of psychotherapy research, there has been an ongoing—and often lively—debate to find out if common ingredients of a treatment, like, e.g. expectations of improvement, or more specific elements—like, e.g. exposure in trauma-therapy—are responsible for psychotherapeutic success. This argument has led to numerous studies, with the question of how to deliver the most efficacious treatment still unanswered [1]. Thus, researchers have recently begun to integrate both sides into one comprehensive model, reflecting the need for a more differentiated adaptation of common and specific treatment

*Correspondence: veronica.kirsch@web.de
^ Deceased
Department of Child and Adolescent Psychiatry and Psychotherapy, University of Ulm, Steinhoevelstr. 5, 89075 Ulm, Germany

aspects, psychiatric disorders and the individuality of the patient, to improve therapeutic success [2, 3].

This integrative approach seems helpful in the context of post-traumatic stress disorder (PTSD), a severe and chronic psychiatric condition leading to profound psychosocial impairment. For instance, both specific and common factors were reported to have substantial and unique impact on treatment success in adults with PTSD [4, 5]. Furthermore, the interplay between these factors may depend on the individual trauma history of the patient and his/her posttraumatic stress symptoms (PTSS; [6]). Traumatic experiences—especially interpersonal ones like sexual or physical violence—often lead to a loss of confidence in oneself, others and the world, so that the affected persons may have difficulties in establishing therapeutic relationships. Moreover, the ability to anticipate a positive outcome is decreased; therefore, patients might become less responsive to common factors. For such patients, evidence based treatment techniques, like exposure to trauma related stimuli, may be more important than common factors in order to facilitate symptom reduction [6, 7]. On the other hand, a good relationship with the therapist and positive outcome expectations seem essential prerequisites to engage patients in challenging exposure techniques, especially patients showing avoidant behavior as usual in PTSD [8], highlighting the importance of common factors.

One of the first advocates for acknowledging the importance of common treatment aspects [9] claimed, that positive outcome expectations were one of the most important factors in symptom change. However, research regarding treatment expectancy (TE), i.e. prognostic beliefs about the consequences of engaging in treatment [10] is rare. For adult patients, the clinical relevance of TE is supported by a meta-analysis indicating a small significant positive effect ($d = 0.24$) on treatment outcome regarding different mental disorders [10]. The authors found that better outcome expectations, assessed at an early stage of treatment, were associated with higher symptom change after treatment completion.

Due to developmental factors and the triangulated relationship with caregivers, findings from research with adults cannot be directly applied to children and adolescents. First of all, their capacity for discerning and verbalizing internal states, as well as—in consequence—TE is limited, and differs from grown-ups [11, 12]. Most of them do not seek help from mental health services on their own, but are sent by adult caretakers [13], and are therefore less likely to expect benefit from treatment or to establish a trustful relationship with the therapist. Additionally, children and adolescents are known to weigh affective aspects of the therapeutic alliance higher than their caregivers do [7, 14]. Therefore, alliance ratings

from children and adolescents and their caregivers or other adults may reflect different sides of a relationship and may not be interchangeable. Secondly—in contrast to adults—psychotherapy in children and adolescents requires active caregivers who, e.g. ensure regular attendance at sessions by accompanying their children to therapy, and who are willing to change their parenting behavior—if necessary—in order to enhance therapeutic success. This triangulates therapeutic relationships and creates further possibilities of therapeutic change. The active participation of caregivers is even more important in Trauma-Focused Cognitive Behavioral Therapy (TF-CBT), as caregivers are involved in each treatment session and are asked to support their children in practicing trauma-related coping skills at home. In fact, a successful involvement of caregivers has repeatedly been shown to be essential for therapeutic improvement in children and adolescents [15, 16]. Thus, results from adult studies are not well applicable to children, and the simultaneous investigation of both patients' and caregivers' common treatment factors is indispensable to understand their contribution to therapeutic improvement.

Although TE is considered a crucial factor for therapeutic success also with children and adolescents [17], almost no empirical research in this domain has been undertaken. In 49 children and adolescents with obsessive compulsive disorders (OCD), patients' self-reported pre-treatment TE, but not caregivers' TE predicted treatment response [18]. Higher TE was associated with high completion rates of exposure based Cognitive Behavioral Therapy (CBT) and symptom reduction. A similar pattern emerged in a large, multisite study about treatment for depression in adolescents. Patients', but not parents', TE predicted self-reported reduction of depressive symptoms immediately after treatment completion [19].

Theoretical models trying to explain TE and its effects on therapeutic improvement often refer to the influence of other common treatment factors, such as patients' collaboration or therapeutic alliance [20, 21]. High prognostic expectations could lead to better collaboration in therapy, e.g. regular homework compliance, and a better working alliance, thus indirectly enhancing therapeutic success (see Fig. 1). Additional common factors should be considered in a process model of therapeutic change, if one wants to understand the TE-outcome link, as these factors are shown to be associated or even to mediate the effect of expectations on therapeutic success.

Working alliance—defined as a consensus between patient and therapist regarding goals, methods and focus of the treatment [22]—might be important to understand the TE-outcome link. In adults, working alliance explains 29% of the variance of treatment outcome, regardless of the number of sessions, the type of treatment, the

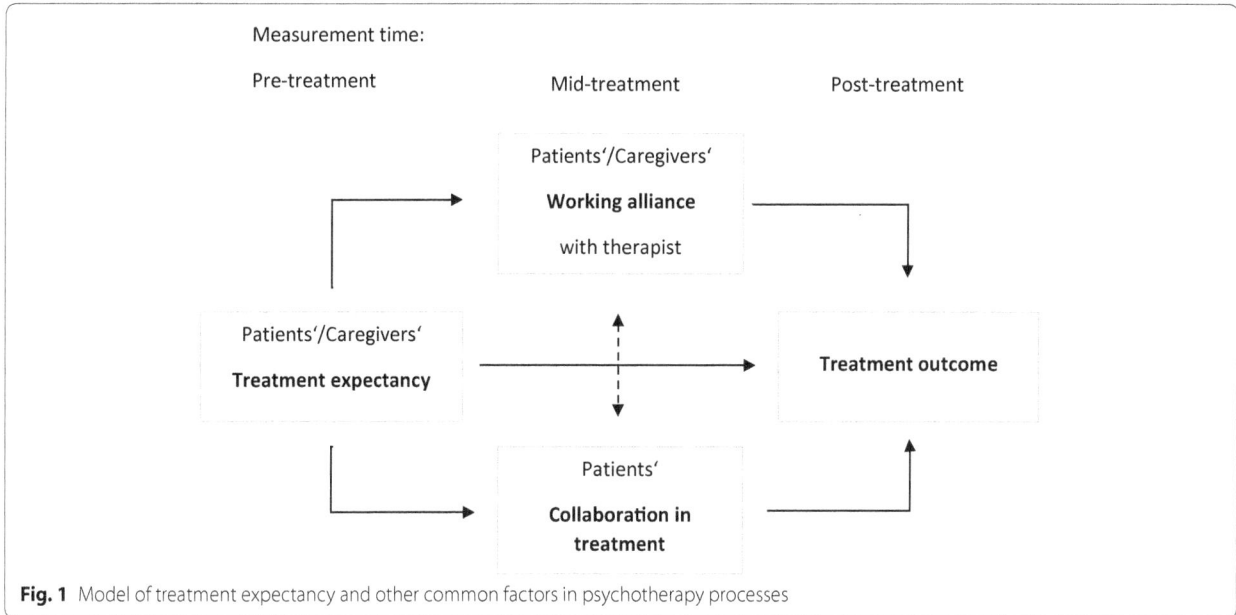

Fig. 1 Model of treatment expectancy and other common factors in psychotherapy processes

specificity of outcomes, or the design of the study [23, 24]. In children and adolescents, slightly smaller effects of alliance are reported ($r = 0.14$, [25]; $r = 0.22$, [26]), and some studies fail to demonstrate the alliance-outcome link [27]. With regard to children and adolescents suffering from PTSS, two randomized controlled trials (RCTs) found positive effects of therapeutic alliance on symptom reduction, especially on internalizing symptoms in the TF-CBT condition [8, 28], whereas another RCT for prolonged exposure in adolescent girls did not find any link between alliance and outcome [29]. Possibly, stronger alliance enhances collaboration and engagement in TF-CBT tasks, which leads to higher symptom reduction, but this was not investigated in children and adolescents with PTSS so far. Thus, knowledge about the association of different common treatment factors with TE and their contribution to treatment success is limited, especially regarding children and adolescents and their caregivers.

It is not clear to date, whether a positive relationship between TE and outcome in children and adolescents with depression or OCD, as well as the insignificance of this link in caregivers, can be generalized to other mental health problems, e.g. PTSS. TE may play an important role in enhancing treatment success in children and adolescents with PTSD. Moreover, caregivers are intensively involved in TF-CBT for children and adolescents, which increases the likelihood of an association of caregivers' TE and treatment outcome. Most recent investigations of common factors in children and adolescents with PTSD focused on working alliance, neglecting TE or a more integrative model of several common factors. Most

of all, recent TF-CBT studies [8, 28, 29] did not include caregivers' rating of common factors, therefore might underestimate their important role in symptom reduction. The current study aims to fill this gap in research on TE in children and adolescents with PTSS and their caregivers. We focused on TE in TF-CBT and investigated direct effects of patients' and caregivers' TE on treatment outcome as well as indirect effects via working alliance and patients' collaboration (see Fig. 1).

We examined the following hypotheses:

1. The patients' as well as the caregivers' TE *directly* affects patients' treatment response to TF-CBT in terms of PTSS score, respectively PTSS reduction after treatment completion.
2. The patients' as well as the caregivers' TE *indirectly* affects treatment response in so far as

   a. the patients' as well as the caregivers' TE affect patients' collaboration *and* at the same time patients' collaboration significantly affects patients' treatment response;
   b. the patients' as well as the caregivers' TE affect patients' and caregivers' working alliance *and* patients' and caregivers' working alliance affects patients' treatment response.

In a complementary analysis, treatment outcome was operationalized by a difference score of pre- and post-treatment symptoms.

Methods

Patients

The present investigation was based on data collected within a randomized controlled effectiveness study (see [30] for more details of procedures and patients). Patients were consecutively recruited at eight German mental health clinics for children and adolescents according to the following inclusion criteria: a history of one or more traumatic event(s) after the age of 3 years and dating back at least 3 months; current age 7–17 years; PTSS as main mental health problem with a total symptom severity score ≥ 35 points on the Clinician Administered PTSD Scale for Children and Adolescents (CAPS-CA; [31]); sufficient knowledge of the German language to respond to questionnaires, clinical interviews and treatment; safe current living circumstances; and the co-operation of at least one non-offending caregiver. Patients with acute suicidal behavior, concurrent psychotherapy, or any change in psychotropic medication within 6 weeks before or during TF-CBT were excluded from the study. Patients whose caregivers had severe psychiatric disorders were also excluded.

Analyses of this study were undertaken with TF-CBT completers ($n = 65$), since data were only available for this subgroup (see Table 1 and [30] for more details). TF-CBT completers were predominantly accompanied by female caregivers ($n = 49$; 75%), mostly a parent or other relative ($n = 46$; 71%) instead of, e.g. an employee of the youth welfare institution. Completers of TF-CBT did not differ from participants dropping out of treatment regarding demographic or clinical variables (see Table 1). Treatment completion was defined as participation in at least 8 sessions TF-CBT ($M = 11.9$; $SD = 1.04$) and the post-treatment assessment. Within the first 8 sessions, the most stimulating components of TF-CBT—psychoeducation, relaxation and gradual exposure in sensu are scheduled to be completed [32]. Patients in the control group who received TF-CBT after completion of the waiting time were not considered for analysis.

Treatment condition

TF-CBT is a component-based manualized treatment including parenting skills, psychoeducation, relaxation, affect modulation, cognitive processing, gradual exposure in sensu (trauma narrative) and in vivo (trauma reminders), conjoint child-caregiver sessions, and the elaboration of strategies for enhancing safety and future development (see [33] for details). Before participating in the study, therapists were carefully trained by experienced clinicians, and certified by an expert TF-CBT trainer, based on videotapes of a training case. Treatment fidelity was supported during the trial by supervision.

Procedure

The local institutional review board approved the study, which was registered under Clinical Trials (NCT01516827). Informed consent of the parents or legal guardians, and informed assent of children and adolescents were obtained. Patients were reimbursed for their time and travel expenses to clinical assessments, but not for participating in treatment sessions. Health insurance companies covered all treatment costs.

Patients were consecutively recruited between February 2012 and January 2015 at eight German mental health clinics for children and adolescents, five of them community clinics and three located at an academic mental health care center. All clinics screened their patients; the

Table 1 Description of the study sample

Variables	TF-CBT completers ($n = 65$)	Tf-CBT dropouts ($n = 11$)	Statistics	p
Female, n (%)	44 (67.7)	9 (81.8)	$\chi^2(1) = 0.89$	0.49
Age (years) M (SD; range)	12.52 (2.90; 7–17)	13.45 (3.01; 8–17)	$t(74) = -0.98$	0.33
Living out of home, n (%)	15 (23.1)	0 (0)	$\chi^2(1) = 3.18$	0.10
Germany as birth country, n (%)	58 (89.2)	10 (90.9)	$\chi^2(1) = 0.85$	1.00
Index trauma, n (%)			$\chi^2(1) = 1.76$	0.42
Sexual violence	25 (38.5)	6 (54.5)		
Physical violence	25 (38.5)	2 (18.2)		
Other (death of a loved one, war, neglect)	15 (23.0)	3 (27.3)		
Full PTSD DSM-IV diagnosis, n (%)	50 (76.9)	7 (63.6)	$\chi^2(1) = 0.89$	0.45
≥ 1 comorbid disorder DSM-IV, n (%)	19 (29.2)	5 (45.5)	$\chi^2(1) = 1.15$	0.31
CAPS-CA total score M (SD; range) pre-treatment	57.86 (16.61; 37–102)	62.36 (22.09; 36–109)	$t(74) = -0.79$	0.43

TF-CBT, Trauma-Focused Cognitive Behavioural Therapy; PTSD, post traumatic stress disorder; CAPS-CA, Clinician Administered PTSD Scale for Children and Adolescents study was additionally announced on the project's website and on the clinics' flyers to promote referrals.

After an initial screening for eligibility, patients and their caregivers underwent a multi-methodical baseline assessment, which comprised measurements of PTSS, other clinical and demographic variables, as well as TE of therapeutic success. TE was assessed separately in patients and their caregivers, e.g. biological parents or employees of the youth welfare system where the patient lived. Children and adolescents were randomized to either 12 sessions TF-CBT à 90 min within 16 weeks or to a waitlist of the same duration. Randomization was performed independently of the project group in a 1:1 ratio; clinics and PTSS severity were treated as strata. At mid-treatment (after 6 sessions), patients and caregivers rated their working alliance with the therapist separately, and the therapist evaluated patients' collaboration in treatment. After treatment, patients' PTSS and working alliances of patients and their caregivers were measured again. All assessments were made by trained, blinded, and independent evaluators. We analyzed the alliance at mid-treatment, since at an early stage of psychotherapeutic processes it proved to be a better predictor of treatment outcome than at treatment completion [23, 34].

Instruments

The Clinician Administered PTSD Scale for Children and Adolescents (CAPS-CA) version for DSM-IV [31] was used to assess treatment outcome. Children and adolescents evaluate both the frequency and intensity of their PTSS over the last month on five-point rating scales (0 = 'None of the time; no symptoms' to 4 = 'daily or almost every day; a whole lot'). Developmentally appropriate language and visual aids for the degrees of symptom frequency and intensity are used. The CAPS-CA provides a total symptom severity score with combined frequency and intensity scores (range 0–152; $\alpha = 0.79$; [31]). Both the post-treatment symptom severity score and a difference score (pre-minus post-treatment symptom severity) were analyzed, the latter with higher scores indicating higher symptom reduction.

TE of patients and their caregivers was each rated by themselves by a single item with a 5-point rating scale (1 = 'I expect this treatment to help me/my child a lot'; 5 = 'I don't expect this treatment to make any difference in my/my child's condition'). The single item format is consistent with prior studies in children and adolescents [18, 19]. The scores were inversed with the result that high scores indicate high TE.

Treatment collaboration was rated by therapists by a single item on a 5-point rating scale (1 = 'Excellent, the patient did his/her homework assiduously and actively participated during session'; 5 = 'None, patient never

finished his/her therapeutic homework and refused any participation during sessions'). To facilitate the judgment of therapists, suitable behavior examples for both ends of the scale were offered. Again, scores were inversed for analyses, and high scores therefore indicate high collaboration.

Patients and caregivers independently completed the short version of the Working Alliance Inventory (WAI-S, [35]) to rate their own alliance with the therapist, comprising 12 items with a 7-point rating scale (1 = 'never'; 7 = 'always'; range 12–84). The WAI is one of the most frequently used instruments with adults [36] and has also been used in research of psychotherapy with children and adolescents [29, 37]. We adapted the patient (WAI-S-P, [35]) version for children and adolescents by translating and back-translating using a systematic process based on recommendations for good practice [38]. The caregiver-therapist version (WAI-S-CT) was adapted with the same items reworded for the use by caregivers. Cronbach's alpha for the adapted German versions total scores were 0.88 (WAI-S-P), and 0.86 (WAI-S-CT).

Statistical analyses

Statistical analyses were performed using IBM SPSS Statistics Version 21 and Mplus Version 7.31 [39]. Variables were inspected for missing values, and single missing raw items of the WAI-S-P and WAI-S-CT were replaced by means of the other items on the respective scale of the respondent (< 1%).

To describe the study sample and to assure comparability, group differences between completers and drop-outs were tested by t-tests for independent samples and χ^2 tests. In preparation of path analysis, the Kolmogorov–Smirnov test was used to test for normal distribution of variables; correlation coefficients between variables were estimated with Kendall's τ, due to their skewed distribution. All statistical tests were two-tailed, and significance levels were set at $p < 0.05$.

In order to test our hypothesis, a path analysis based on structural equation modeling (SEM) was used to determine the direct and indirect effects of treatment expectancy on treatment outcome. The model was estimated with the Maximum Likelihood Robust (MLR) estimator, since the data were not normally distributed. TE served as the independent variable (IV), and working alliance, collaboration, and PTSS after treatment completion, respectively PTSS difference score as dependent variables (DV). The assumed directions of relationships in the hypothesized model are depicted in Fig. 1, correlations are indicated by lines with arrows on both ends. Path analyses were conducted and presented in accordance to guidelines [40, 41]. Model fit is perfect by definition as the model includes all possible paths between variables.

Standardized parameter estimates were used for comparisons within the model.

Results
Preliminary analyses
Descriptive values and correlation coefficients between patients' and caregivers' common factors and CAPS-CA total symptom severity after completion of treatment are displayed in Table 2. None of the common variables was significantly correlated with treatment outcome ($\tau = 0.01–0.15$). PTSS post-treatment, as well as common factors of patients and caregivers, were not normally distributed. The PTSS pre-post difference score was $M = 32.31$ ($SD = 21.44$).

Direct effects of TE on outcome
Neither the patients' ($\beta = -0.026$, ns; see Table 3) nor the caregivers' TE directly predicted the treatment outcome ($\beta = 0.183$, ns). The same applies to the prediction of PTSS difference scores by patients' ($B = 1.042$, SE $B = 2.851$, $\beta = 0.045$, $p = 0.713$) or caregivers' TE ($B = -2.082$, SE $B = 5.688$, $\beta = -0.064$, $p = 0.655$).

Indirect effects
Neither patients' nor caregivers' TE had an indirect effect on PTSS score post-treatment via collaboration. TE did neither affect patients' collaboration ($\beta = 0.010–0.217$; ns) nor did the latter predict the post-treatment outcome ($\beta = 0.039$; ns; difference score $B = 1.061$, SE $B = 2.757$, $\beta = -0.045$, $p = 0.697$.

Patients' TE predicted patients' working alliance ($\beta = 0.514$, $p < 0.001$), but only caregivers' working alliance was related to post-treatment outcome ($\beta = -0.533$, $p < 0.001$; difference score $B = 1.100$, SE $B = 0.522$, $\beta = 0.335$, $p = 0.031$). Working alliances of patients and their caregivers were significantly correlated ($\beta = 0.446$, $p < 0.001$; see Fig. 2).

Table 3 Unstandardized and standardized effects, and standard errors from path analysis

Effect	B	SE B	β	p
Post-treatment PTSS on				
TE patients	− 0.659	3.409	− 0.026	0.846
TE caregivers	6.418	5.429	0.183	0.221
WAI patients	0.620	0.379	0.286	0.153
WAI caregivers	− 1.946	0.493	− 0.553	0.000
Collaboration	0.999	2.945	0.039	0.732
WAI patients on				
TE patients	5.936	1.875	0.514	0.000
TE caregivers	− 0.883	2.325	− 0.055	0.694
WAI caregivers on				
TE patients	1.201	0.914	0.169	0.175
TE caregivers	1.996	1.385	0.200	0.131
Collaboration on				
TE patients	0.212	0.208	0.217	0.281
TE caregivers	0.014	0.170	0.010	0.934
WAI caregiver with WAI patients	25.564	7.091	0.446	0.000
Collaboration with WAI patients	1.732	1.352	0.217	0.234
Collaboration with WAI caregiver	1.502	0.916	0.273	0.078
TE patients with TE caregivers	0.079	0.066	0.131	0.243

TE, treatment expectancy; WAI, Working Alliance Inventory; B, unstandardized path coefficient; SE, standard error; β, standardized path coefficient

Discussion
This study investigated direct and indirect effects of treatment expectancy on outcome of TF-CBT in children and adolescents with PTSS and their caregivers. Neither the patients' nor the caregivers' treatment expectancy did affect the treatment outcome directly, nor did TE affect the outcome indirectly via treatment collaboration or working alliance. These findings are confirmed when treatment outcome is defined as symptom reduction. However, caregivers' working alliance emerged as a factor with a significant positive effect on treatment outcome.

Table 2 Medians, first quartiles and correlation coefficients (n = 65)

Variables	Kendall's τ					Median	First quartile
	1	2	3	4	5		
1. Treatment expectancy patients	–					4.00	4.00
2. Treatment expectancy caregivers	0.18	–				4.00	4.00
3. Working alliance patients	0.33*	0.04	–			74.00	65.00
4. Working alliance caregivers	0.08	0.15	0.31*	–		78.00	72.50
5. Collaboration	0.18	0.04	0.16	0.22	–	4.00	3.00
6. Post-treatment PTSS	0.03	0.04	− 0.01	− 0.15	− 0.01	17.00	7.75

* p < 0.05

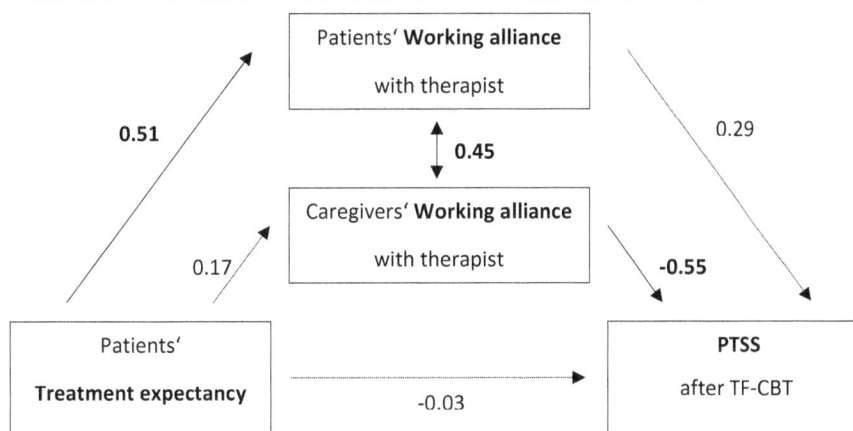

Fig. 2 Standardized path coefficients of the model including TE, working alliance and outcome. Numbers in bold are statistically significant. PTSS posttraumatic stress symptoms; TF-CBT, Trauma-Focused Cognitive Behavioral Therapy

Contrary to most findings in adults [10] and preliminary results concerning children and adolescents with OCD [18] or depression [19], treatment outcome in this TF-CBT study was not predicted by TE of patients with PTSS or their caregivers. Possibly, the TE-outcome link is less pronounced in children and adolescents compared to adult patients, which refers to a developmental effect that is also reported for the association between working alliance and treatment success [25, 42]. In comparison to adult patients, developmentally defined characteristics may limit children's social, emotional and cognitive abilities to perceive, evaluate and report expectations and working alliance, which, as a consequence, weakens the association with symptom reduction. Alternatively, children and adolescents might have an even more vague and imprecise concept of psychotherapy than adult patients, leading to unspecific expectations which are not associated with outcome. Additionally, the intensity of the TE-outcome link might depend on whatever psychiatric disorder the patients have. It is quite conceivable that the impact of expectations might differ for patients suffering from, e.g. OCD, in comparison with children and adolescents predominantly suffering from a primary depression or PTSS. Cognitive distortions and negative expectations about oneself, the world and the future are inherent to depressive disorders and PTSS, and positive expectations regarding future treatment success may have a big impact on both. In PTSS, dysfunctional cognitions are known to be an important driver in both symptom development [43] and symptom reduction [44, 45]. Although depression is the most common comorbid condition in PTSS, knowledge of the association of these two is limited. Results point to divergent ways of therapeutic change as a function of different subtypes of comorbid PTSS and depression [46, 47]. Thus, also TE may

influence treatment outcome depending on the subtype of comorbid PTSS and depression. Additionally, the conceptualization of TE as a dynamic, changeable variable seems more suitable, especially in the treatment of PTSS. Trauma-focused interventions, reported to have the best evidence for PTSS in children and adolescents [48], include the steady commitment of patients during treatment to counteract avoidance behavior. Repeated motivational techniques or psychoeducational elements may thus change TE during treatment. It is possible that TE measured later in treatment may have a stronger association with outcome than pre-treatment TE, as assessed in our study. Though, even if TE is likely to be highly influenced by the first meeting with the therapist and the presentation of the treatment model, naïve TE—i.e. TE assessed before patients ever met their therapists—was reported to be significantly associated with outcome in children and adolescents with depression or OCD in children and adolescents [19, 25] and adults [10]. Furthermore, the TE-outcome link might be more complex than we expected in our model, as associations may depend on how patients' expectancies and therapists' attitudes match during the first sessions [10, 49]. Also, associations might be nonlinear, with the best treatment outcome in patients with medium treatment expectations [20].

Our results are partly consistent with the well-known pathway from TE over working alliance to treatment outcome in adults [50]. Children and adolescents' TE significantly increased their working alliance, which was positively associated with their caregivers' working alliance and by this pathway suggests an indirect prediction of treatment outcome. Recently, the adolescents' perception of their caregivers' approval of TF-CBT was reported to be more important than their own alliance with the therapist to continue treatment protocol [51].

These findings emphasize the importance of caregiver participation in TF-CBT [25, 52]. Caregivers ensure a continuous treatment participation, which is especially important in PTSS, where avoidant behavior may interrupt the therapeutic exposure with traumatic memories. Therefore, caregivers willingness to actively support their child's treatment participation is necessary to ensure treatment success [53]. Additionally, a good alliance with the therapist motivates caregivers to improve their parenting behavior, as taught in TF-CBT. This treatment component seems especially important in PTSS, as the difficulties mentioned above often challenge caregivers' skills, leading to vicious circles of negative communication and behavior [54].

Limitations

Several limitations apply due to the characteristics of this study. First of all, the sample size was slightly too small for investigations of TE, and statistical power was not sufficient to detect small effects of TE on outcome. However, the sample size can be regarded as sufficient for path analyses [41]. Secondly, TE was measured only once pretreatment by a single item to avoid additional strain on patients and their caregivers, given the elaborated psychometric assessments within the study. Although former investigations [18, 19] using single items measured before start of treatment reported positive associations of TE and outcome, a more differentiated, repeated assessment of TE might have influenced results. Additionally, findings might depend on instruments, as we used an age appropriate adaptation of the WAI-S, whereas others applied, e.g. the Therapeutic Alliance Scale for Children (TASC; [55]). However, the alliance-outcome link is reported to be free from effects of the instruments used with adult patients [36], as well as with children and adolescents [25]. Moreover, ceiling effects in our variables—probably due to a positive selection of motivated study participants—limited our statistical analyses and might explain the nonsignificant findings.

Conclusions

The influence of TE on the success of CBT in children and adolescents seems rather limited. Future studies should conceptualize TE as a dynamic construct, which may be adjusted during treatment and influence outcome together with other common factors like working alliance. TE and working alliance should be assessed repeatedly at the beginning and during psychotherapy from different perspectives, in a larger sample, and—if possible—also including patients with lower TE. Additionally, more efforts should be made to understand the role of caregivers in the treatment of PTSS in children and adolescents, as the inclusion of a supportive caregiver can be regarded as essential for therapy success in this population.

Abbreviations

CAPS-CA: Clinician Administered PTSD Scale for Children and Adolescents; CBT: Cognitive Behavioral Therapy; OCD: obsessive-compulsive disorder; PTSS/D: posttraumatic stress symptoms/disorder; RCT: randomized controlled trial; TASC: Therapeutic Alliance Scale for Children; TE: treatment expectancy; TF-CBT: Trauma-Focused Cognitive Behavioral Therapy; WAI: Working Alliance Inventory.

Authors' contributions

VK and LG conceived and designed the study; VK drafted the manuscript; DT analyzed the data; FK gave statistical support; All authors participated in the revision of the manuscript. VK, FK and DT read and approved the final manuscript, as LG passed away before its completion.

Acknowledgements

The authors wish to thank Professor Paul Plener for his great support and assistance in the completion of the manuscript.

Competing interests

The authors declare that they have no competing interests.

Funding

The present investigation was not funded; the main RCT was funded by the German Ministry of Education and Research (01GY1141).

References

1. Norcross JC, Lambert MJ. Psychotherapy relationships that work II. Psychotherapy. 2011;48:4–8. https://doi.org/10.1037/a0022180.
2. Hofmann SG, Barlow DH. Evidence-based psychological interventions and the common factors approach: the beginnings of a rapprochement? Psychotherapy. 2014. https://doi.org/10.1037/a0037045.
3. Wampold BE. How important are the common factors in psychotherapy? An update. World Psychiatry. 2015;14:270–7.
4. Benish SG, Imel ZE, Wampold BE. The relative efficacy of bona fide psychotherapies for treating post-traumatic stress disorder: a meta-analysis of direct comparisons. Clin Psychol Rev. 2008;28:746–58.
5. Wampold BE, Imel ZE, Laska KM, Benish SG, Miller ME, Flückinger C, Budge S. Determining what works in the treatment of PTSD. Clin Psychol Rev. 2010;30:923–33. https://doi.org/10.1016/j.cpr.2010.06.005.
6. Ehlers A, Bisson J, Clark DM, Creamer M, Pilling S, Richards D, Yule W. Do all psychological treatments really work the same in posttraumatic stress

disorder? Clin Psychol Rev. 2010;30:269–76. https://doi.org/10.1016/j.cpr.2009.12.001.

7. Shirk SR, Karver M. Prediction of treatment outcome from relationship variables in child and adolescent therapy: a meta analytic review. J Consult Clin Psychol. 2003;71:452–64. https://doi.org/10.1037/0022-006X.71.3.452.

8. Ormhaug SM, Jensen TK, Wentzel-Larsen T, Shirk SR. The therapeutic alliance in treatment of traumatized youth: relation to outcome in a randomized controlled trial. J Consult Clin Psychol. 2014;82:52–64. https://doi.org/10.1037/a0033884.

9. Frank JD, Frank JB. Persuasion and Healing. A comparative study of psychotherapy. 3rd ed. Baltimore: The John Hopkins University Press; 1991.

10. Constantino M, Arnkoff D, Glass C, Ametrano R, Smith JZ. Expectations. J Clin Psychol. 2011;67:184–92.

11. Compas B, Connor-Smith J, Saltzman H, Thomsen A, Wadsworth M. Coping with stress during childhood and adolescence: problems, progress, and potential in theory and research. Psychol Bull. 2001;127:87–127.

12. Veneziano E. Language and internal states: a long developmental history at different levels of functioning. Rivista di psicolinguistica applicata. 2009;9:15–34. https://doi.org/10.1400/122907.

13. Schonert-Reichl K, Muller J. Correlates of help-seeking in adolescence. J Youth Adolesc. 1996;25:705–31.

14. Ormhaug SM, Shirk SR, Wentzel-Larsen T. Therapist and client perspectives on the alliance in the treatment of traumatized adolescents. Eur J Psychotraumatol. 2015;6:27705. https://doi.org/10.3402/ejpt.v6.27705.

15. Cohen J. Factors that mediate treatment outcome of sexually abused preschool children. J Am Acad Child Adolesc Psychiatry. 1996;35:1402–10.

16. Haine-Schlagel R, Walsh N. A review of parent participation in child and family mental health treatment. Clin Child Fam Psychol Rev. 2015;18:133–50. https://doi.org/10.1007/s10567-015-0182-x.

17. DeFife J, Hilsenroth MJ. Starting off the right foot: common factor elements in early psychotherapy process. J Psychother Integr. 2011;21:172–91. https://doi.org/10.1037/a0023889.

18. Lewin AB, Peris TS, Bergman RL, McCracken JT, Piacentini J. The role of treatment expectancy in youth receiving exposure-based CBT for obsessive compulsive disorder. Behav Res Ther. 2011;49:536–43. https://doi.org/10.1016/j.brat.2011.06.001.

19. Curry J, Rohde P, Simons A, Silva S, Vitiello B, Kratochvil C, Reinecke M, Feeny N, Wells K, Pathak S, Weller E. Predictors and moderators of acute outcome in the Treatment for Adolescents with Depression Study (TADS). J Am Acad Child Adolesc Psychiatry. 2006;45:1427–39. https://doi.org/10.1097/01.chi.0000240838.78984.e2.

20. Bohart A and Wade S. The client in psychotherapy. In: Bergin and Garfield's Handbook of psychotherapy and behavior change, 6th edn. Hoboken: Wiley; 2013. p. 219–57.

21. McClintock A, Anderson T, Petrarca A. Treatment expectations, alliance, session positivity, and outcome: an investigation of a three-path mediation model. J Clin Psychol. 2016;71:41–9.

22. Bordin E. The generaliziability of the psychoanalytic concept of the working alliance. Psychother Theory Res Pract. 1979;16:252–60.

23. Flückinger C, Del Re AC, Wampold BE, Symonds D, Horvath AO. How central is the alliance in psychotherapy? A multilevel longitudinal meta-analysis. J Counc Psychol. 2012;59:10–7. https://doi.org/10.1037/a0025749.

24. Martin D, Garske JDM. Relation of the therapeutic alliance with outcome and other variables: a meta-analytic review. J Consult Clin Psychol. 2000;68:438–50. https://doi.org/10.1037/0022-006X.68.3.438.

25. McLeod BD. Relation of the alliance with outcomes in youth psychotherapy: a meta-analysis. Clin Psychol Rev. 2011;31:603–16. https://doi.org/10.1016/j.cpr.2011.02.001.

26. Shirk SR, Karver MS, Brown R. The alliance in child and adolescent psychotherapy. Psychotherapy. 2011;48:17–24. https://doi.org/10.1037/a0022181.

27. Abrishami GF, Warren JS. Therapeutic alliance and outcomes in children and adolescents served in a community mental health system. J Child Adolesc Behav 2013;1:110. https://doi.org/10.4172/jcalb.1000110.

28. Zorzella KM, Muller RT, Cribbie RA. The relationships between therapeutic alliance an internalizing and externalizing symptoms in Trauma-Focused Cognitive Behavioral Therapy. Child Abuse Negl. 2015;50:171–81.

29. Capaldi S, Asnaani A, Zandberg LJ, Carpenter JK, Foa EB. Therapeutic alliance during prolonged exposure versus client-centered therapy for adolescent posttraumatic stress disorder. J Clin Psychol. 2016;72:1026–36.

30. Goldbeck L, Muche R, Sachser C, Tutus D, Rosner R. Effectiveness of Trauma-Focused Cognitive Behavioral Therapy for children and adolescents: a randomized controlled trial in eight german mental health clinics. Psychother Psychosom. 2016;85:159–70. https://doi.org/10.1159/000442824.

31. Nader K, Kriegler J, Blake D. The clinician-administered PTSD scale for children and adolescents for DSM-IV (CAPS-CA). White River Junction: National Centre for PTSD; 2002.

32. Miller-Graff L, Campion K. Interventions for posttraumatic stress with children exposed to violence: factors associated with treatment success. J Clin Psychol. 2015;72:226–48.

33. Cohen J, Mannarino AP, Deblinger E. Treating trauma and traumatic grief in children and adolescents. New York: Guilford Press; 2006.

34. Klein D, Schwartz J, Santiago N, Vivian D, Vocisano C, Castonguay L, Arnow B, Blalock JA, Manber R, Markowitz J. Therapeutic alliance in depression treatment: controlling for prior change and patient characteristics. J Consult Clin Psychol. 2003;71:997–1006. https://doi.org/10.1037/0022-006X.71.6.997.

35. Tracey T, Kokotovic A. Factor structure of the Working Alliance Inventory. Psychol Assess. 1989;1:207–10.

36. Flückinger C, Horvath AO, DelRe AC, Symonds D, Holzer C. Die Bedeutung der Arbeitsallianz in der Psychotherapie—Übersicht aktueller Metaanalysen. Psychotherapeut. 2015. https://doi.org/10.1007/s00278-015-0020-0.

37. Anderson RE, Spence SH, Donovan CL, March S, Prosser S, Kenardy J. Working alliance in online cognitive behavior therapy for anxiety disorders in youth: comparison with clinic delivery and its role in predicting outcome. J Med Internet Res. 2012;14(3):e88. https://doi.org/10.2196/jmir.1848.

38. Wild D, Grove A, Martin M, Eremenco S, McElroy S, Verjee-Lorenz A, Erikson P. Principles of good practice for the translation and cultural adaptation process for patient-reported outcomes (PRO) measures: report of the ISPOR task force for translation and cultural adaptation. Value Health. 2005;8(2):94–104.

39. Muthén L, Muthén B. MPlus user's guide, version 7. Los Angeles: Muthén & Muthén; 2015.

40. McDonald R, Ho M-HR. Principles and practice in reporting structural equation analyses. Psychol Methods. 2002;7:64–82.

41. Stage F, Carter H, Nora A. Path analysis: an introduction and analysis of a decade of research. J Educ Res. 2010;98:5–13.

42. Kaufman N, Rohde P, Seeley J, Clarke G, Stice E. Potential mediators of cognitive-behavioral therapy for adolescents with co-morbid major depression and conduct disorder. J Consult Clin Psychol. 2005;73:38–46. https://doi.org/10.1037/0022-006X.73.1.38.

43. Ehlers A, Clark DM. A cognitive model of posttraumatic stress disorder. Behav Res Ther. 2000;38:319–45.

44. Kleim B, Grey N, Wild J, Nussbech FW, Stott R, Hackmann A, Ehlers A. Cognitive change predicts symptom reduction with cognitive therapy for posttraumatic stress disorder. J Consult Clin Psychol. 2013;81:383–93.

45. Kumpula MJ, Rentel KZ, Foa EB, LeBlanc NJ, Bui E, McSweeney LB, Knowles K, Bosley H, Simon NM, Rauch SA. Temporal sequencing of change in posttraumatic cognitions and PTSD symptom reduction during prolonged exposure therapy. Behav Ther. 2017;48:561–651.

46. Contractor A, Roley-Roberts M, Lagdon S, Armour C. Heterogeneity in patterns of DSM5 posttraumatic stress disorder and depression symptoms: latent profile analyses. J Affect Disord. 2017;212:17–24.

47. Flor J, Yehuda R. Comorbidity between post-traumatic stress disorder and major depressive disorder: alternative explanations and treatment considerations. Dialogues Clin Neurosci. 2015;17:141–50.

48. Ramirez de Arellano MA, Lyman DR, Jobe-Shields L, George P, Dougherty RH, Daniels AS, Huang L, Delphin-Rittmon ME. Trauma-Focused Cognitive Behavioral Therapy: assessing the evidence. Psychiatr Serv (Washington, D.C.). 2014;65(5):591–602. https://doi.org/10.1176/appi.ps.201300255.

49. Ahmed M, Westra H. Impact of a treatment rationale on expectancy and engagement in cognitive behavioural therapy for social anxiety. Cogn Ther Res. 2009;33:314–22. https://doi.org/10.1007/s10608-008-9182-1.

50. Meyer B, Pilkonis P, Krupnick J, Egan M, Simmens S, Sotsky S. Treatment expectancies, patient alliance, and outcome: further analyses from the National institute of Mental Health Treatment of Depression Collaborative Research Program. J Consult Clin Psychol. 2002;70:1051–5. https://doi.org/10.1037/0022-006X.70.4.1051.

51. Ormhaug SM and Jensen TK. Investigating treatment characteristics and first-session relationship variables as predictors of dropout in the treatment of traumatized youth. Psychother Res. 2018;28(2). 235–249https://doi.org/10.1080/10503307.2016.1189617.

52. Loos S and Goldbeck L. Working alliance and its association with treatment outcome in Trauma-Focused Cognitive Behavioral Therapy with children and adolescents. 2017 (**submitted manuscript**).

53. Glickman K, Shear M, Wall M. Mediators of outcome in complicated grief. J Clin Psychol. 2016;73:817–28. https://doi.org/10.1002/jclp.22384.

54. Samuelson K, Wilson C, Padrón E, Lee S, Gavron L. Maternal PTSD and children's adjustment: parenting stress and emotional availability as proposed mediators. J Clin Psychol. 2016;73:693–706. https://doi.org/10.1002/jclp.22369.

55. Shirk SR, Saiz CC. Clinical, empirical, and developmental perspectives on the therapeutic relationship in child psychotherapy. Dev Psychopathol. 1992;4:713–28. https://doi.org/10.1017/S0954579400004946.

8

Child Protection Service interference in childhood and the relation with mental health problems and delinquency in young adulthood: a latent class analysis study

Laura van Duin[1][*][†], Floor Bevaart[1][†], Carmen H. Paalman[1], Marie-Jolette A. Luijks[1], Josjan Zijlmans[1], Reshmi Marhe[1], Arjan A. J. Blokland[2], Theo A. H. Doreleijers[1] and Arne Popma[1]

Abstract

Background: Most multi-problem young adults (18–27 years old) have been exposed to childhood maltreatment and/or have been involved in juvenile delinquency and, therefore, could have had Child Protection Service (CPS) interference during childhood. The extent to which their childhood problems persist and evolve into young adulthood may differ substantially among cases. This might indicate heterogeneous profiles of CPS risk factors. These profiles may identify combinations of closely interrelated childhood problems which may warrant specific approaches for problem recognition and intervention in clinical practice. The aim of this study was to retrospectively identify distinct statistical classes based on CPS data of multi-problem young adults in The Netherlands and to explore whether these classes were related to current psychological dysfunctioning and delinquent behaviour.

Methods: Age at first CPS interference, numbers and types of investigations, age at first offence, mention of child maltreatment, and family supervision order measures (Dutch: ondertoezichtstelling; OTS) were extracted from the CPS records of 390 multi-problem young adult males aged 18–27 (mean age 21.7). A latent class analysis (LCA) was conducted and one-way analyses of variance and post-hoc t-tests examined whether LCA class membership was related to current self-reported psychological dysfunctioning and delinquent behaviour.

Results: Four latent classes were identified: (1) *late CPS/penal investigation group* (44.9%), (2) *early CPS/multiple investigation group* (30.8%), (3) *late CPS interference without investigation group* (14.6%), and (4) *early CPS/family investigation group* (9.7%). The early CPS/family investigation group reported the highest mean anxiousness/depression and substance use scores in young adulthood. No differences were found between class membership and current delinquent behaviour.

Conclusions: This study extends the concept that distinct pathways are present in multi-problem young adults who underwent CPS interference in their youth. Insight into the distinct combinations of CPS risk factors in the identified subgroups may guide interventions to tailor their treatment to the specific needs of these children. Specifically, treatment of internalizing problems in children with an early onset of severe family problems and for which CPS interference is carried out should receive priority from both policy makers and clinical practice.

Keywords: Child Protection Service, Latent classes, Multi-problem, Young adults, Delinquency

*Correspondence: l.vanduin@vumc.nl
[†]Laura van Duin (1st author) and Floor Bevaart (1st author) collaborated on the first draft of the manuscript
[1] Department of Child and Adolescent Psychiatry, VU University Medical Center, Meibergdreef 5, 1105 AZ Amsterdam, The Netherlands
Full list of author information is available at the end of the article

Background

Childhood onset of delinquent behaviour and severe family problems, including child maltreatment and neglect, are associated with a variety of adverse outcomes in young adulthood [1–6]. These childhood problems are important risk factors for later delinquent behaviour and hamper psychological functioning [1, 3, 4, 7–17]. So far, childhood risk factors of adulthood problems have been studied either within delinquent populations [1–3, 9, 13, 18–21] or in populations of young adults who experienced maltreatment and out-of-home placements in their childhood [3, 22]. These studies focused predominantly on the severity, age of onset and persistence of delinquent behaviour and on maltreatment and family interferences by, for example, the Child Protection Services (CPS; Dutch: *Raad voor de Kinderbescherming*). However, such childhood problems are closely interrelated and the presence of multiple problems in childhood drastically increases the probability of adverse adult outcomes [19, 23, 24]. Therefore, studies should focus on combinations of risk factors in young children [13, 25, 26], instead of focusing on single risk factors, and assess to what extent these combinations can predict outcomes later in life. In this way, it may be possible to distinguish among youth risk profiles which may help tailor primary, secondary and tertiary prevention strategies. The present study tackled these issues by retrospectively studying combined risk factors and long-term outcomes of both childhood judicial and civil CPS interferences in multi-problem young adults.

Young adulthood is considered a distinct developmental stage comprising major psychological [27–29], social [27] and neurobiological [30] changes that are critical for a healthy transition towards adulthood [31–33]. In most cases, young adults (aged 18–27) who experienced severe psychological, family and judicial problems since childhood encounter difficulties during this transition in becoming self-sufficient adults [32–35]. Previous studies have provided evidence that these vulnerable young adults are at high risk of an accumulation of several problems such as unemployment, psychological problems, early parenthood, and court involvement [34, 36–38]. Furthermore, a majority of these young adults suffer from substance use disorder [39, 40], and lack social support [33, 34]. This group with multiple and intertwined problems has been called multi-problem young adults, and is increasingly recognized as warranting specific scientific attention in order to inform and help improve professional support [33, 41]. An important aspect in this respect is to understand the development of the childhood problems that culminate in these multi-problem young adults.

In general, childhood problems as risk factors of later delinquent behaviour and mental health problems are widely studied. These risk factors are often distinguished on the individual and family level [2, 9, 12, 13]. Individual risk factors as intellectual disability, disruptive behaviour, psychological problems and an early onset of substance use are related to the development of antisocial behaviour [2, 42–44] later in life, and to mental health problems in adulthood as well [45]. Other risk factors in this respect are low school achievement and truancy [46, 47]. Important risk factors on the family level are inadequate parenting, low social economic status, maltreatment and neglect, mental health problems and substance abuse of parents [12]. All these factors may have contributed in their own unique way to the various problems of young adults.

Many multi-problem young adults have demonstrated delinquent behaviour and severe family problems during childhood [1, 22, 48–50] and, therefore, are likely to have underwent CPS interference during their youth. In The Netherlands, there are two main reasons for a child to receive a CPS investigation: to request a civil or a penal measure. It is not uncommon for children to receive multiple CPS interferences during their lives [3]. Therefore, the characteristics of CPS interference differ among children [21, 51–53]. Multi-problem young adults are likely to have experienced several judicial, school and family problems simultaneously [19, 23, 24], for which the timing, the number and the intensity of CPS investigations may vary [3]. CPS characteristics can be seen as static risk factors [54] for deviant development since children who underwent CPS interference have an elevated risk of developing delinquent behaviour and mental health problems in young adulthood [1, 3, 8, 21, 48, 55, 56]. The annual arrest rate for young adults who as children had been referred to CPS is more than four times higher than the national rate for 18- to 24-year olds [57] and 50% of this young adult population have experienced mental health problems [57].

Whereas all children who were exposed to severe family problems and/or who were involved in juvenile delinquency have an elevated risk of adult problem behaviour [1, 6, 15, 50, 58–61], the extent to which these problems persist and evolve into young adulthood differs substantially [7, 61, 62]. This might indicate heterogeneous profiles of the concurrent childhood problems. Several studies investigated and aimed to reduce the heterogeneity of problems within comparable populations of high-risk youths by exploring profiles [9, 13]. A study by Haapasalo found two groups of young adult offenders with CPS interventions: an early onset multiple intervention group and a late onset group who had fewer interventions [3]. A study by Dembo et al. [9] in high-risk youths reported two classes based on self-report data; one with a low prevalence and the other with a high prevalence of problems in family and peer relations, psychological functioning and education [9]. Furthermore, Geluk et al. [13] distinguished three profiles in childhood arrestees, differing in the extent of problems in peer relations, psychological functioning and authority conflicts. So, exploring profiles proved useful in ordering these childhood problems into several homogenous classes concerning the onset, the prevalence and the extent of the problems. However, these studies did not explore specifically if and how these childhood classes may contribute to a deviant development into (young) adulthood.

Although CPS does not provide treatment, CPS interference is directly related to extensive contact with judicial, mental health and social services [48, 63] and CPS may refer their clients to appropriate care, if necessary. However, many (young) adults with a childhood history of CPS interference still experience serious problems, even after repeated intervention [3, 48, 49, 64, 65]. As such, it seems that the effectiveness of current secondary prevention and intervention practices during childhood is limited in this population. Therefore, retrospectively identifying classes of interrelated static risk factors of CPS interference within a relatively unstudied population of multi-problem young adults may prove useful for more effective problem recognition and screening purposes in childhood [26, 54]. Finally, relating these childhood classes to delinquency and mental health problems in young adulthood may give useful indications for the prevention of the escalation of these problems to clinical practice [48, 49].

The present study aims to explore whether groups of CPS characteristics in childhood can be identified within a sample of multi-problem young adults. Furthermore, the associations between class membership and both self-reported delinquency and psychological functioning in young adulthood are investigated. Based on the literature, we expect multi-problem young adults to have a significant prevalence of CPS interference. Within this group we expect to find distinct latent classes differing in the onset, number and intensity of judicial and civil interferences [3] and in the extent of family problems [7, 9]. Lastly, it is hypothesized that classes of CPS interference in youths relate differently to current psychological dysfunctioning and current severity of delinquent behaviour in multi-problem young adults [1, 65, 66].

Methods
Study sample
In 2014–2016 a total of 596 multi-problem young adults were recruited in Rotterdam, The Netherlands. All participants were male, between 18 and 27 years old (mean age 21.7), and had sufficient knowledge of the Dutch language to understand the study procedure and the questionnaires. This study was part of a larger study in which participants were recruited from two sites. The first site was a municipal agency (Dutch: *Jongerenloket*) where young adults between the ages of 18 and 27 can apply for

social welfare. Every year over 4000 intakes are carried out by so-called youth coaches [67]. During this intake, the level of self-sufficiency of the young adult is assessed on eleven life domains with the validated Self-Sufficiency Matrix—Dutch version (SSM-D) [68–70], based on the American version of the SSM [71], on a five-point scale with scores ranging from 1 (acute problems) to 5 (completely self-sufficient). Participants were eligible when they adhered to the following definition: (a) a score of 1 or 2 on the domains Income and Daytime Activities, (b) a maximum score of 3 on at least one of the following domains: Addiction, Mental health, Social network, Justice and (c) a minimum score of 3 on the domain Physical health [72]. Eligible young adults were asked to cooperate voluntarily. As a part of a larger study, $N = 436$ participants were recruited in this way [72]. The second site was multimodal day treatment program *New Opportunities* (Dutch: *De Nieuwe Kans*; DNK). Multi-problem young adults also signed up to DNK themselves or were referred to DNK directly by youth care, probation services, mental health services or social organizations. Therefore, additional participants were recruited directly from DNK ($N = 160$). From the total study sample ($N = 596$), 99.3% ($N = 592$) gave informed consent to conduct the register and record research. Of the $N = 592$, 65.9% ($N = 390$) was matched to a record in the CPS system.

Procedure
The study was performed by the VU University Medical Center Department of Child and Adolescent Psychiatry and approved by the Medical Ethics Review Committee of VU University Medical Center.[1] Participants gave informed consent before voluntary participation after a member of the research team had provided oral information accompanied by written information. After informed consent, trained (junior) researchers administered questionnaires.

Interference with CPS was checked in the CPS system *Kinderbescherming Bedrijfs Processen Systeem* (KBPS) using first names, surname and date of birth of the participants. This resulted in a match of 65.9% (N = 390) of the total sample (N = 592); 34.1% (N = 202) did not match to a record in the system. For a part of the latter group it is uncertain whether they truly never had CPS contact or whether their record has been destroyed, since CPS is legally required to destroy records of clients that reach age 24. This applies to N = 98 of the N = 202 that did not match to a record in the system. For the other N = 104 (51.5% of N = 202), it was certain that they did not have CPS interference, since they were younger than 24 years old. The CPS files consist of

---

[1] Registration number: 2013.422—NL46906.029.13.

all documents received and sent by the CPS concerning the child and a selection of judicial and police report data [73]. Data were extracted from April 2015 to August 2016 by trained (junior) researchers. To test the inter-rater reliability, 19 randomly selected files were scored by two independent raters, showing a substantial inter-rater reliability (κ = 0.72) [74, 75].

Context

The register and record research was conducted at CPS and the data were extracted between April 2015 and August 2016. CPS monitors children between 0 and 18 years old when there are serious concerns regarding their home situation and upbringing. In families with severe parenting problems a child welfare investigator can perform a civil protection investigation of the home environment of the child, at the request of CPS. At the request of the court, CPS mediates when parents break up and disagree about arrangements concerning their children. Moreover, CPS can initiate a judicial or truancy investigation for youth suspected of an offence or truancy. The investigation report with recommendations on (mandatory) service use or a suitable penalization is delivered to the court [73].

Measurements

Socio-demographic characteristics

Socio-demographic characteristics were assessed with a structured self-report questionnaire. *Ethnicity* was based on the country of birth of the respondent and at least one of his parents. A respondent was classified as non-Dutch if he or one of his parents was not born in The Netherlands [76]. Ethnicity was recoded into a dichotomous variable (Dutch ethnicity vs. other ethnicity). *Educational level* was classified into three levels: maximum primary education, achievement of junior secondary education and senior secondary education attainment. *Family problems in youth* were assessed with the single item 'Did you suffer from problems that existed in the family you grew up with? (Yes/No)'. *Police contact of family members in youth* was assessed with the single item 'Did family members you grew up with have police contact? (Yes/No)'. *Prior service use* was assessed with the single item 'Did you previously use services? (Yes/No)'. *Frequency of service use* was assessed with the single item 'Which services did you have contact with?' (e.g., youth care, probation services, child protection services). This was recoded into a frequency score defined as the number of self-reported services.

CPS variables

Several variables were obtained from the CPS records. All variables were divided into categories to perform the latent class analysis (LCA), as it is a condition for this analysis to use categorical variables. The variables Age of first CPS report, Type of investigation, Number of investigations, Child maltreatment, Age of onset of delinquent behaviour and Family supervision order were used as indicators to execute the LCA. *Age of first CPS report* in which date of the first CPS investigation was recoded into four categories: no report, below age 13, 13 or 14 years old, age 15 up to 18. The CPS records provided information on three types of investigations: offence investigation, protection investigation and truancy investigation. *Type of investigation* was recoded into a variable that contained five categories: no investigation, protection investigation, offence investigation, truancy investigation, several types of investigations. *Number of CPS investigations* was recoded into three categories: no investigation, one or two investigations, at least three investigations. *Child maltreatment* was extracted from the record when a professional ascertained child maltreatment (Yes/No). *Domestic violence* was observed and registered by a professional (Yes/No). The verdict of the court to impose a *family supervision order* was included in the record (Yes/No). *Out-of-home placement* was also included in the record in the verdict of the court (Yes/No). *Age of onset of delinquent behaviour*: the date of the first offence was registered based on the police report. Using this date combined with the date of birth, the age of first offence was computed. This variable was recoded into four categories: no offence, first offence below age thirteen, first offence between 13 and 14 years of age, and first offence at age 15 or older.

Current psychological functioning

The Dutch version of the Adult Self Report (ASR) [77] was assessed orally and filled out by the researcher to obtain current psychological functioning. ASR part VIII consists of 123 items on internalizing and externalizing problems during the previous 6 months. The reliability of the questionnaire is good, with a Cronbach's α of 0.83. In this study the ASR total problem score and the scores of nine subscales were used as outcome measures. The subscales are: anxious/depressed, withdrawn, somatic complaints (internalizing problems); intrusive, rule-breaking and aggressive behaviour (externalizing problems); thought problems, attention problems and substance use. The prevalence of serious dysfunctioning on all subscales is presented in Table 1. The mean scale scores per class as outcome measure are based on percentile scores [78] (Table 5).

Delinquent behaviour

The frequency and seriousness of delinquent behaviour were investigated orally and filled out by a researcher using the Dutch version [79] of the Self-report Delinquency Scale (SRD) [80]. This questionnaire has 29 items

Table 1 **Descriptive characteristics in percentages (N = 390)**

Socio-demographic characteristics	
Mean age	21.7 years old
Born in The Netherlands	
Yes	76.6
Dutch ethnicity	
Yes	12.6
Educational level	
Primary	36.5
Junior secondary	44.7
Senior secondary	17.5
Other	1.3
Family characteristics	
Family problems in youth	
Yes	63.2
Police contact of family members in youth	
Yes	19.0
Service use	
Service use	
Yes	83.3
Frequency of service use	
None	16.2
Once	28.0
2 or 3	36.5
4 or more	19.3

	Prevalence serious dysfunctioning (%)[a]
Psychological functioning previous 6 months (ASR)	
Total problems	29.8
Anxious/depressed	30.8
Withdrawn	51.2
Somatic complaints	29.3
Intrusive	7.7
Rule-breaking behaviour	44.7
Aggressive behaviour	28.0
Attention problems	30.6
Thought problems	34.2
Substance use	53.0
Delinquent behaviour from onset till young adulthood (SRD)	
Committed at least one offence	
Yes	93.3
Destruction/public order offence	
Yes	62.6
Property offence	
Yes	85.9
Aggression/violent offence	
Yes	73.1
Drug offence	
Yes	59.2

Table 1 **continued**

	Prevalence serious dysfunctioning (%)[a]
Delinquent behaviour previous 6 months (SRD) (N = 179)[b]	
Committed at least one offence	
Yes	63.0
Destruction/public order offence	
Yes	10.8
Property offence	
Yes	27.1
Aggression/violent offence	
Yes	21.6
Drug offence	
Yes	21.0

[a] Prevalence of serious dysfunctioning is based on percentile scores in the borderline (between the 84th and 90th percentiles) and clinical range (above the 90th percentile) [78]

[b] Self-reported delinquency in the previous 6 months has been added during the study and measured in 179 participants

(including two items of violation: fare dodging and lighting fireworks when prohibited) and the internal consistency of the total score is excellent with Cronbach's $\alpha = 0.85$ [79, 81]. The questionnaire explored the frequency of offences committed both during the respondent's lifetime and in the previous 6 months. In addition, the items were also divided into four different offence categories: destruction/public order offences (5 items, Cronbach's $\alpha = 0.64$), property offences (11 items, Cronbach's $\alpha = 0.79$), aggression/violent offences (8 items, Cronbach's $\alpha = 0.7$) and drug offences (3 items, Cronbach's $\alpha = 0.72$) [79]. The frequencies per offence category were recoded into dichotomous variables (Yes/No), due to the skewed distribution of the data. Lifetime and previous 6 months' prevalence are presented in Table 1. Mean scores based on the frequencies of offences in the previous 6 months were used as outcome measure (see Table 5). The 27 items (excluding two items of violation) add up to one total delinquency score reflecting the multiplication of the seriousness of the offences and their frequency. The seriousness is divided into minor and serious offences based on applicable legal penalties; minor offences have a maximum custodial sentence of 48 months (score 1) and serious offences have a minimum custodial sentence of 48 months (score 2) [79, 80].

Data analysis

In order to detect classes of childhood correlates Latent Class Analysis (LCA) was performed. LCA is a useful method for analysing the relationships among observed variables, when each observed variable is categorical, in a heterogeneous population assumed to be comprised of a set of latent classes [82]. LCA was performed with the program Statistical Analysis System (SAS) version 9.3. The six CPS childhood indicators mentioned above were entered into the LCA. Analyses were conducted using PROC LCA 1.2.6 for SAS 9.3 [83]. Good qualification quality was established taking into account the Bayesian information criterion (BIC), entropy and Akaike information criterion (AIC) [82]. The entropy value ranges between 0 and 1; a value approaching 1 indicates a clear description of the classes [84]. Subsequently, item response probability scores on all indicators were used to interpret the classes. Lastly, to explore differences among classes derived from the LCA on current psychological functioning and delinquent behaviour, One-Way Analyses of Variance and Post Hoc t-tests with Bonferroni correction were performed with Statistical Packages for the Social Sciences, version 22 for Windows [85].

Results

Table 1 shows the self-reported socio-demographic and family characteristics, service use, current psychological functioning and delinquent behaviour of multi-problem young adults with CPS interference in youth. It shows that many young adults had problems in youth; 63.2% had problems in their family, 83.3% reported prior service use and 93.3% committed an offence. During the previous 6 months, 53.0% had serious substance use problems and 63.0% committed an offence.

Childhood correlates of the CPS records

Table 2 shows the descriptive results of the childhood CPS correlates in percentages. After referral to CPS, 84.9% of participants were investigated. In 21.0% of the participants the first CPS investigation was below the age of thirteen and 39.0% had their first investigation at age fifteen or older. Almost half of the group (43.9%) had one or two CPS investigations and 41.5% had at least three CPS investigations. Judicial investigations were conducted in 75.0% of the group and protection investigations in 40.0% of participants. Multiple types of investigations were conducted in 32.6% of participants of which 50.0% first had a protection investigation and 40.0% first had a judicial investigation. Truancy investigations rarely occurred separately (1.8%). Child maltreatment was registered in 29.5% of the CPS reports and the CPS records reported domestic violence in 16.4% of the cases. Protection measures taken by the juvenile court were investigated as well; 33.6% of participants underwent a family supervision order and 22.1% an out-of-home placement. In 88.5% of the CPS records childhood delinquency was

Table 2 Frequencies of childhood correlates CPS records (N = 390)

	%
Age of the first CPS report	
No report	15.1
First report below age 13	21.0
First report age 13 or 14	24.9
First report age 15 or older	39.0
Number of CPS investigations	
None	14.6
1 or 2	43.9
3 or more	41.5
Type of CPS investigation	
No investigation	14.9
Protection investigation	8.0
Judicial investigation	42.7
Truancy investigation	1.8
Multiple types of investigations	32.6
Registered child maltreatment	
Yes	29.5
Domestic violence	
Yes	16.4
Family supervision order	
Yes	33.6
Out-of-home placement	
Yes	22.1
Age at onset of delinquent behaviour	
No offence	10.5
Below age 13	23.3
Age 13 or 14	33.6
Age 15 or older	32.6

Table 3 Model fit sizes of latent class analysis of childhood correlates (N = 390)

Model	Entropy	AIC	BIC	Df
2	1.00	1009.57	1124.58	930
3	0.93	597.93	772.44	915
4	0.95	458.02	692.03	900
5	0.91	417.74	711.24	885

AIC Akaike information criteria, BIC Bayesian information criteria; Df degrees of freedom

registered and 23.3% committed their first offence below age 13.

Identification of childhood correlate classes (Latent Class Analysis)

The first step conducted for the LCA involved identifying the number of latent classes that best fit the data on six childhood indicators. Table 3 presents the fit indices after

Table 4 Item response probabilities LCA ($N = 390$)

Class	1 ($N = 175$)	2 ($N = 120$)	3 ($N = 57$)	4 ($N = 38$)
Class size proportions	44.9%	30.8%	14.6%	9.7%
Family supervision order				
Yes	0.02	0.84	0.02	0.70
No	0.98	0.16	0.98	0.30
Registered child maltreatment				
Yes	0.14	0.57	0.02	0.59
No	0.86	0.43	0.98	0.41
Age at onset of delinquent behaviour				
No offence	0.00	0.00	0.31	0.62
Below age 13	0.20	0.42	0.05	0.10
Age 13 or 14	0.41	0.37	0.18	0.11
Age 15 or older	0.39	0.21	0.46	0.18
Age of the first CPS report				
No report	0.01	0.01	0.997	0.00
First report below age 13	0.04	0.44	0.00	0.60
First report age 13 or 14	0.29	0.34	0.00	0.15
First report age 15 or older	0.67	0.21	0.00	0.25
Number of CPS investigations				
None	0.00	0.00	0.997	0.00
1 or 2	0.68	0.13	0.00	0.94
3 or more	0.32	0.87	0.00	0.06
Type of CPS investigation				
No investigation	0.00	0.00	0.997	0.03
Protection investigation	0.00	0.00	0.00	0.85
Judicial investigation	0.89	0.04	0.00	0.12
Truancy investigation	0.04	0.00	0.00	0.00
Multiple types of investigations	0.07	0.95	0.00	0.00

Current psychological functioning and delinquent behaviour per group

carrying out several class models. Based on the entropy (0.95) and the BIC value (692.03), the four-class models fitted best. The five-class model, however, had the lowest value of the AIC (417.74). Models distinguishing six or more classes all performed worse on all indicators. Based on these findings and the interpretability of the resulting latent class model, we decided that the four-class model had the best fit for these data.

In order to interpret the latent classes, item response probabilities of the indicators were examined for each latent class. Table 4 presents the item-response probabilities and the proportions of the classes.

The first class, labelled as the *late CPS/penal investigation group* (44.9%) (Fig. 1), did not experience maltreatment or a family supervision order in childhood. They all committed at least one offence[2] and their first offence

was at age 13 or 14. Their first judicial CPS report was executed at age fifteen or older (late CPS interference) and they had a maximum of two, solely judicial, reports.

A majority of the second class, labelled as the *early CPS/multiple investigation group* (30.8%) (Fig. 2), experienced maltreatment in childhood which often resulted in at least one family supervision order pronounced by the court. They had their first report at a young age, below age 13 (early CPS interference) and had three or more CPS investigations, due to various causes (judicial and/or family and/or truancy investigations), since they often committed their first offence below age thirteen.

The third class, labelled as the *late CPS interference without investigation group* (14.6%) (Fig. 3), did not experience any severe family problems such as maltreatment or family supervision orders. If they committed an offence, it was at age 15 or older (late CPS interference). CPS decided mostly not to investigate the child and they often did not have any reports in their record.

---

[2] Those who committed no offence in youth, have not (yet) experienced the onset of delinquency. Therefore, the category 'no offence' is mentioned in Table 4. For classes 1 and 2 this translates into all respondents in these classes having committed at least one offence.

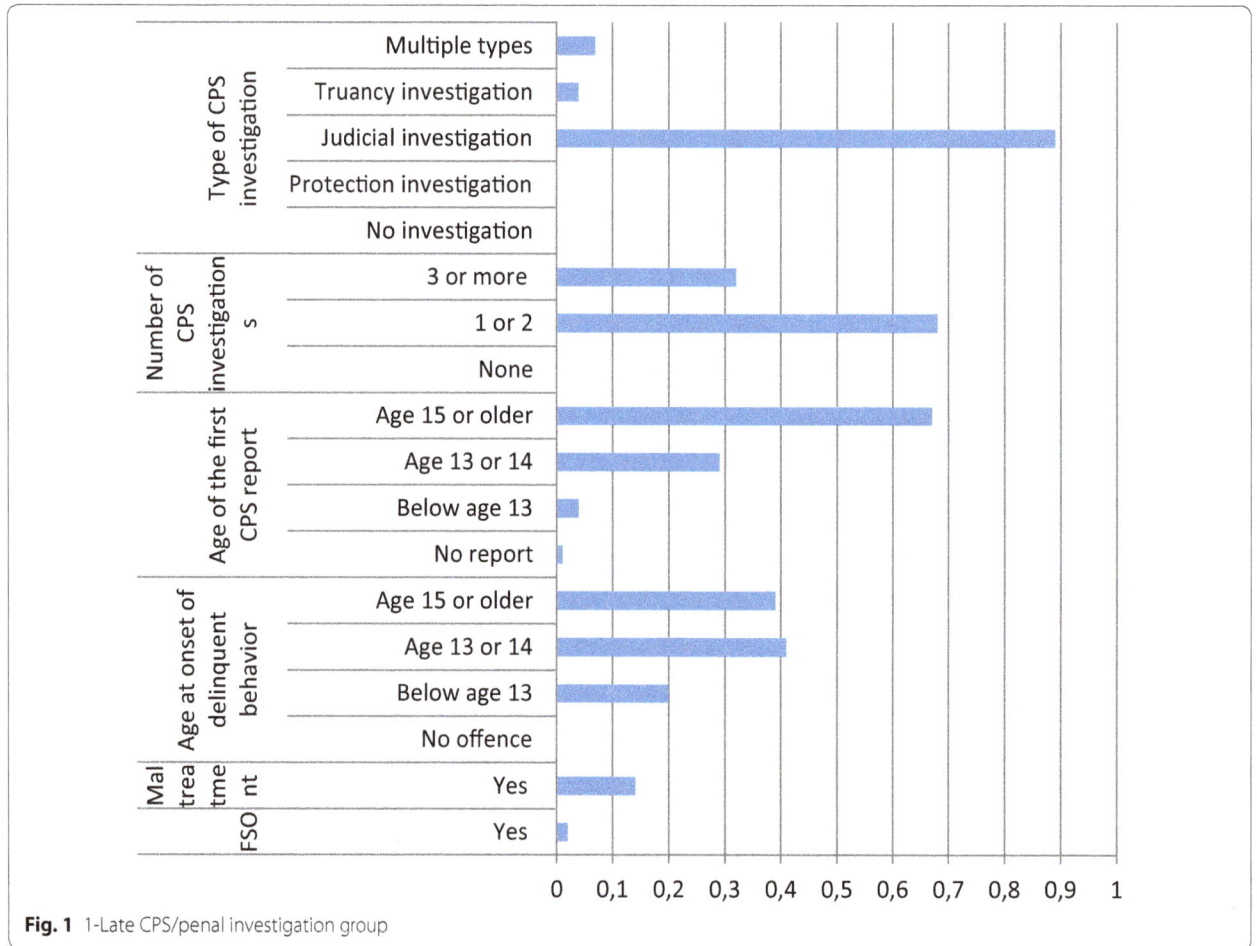

Fig. 1 1-Late CPS/penal investigation group

The fourth class, labelled as the *early CPS/family investigation group* (9.7%) (Fig. 4), had early CPS interference below age thirteen (early CPS interference), due to severe family problems such as maltreatment which resulted mostly in at least one family supervision order. CPS decided to investigate their situations once or twice, which were specifically protection investigations. Participants in this group were not likely to commit any offence.

Table 5 presents results of the ANOVA and post hoc comparisons between LCA class membership on current psychological functioning. There was a significant difference among classes on anxious/depressive problems ($p = 0.035$), a borderline significant difference on intrusive problems ($p = 0.056$) and a significant difference on substance use ($p = 0.029$). The post hoc test showed that participants of the early CPS/family investigation group reported significantly more anxious/depressive problems than participants of the early CPS/multiple investigation group ($p = 0.022$). Moreover, the early CPS/family investigation group reported more substance abuse than the late CPS interference without investigation group (borderline significant; $p = 0.056$).

No significant differences among LCA classes were found on self-reported current delinquent behaviour (Table 5).

Discussion
The purpose of this study was twofold. The first aim was to retrospectively identify distinct classes in multiproblem young adults based on childhood CPS characteristics. This resulted in four latent classes: a late CPS/penal investigation group (44.9%), an early CPS/multiple investigation group (30.8%), a late CPS interference without investigation group (14.6%) and an early CPS/family investigation group (9.7%). The second aim was to explore whether these classes differed on current young adult psychological functioning and delinquent behaviour. The early CPS/family investigation group reported significantly more problematic anxiousness/depression problems than the other groups. Substance use differed significantly among groups, although post hoc tests only revealed borderline significant differences. No differences in current delinquent behaviour were reported among the classes.

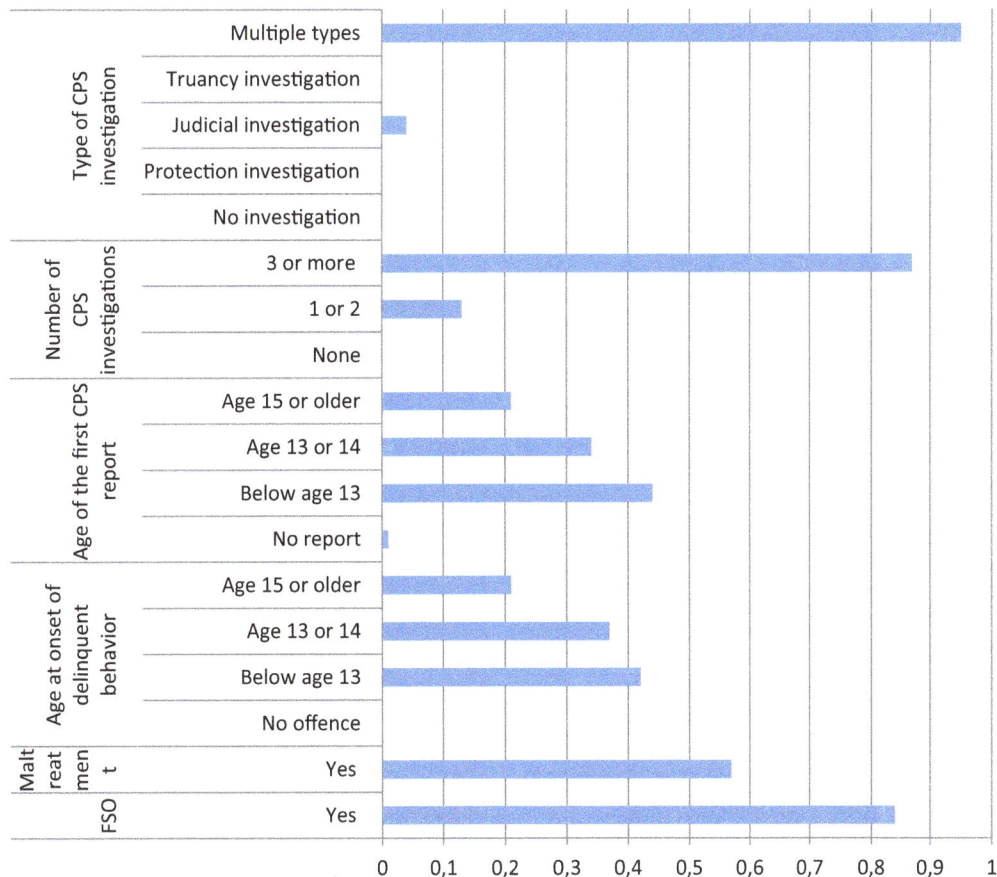

Fig. 2 2-Early CPS/multiple investigation group

In our sample of multi-problem young adults, 65.9% had one or more CPS interference(s) during their childhood versus 1% of the total population of Dutch children in 2016 [86]. Furthermore, 29.5% in the current sample underwent maltreatment versus 3% of Dutch youth that was in danger of any type of maltreatment in 2010 [87]. Thus, the prevalence of CPS interferences and severe family problems is, as expected, clearly higher in this population of multi-problem young adults than in the general population. One should note, however, that these percentages are not completely comparable, since the prevalence in the current study was not limited to 1 year. The high prevalence of CPS interference in multi-problem young adults matches their self-reported problems in childhood quite adequately: 83.3% reported service use in their youth and 63.2% reported family problems. As expected, multi-problem young adults also experience heterogeneous problems in their current functioning. This extends findings in other studies [88–90] that argue that different forms of problem behaviour (such as mental health problems, delinquency and substance use) with an onset in childhood are interrelated and may be seen as symptoms of a general disposition toward deviant behaviour through life, by some referred to as problem behaviour syndrome (PBS) [91]. How PBS is expressed may vary over time and across contexts. For children with PBS, the transition to adulthood typically occurs in the context of severe family problems and interference by multiple justice/care/and child welfare systems [41, 66]. Therefore, they may experience a differential pathway into adulthood in which more tailor-made specialized care is needed to support their adopting adult responsibilities such as independent living [41]. This way, they may be prevented from growing into multi-problem young adults. Our first findings underline the importance of gaining more insight into the childhood onset of the problem heterogeneity of multi-problem young adults in order to enhance effective tailor-made intervention.

The present study confirmed several distinct classes of risk factors for adult problem behaviour in addition to earlier studies [3, 9, 13]. Dembo et al. 9 and Geluk et al. 13 identified two and three classes, respectively, differing in the extent of problem behaviour; Haapasalo [3] reported two classes differing in age of onset and number

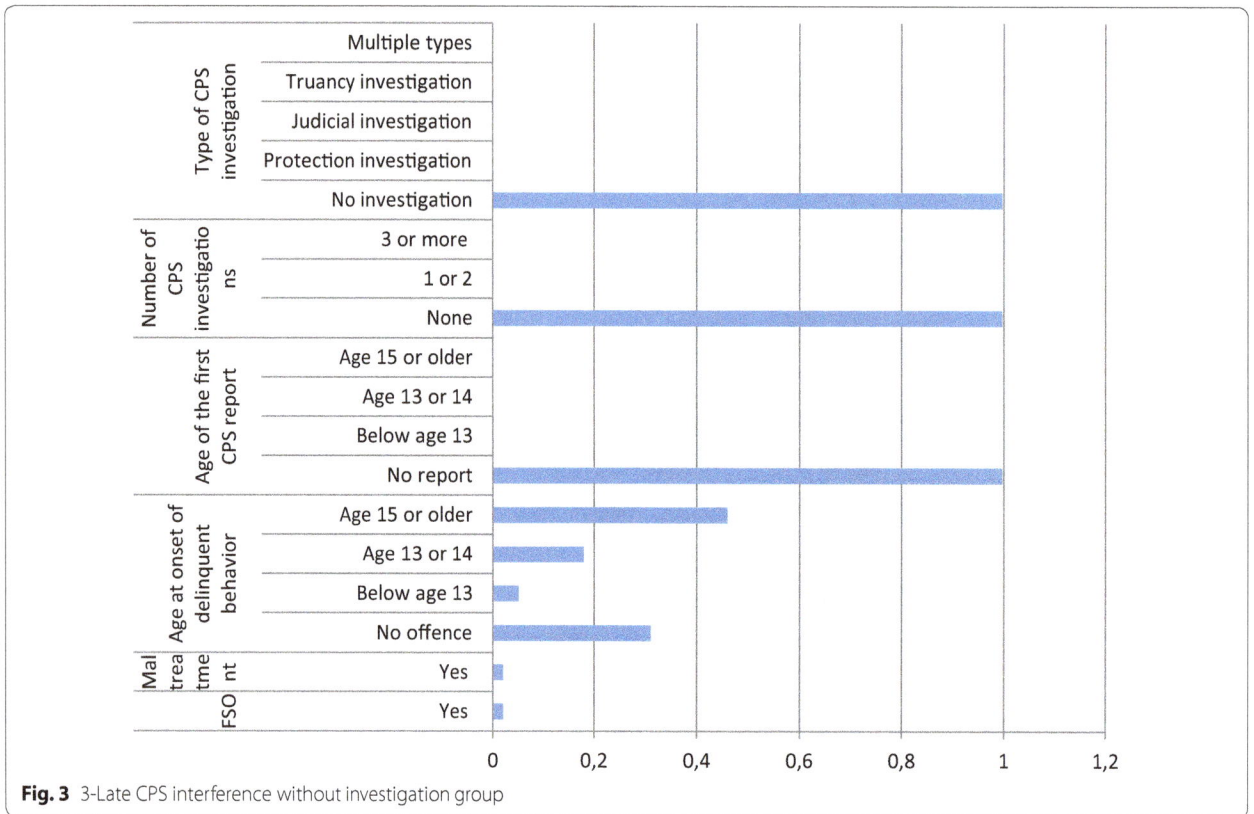

Fig. 3 3-Late CPS interference without investigation group

of CPS interventions. A first distinction in the identified classes in the current study indeed occurred between early (below age 13) and late (from age 15) CPS involvement. The early CPS/multiple investigation group had the earliest onset of delinquent behaviour (below age 13). Several studies show that early onset delinquents are more at risk for problems in young adulthood, such as mental health problems, substance abuse, drug related and violent delinquent behaviour, than later onset delinquents [20, 61]. Furthermore, the early CPS/multiple investigation group underwent the most CPS investigations and is, therefore, also comparable to the early onset group in the Haapasalo study [3], in which the offenders demonstrated more problems during their youth and were in greater need of CPS interventions such as placement in foster care.

Regarding the long term outcomes of childhood CPS interference specifically, the early CPS/family investigation group reported the most anxious/depression problems and the most substance abuse in young adulthood. Maltreatment, family supervision and other severe family problems in childhood have repeatedly been shown to be robust risk factors for mental health problems in (young) adulthood [7, 16]. For example, according to Thornberry et al. [15], childhood maltreatment is indeed strongly related to later substance abuse and internalizing

problems. Although the early CPS/family investigation was the smallest identified group (9.7%), they seem to have followed the most adverse developmental pathway into young adulthood. It is possible that CPS failed to provide appropriate interventions for this group, since the CPS involvement was not as intensive as for the early onset/multiple investigation group. Moreover, the early CPS/family group was the only group that did not engage in delinquent behaviour in childhood/adolescence. This may have caused them to stay unnoticed for a longer period of time. However, traumatic events in the child's family environment may have already occurred long before the first CPS interference and are associated with an increased likelihood of adverse adult outcomes [7, 16]. Besides a broader focus on the problems of the child itself, children with solely civil CPS interference may benefit from more attention to treatment of the problems of the parents. Interventions could be aimed at strengthening their parenting capabilities and resources. Adopting such a 'two-generation approach' has shown promising results in preventing family and childhood problems from growing worse [92].

No significant differences among classes in current delinquent behaviour were found among groups. The late CPS/penal group was the largest group in our sample (44.9%); their first CPS investigation was at age 15 or

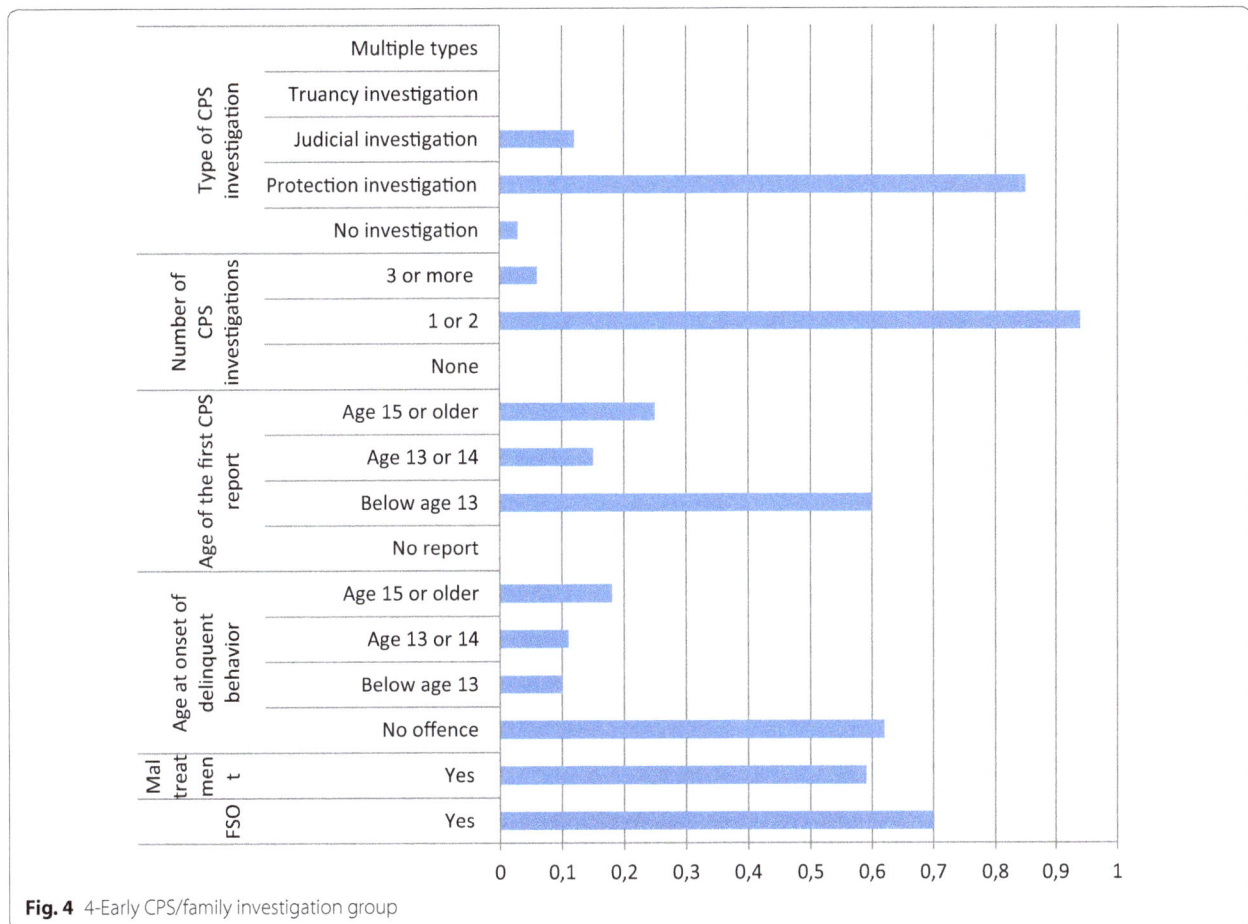

Fig. 4 4-Early CPS/family investigation group

older and the age of onset of their delinquent behaviour varied between ages 13 and 15. All multi-problem young adults showed a strong tendency for persisting in and/or developing criminal behaviour into adulthood, notwithstanding their distinct childhood histories. Moreover, since the group without CPS investigations also reported delinquent behaviour in adulthood, all forms of CPS interference (even marginal contact) should be considered risk factors for later antisocial behaviour. In addition, the late CPS/penal children proved to be a group without severe family problems, at least according to the CPS data. Steinberg [17] noted that adolescent onset offenders often manifest less severe patterns of family pathology and mental health problems than life course persistent offenders [61]. In our sample, both late onset CPS groups indeed reported fewer mental health problems in young adulthood than the early onset groups. A follow-up study should be conducted to explore whether these differences in problem behaviour among groups still persist into (middle) adulthood. Finally, since all groups persisted in their delinquent behaviour, children with CPS interference should be targeted as a high-risk

population in need of specialized interventions aimed at reducing the criminogenic risk factors associated with recidivism.

Limitations

Like any other study, this study has some limitations. First, the CPS record investigation in the current study was not performed using a validated instrument, because an applicable instrument was not available. However, CPS investigations are standardized and in order to optimize and monitor the quality of the data, inter-rater reliability was analysed and found to be substantial. Second, registered offence data, and in particular data on the first offence, is likely to be under reported, as a minority of juvenile delinquents is actually convicted [24]. Still, in this sample officially recorded and self-reported delinquency data are, while not exactly similar, quite comparable, both showing a high prevalence of delinquent behaviour. Third, in this study, self-report questionnaires were also used to investigate socio-demographic characteristics and psychological functioning. To achieve good reliability, a validated self-report psychological

Table 5 Results of ANOVA comparisons among classes on current self-reported psychological functioning and delinquent behaviour ($N = 390$)

Class	1 ($N = 175$)	2 ($N = 120$)	3 ($N = 57$)	4 ($N = 38$)	F	p
	M (SD)	M (SD)	M (SD)	M (SD)		
Psychological functioning[a]						
Total psychological problems	61.4 (26.0)	61.5 (25.8)	59.8 (28.2)	71.1 (22.8)	1.71	0.164
Anxious/depressed	69.2 (18)	66.3 (16)	69.4 (18)	75.8 (18)	2.88[b]	0.035**
Withdrawn	79.0 (17.2)	78.1 (16.8)	73.2 (18.7)	80.8 (16.6)	1.97	0.118
Somatic complaints	68.1 (16.4)	67.8 (16.1)	69.2 (17.4)	72.6 (16.7)	0.90	0.439
Intrusive	55.7 (1)	59.3 (1)	55.7 (1)	57.8 (2)	2.55[c]	0.056*
Rule-breaking behaviour	78.6 (16.8)	79.9 (16.8)	78.4 (16.2)	82.6 (17.6)	0.71	0.549
Aggressive behaviour	67.7 (16.1)	67.2 (15.5)	68.5 (17)	74.2 (16.9)	1.97	0.118
Attention problems	73.4 (14.3)	74 (14.5)	72.3 (14.5)	77.7 (14.7)	1.18	0.317
Thought problems	74.3 (17.5)	73.2 (16.3)	72.1 (17.3)	79.2 (16.5)	1.52	0.208
Substance use[d]	78.0 (18)	81 (19)	73.9 (19)	83.9 (18)	3.04[e]	0.029**

Class	1 ($N = 74$)	2 ($N = 59$)	3 ($N = 25$)	4 ($N = 21$)	F	p
	M (SD)	M (SD)	M (SD)	M (SD)		
Delinquency previous 6 months						
Total delinquency	3.5 (8.1)	7.1 (11.5)	6.0 (13.2)	2.2 (5.3)	2.1	0.101
Destruction/public order offence	0.09 (0.3)	0.14 (0.4)	0.00 (0)	0.19 (0.4)	1.89	0.133
Property offence	0.22 (0.4)	0.37 (0.5)	0.27 (0.5)	0.18 (0.4)	1.72	0.165
Aggression/violent offence	0.20 (0.4)	0.27 (0.4)	0.15 (0.4)	0.23 (0.4)	0.61	0.609
Drug offence	0.57 (0.5)	0.65 (0.5)	0.54 (0.5)	0.61 (0.5)	1.35	0.261

[a] Normal functioning (score < 84), borderline range (score 84-90), clinical range (above 90) [78]

[b] Significant difference between early CPS/family investigation group and early CPS/multiple investigation group

[c] Significant difference between early CPS/multiple investigation group and late CPS/penal investigation group

[d] Class 1; $N = 174$

[e] Significant difference between early CPS/family investigation group and late CPS interference without investigation group

* $p < 0.10$, ** $p < 0.05$, *** $p < 0.01$

functioning questionnaire is used and anonymity and privacy of participants was emphasized before and during the assessment of questionnaires. Fourth, a majority of 87.4% of participants in this study have a non-Dutch ethnicity. In our case, non-Dutch ethnicity refers to an amalgam of cultural backgrounds, for example Surinamese, Antillean, Moroccan and Turkish. However, due to small sample sizes per ethnic subgroup, it was not possible to perform separate analyses. Fifth, generalizability of study results to an international context is not straightforward, because of different service system organizations. In Great-Britain and the United States of America, for example, child protection service and the judicial youth system are more separate systems than in The Netherlands [93, 94]. Scandinavian countries have more comparable systems to the Dutch system, although those systems are more based on prevention. For instance, in Sweden voluntary and involuntary services are not divided as in The Netherlands [95]. And lastly, LCA is an exploratory data-driven method and the findings per class represent probabilities on latent indicators.

Conclusions

This study adds to the concept that even in a highly complex sample of multi-problem young adults who underwent CPS interference in their youth distinct developmental pathways, at least for mental health problems, can be distinguished. Although this exploratory study was not intended to produce definite ideas on how the underlying latent subgroups may experience differential treatment effects, our findings do suggest that members of the groups might benefit from interventions specifically tailored to their differing patterns of problems. The development of specific secondary and tertiary prevention programmes for children with an early onset of CPS interference and severe family problems should receive priority from both policy makers and clinical practice. In addition, evidence based interventions should be developed to prevent problem behaviour of all children that underwent CPS interference in their youth to prevent mental health problems and the persistence of delinquent behaviour into (young) adulthood.

Abbreviations

AIC: akaike information criterion; ANOVA: analysis of variance; ASR: adult self report; BIC: Bayesian information criterion; CAU: care as usual; CPS: Child Protection Services; Df: degrees of freedom; DNK: New Opportunities (Dutch: *De Nieuwe Kans*); KBPS: Kinderbescherming Bedrijfs Processen System (*CPS system*); LCA: latent class analysis; M: mean; SAS: Statistical Analysis System; SD: standard deviation; SPSS: Statistical Packages for the Social Sciences; SRD: Self-Report Delinquency Scale; SSM-D: Self-Sufficiency Matrix-Dutch Version.

Authors' contributions

TD and AP are the principal investigators and obtained funding for the study. LD coordinate the record and register research and, together with JZ and ML, the data collection during the study. LD and FB drafted the manuscript with important contributions from CP, ML, JZ, RM, AB, TD, and AP. LD and AB together performed the data analysis. All authors read and approved the final manuscript.

Author details

¹ Department of Child and Adolescent Psychiatry, VU University Medical Center, Meibergdreef 5, 1105 AZ Amsterdam, The Netherlands. ² Leiden Law School, Leiden University, Institute of Criminal Law and Criminology, PO Box 9520, 2300 RA Leiden, The Netherlands.

Acknowledgements

The data that support the findings of this study are available from VU University Medical Center but restrictions apply to the availability of these data, which were used under license for the current study, and so are not publicly available. Data are however available from the authors reasonable request and with permission of VU University Medical Center. We would like to thank the social welfare agency (Jongerenloket) in Rotterdam, DNK, The Child Care and Protection Service for their cooperation with this study.

Competing interests

The authors declare that they have no competing interests.

Funding

This research project is funded by De Verre Bergen foundation. De Verre Bergen foundation is a venture philanthropy organization that aims to build a better Rotterdam through substantial investments in innovative, impactful social ventures. The financer is not involved in the design of the study nor the drafting of the manuscript. Furthermore, the financer is not and shall not be involved in the subsequent process of data collection, analysis and interpretation. Contact information: Nanne Boonstra, Parklaan 22, 3016 BB Rotterdam, The Netherlands; Tel: 0031 10 209 2000; E-mail: nboonstra@sdvb.com.

References

1. Barrett DE, Katsiyannis A, Zhang D, Zhang D. Delinquency and recidivism: a Multicohort, Matched-Control Study of the Role of Early Adverse Experiences, Mental Health Problems, and Disabilities. J Emot Behav Disord. 2014;22:3–15.

2. Barrett DE, Katsiyannis A. Juvenile offending and crime in early adulthood: a large sample analysis. J Child Fam Stud. 2016;25:1086–97.

3. Haapasalo J. Young offenders' experiences of Child Protection Services. J Youth Adolesc. 2000;29:355–71.

4. Edwards VJ, Holden GW, Felitti VJ, Anda RF. Relationship between multiple forms of childhood maltreatment and adult mental health in community respondents: results from the Adverse Childhood Experiences Study. Am J Psychiatry. 2003;160:1453–60.

5. Pecora PJ, Kessler RC, O'Brien K, White CR, Williams J, Hiripi E, et al. Educational and employment outcomes of adults formerly placed in foster care: results from the Northwest Foster Care Alumni Study. Child Youth Serv Rev. 2006;28:1459–81.

6. Braga T, Gonçalves LC, Basto-Pereira M, Maia Â. Unraveling the link between maltreatment and juvenile antisocial behavior: a meta-analysis of prospective longitudinal studies. Aggress Violent Behav. 2017;33:37–50.

7. Widom CS. The cycle of violence. Science. 1989;244:160–6.

8. DeGue S, Widom CS. Does out-of-home placement mediate the relationship between child maltreatment and adult criminality? Child Maltreat. 2009;14:344–55.

9. Dembo R, Wareham J, Poythress N, Meyers K, Schmeidler J. Psychosocial functioning problems over time among high-risk youths. Crime Delinq. 2008;54:644–70.

10. King DC, Abram KM, Romero EG, Washburn JJ, Welty LJ, Teplin LA. Childhood maltreatment and psychiatric disorders among detained youths. Psychiatr Serv. 2011;62:1430–8.

11. Haapasalo J, Pokela E. Child-rearing and child abuse antecedents of criminality. Aggress Violent Behav. 1999;4:107–27.

12. Moffitt TE, Caspi A. Childhood predictors differentiate life-course persistent and adolescence-limited antisocial pathways among males and females. Dev Psychopathol. 2001;13:355–75.

13. Geluk CAML, Van Domburgh L, Doreleijers TAH, Jansen LMC, Bouwmeester S, Garre FG, et al. Identifying Children at risk of problematic development: latent clusters among childhood arrestees. J Abnorm Child Psychol. 2014;42:669–80.

14. van Domburgh L, Loeber R, Bezemer D, Stallings R, Stouthamer-Loeber M. Childhood predictors of desistance and level of persistence in offending in early onset offenders. J Abnorm Child Psychol. 2009;37:967–80.

15. Thornberry TP, Henry KL, Ireland TO, Smith CA. The causal impact of childhood-limited maltreatment and adolescent maltreatment on early adult adjustment. J Adolesc Health. 2010;46:359–65.

16. Horwitz AV, Widom CS, McLaughlin J, White HR. The impact of childhood abuse and neglect on adult mental health: a Prospective Study. J Health Soc Behav. 2001;42:184–201.

17. Steinberg L. Adolescence. 10th ed. New York: McGraw-Hill; 2014.

18. Potter CC, Jenson JM. Cluster profiles of multiple problem youth: mental health problem symptoms, substance use, and delinquent conduct. Crim Justice Behav. 2003;30:230–50.

19. Van der Geest V, Bijleveld C, Blokland A. Ontwikkelingspaden van delinquent gedrag bij hoog-risicojongeren. Tijdschr. Voor Criminol. 2007;49:351–69.

20. Odgers CL, Moffitt TE, Broadbent JM, Dickson N, Hancox RJ, Harrington H, et al. Female and male antisocial trajectories: from childhood origins to adult outcomes. Dev Psychopathol. 2008;20:673–716.

21. Van Domburgh L, Vermeiren R, Blokland AA, Doreleijers TA. Delinquent development in dutch childhood arrestees: developmental trajectories, risk factors and co-morbidity with adverse outcomes during adolescence. J Abnorm Child Psychol. 2009;37:93–105.

22. Colman RA, Mitchell-Herzfeld S, Kim DH, Shady TA. From delinquency to the perpetration of child maltreatment: examining the early adult criminal justice and child welfare involvement of youth released from juvenile justice facilities. Child Youth Serv Rev. 2010;32:1410–7. https://doi.org/10.1016/j.childyouth.2010.06.010.

23. Shaw DS, Hyde LW, Brennan LM. Early predictors of boys' antisocial trajectories. Dev Psychopathol. 2012;24:871–88.

24. Geest, Van der V, Blokland A, Bijleveld C. Delinquent development in a sample of high-risk youth: shape, content, and predictors of delinquent trajectories from age 12 to 32. J Res Crime Delinq. 2009;46:111–43. http://jrc.sagepub.com/content/46/2/111.abstract.

25. DeLisi M, Neppl TK, Lohman BJ, Vaughn MG, Shook JJ. Early starters: which type of criminal onset matters most for delinquent careers? J Crim Justice. 2013;41:12–7.

26. Loeber R, Burke JD. Developmental pathways in Juvenile externalizing and internalizing problems. J Res Adolesc. 2011;21:34–46.

27. Blokland A, Palmen H, San Van M. Crimineel gedrag in de jongvolwassen-heid. Tijdschr Voor Criminol. 2012;54:85–98.

28. Doreleijers TH, Fokkens JW. Minderjarigen en jongvolwassenen: Pleidooi voor een evidence based strafrecht. Rechtstreeks. 2010;2:9–47.

29. Lamet W, James C, Dirkzwager A, Van der Laan P. Reclasseringstoezicht en jongvolwassenen. PROCES. 2010;89:371–83.

30. Crone EA. Executive functions in adolescence: inferences from brain and behavior. Dev Sci. 2009;12:825–30.

31. Arnett JJ. Emerging adulthood: a theory of development from the late teens through the twenties. Am Psychol. 2000;55:469–80.

32. Arnett JJ. Emerging adulthood : what is it, and What is it good for ? Child Dev Perspect. 2007;1:68–73.

33. D'Oosterlinck F, Broekaert E, Vander Haeghen C. Probleemjongeren te vroeg het te-huis uit? voor Orthop Kinderpsychiatrie, en Klin Kinderpsy-chologie. 2006;31:58–68.

34. Berzin SC. Difficulties in the transition to adulthood: using propensity scoring to understand what makes foster youth vulnerable. Soc Serv Rev. 2008;82:171–96.

35. Collins ME. Transition to adulthood for vulnerable youths: a review of research and implications for policy. Soc Serv Rev. 2001;72:271–91.

36. Bullis M, Yovanoff P. Those who do not return: correlates of the work and school engagemtnt of formerly incarcerated youth who remain in the community. J Emot Behav Disord. 2002;10:66–78.

37. Fagan J, Freeman R. Crime and work. Crime Justice. 1999;25:225–90.

38. Ahrens KR, Garrison MM, Courtney ME. Health outcomes in young adults from foster care and economically diverse backgrounds. Pediatrics. 2014;134:1067–74.

39. Copeland WE, Miller-Johnson S, Keeler G, Angold A, Costello EJ. Child-hood psychiatric disorders and young adult crime: a prospective population-based study. Am J Psychiatry. 2007;164:1668–75.

40. Arnett JJ. The developmental context of substance use in emerging adulthood. J Drug Issues. 2005;35:235–53.

41. Osgood DW, Foster EM, Flanagan C, Gretchen RR, Courtney ME, Heuring DH, et al. On your own without a net: the transition to adulthood for vulnerable populations. Osgood DW, Foster EM, Flanagan C, Ruth GR, editors. Chicago: The University of Chicago; 2005.

42. Fergusson DM, Horwood LJ. Early onset cannabis use and psychosocial adjustment in young adults. Addiction. 1997;92:279–96.

43. Loeber R, Farrington DP. Young children who commit crime: epidemiol-ogy, developmental origins, risk factors, early interventions, and policy implications. Dev Psychopathol. 2000;12:737–62.

44. Barron P, Hassiotis A, Banes J. Offenders with intellectual disability: a prospective comparative study. J Intellect Disabil Res. 2004;48:69–76.

45. Mun EY, Windle M, Schainker LM. A model-based cluster analysis approach to adolescent problem behaviors and young adult outcomes. Dev Psychopathol. 2008;20:291–318.

46. Murray J, Farrington DP. Risk factors for conduct disorder and delin-quency: key findings from longitudinal studies. Can J Psychiatry. 2010;55:633–42.

47. Kearney CA. School absenteeism and school refusal behavior in youth: a contemporary review. Clin Psychol Rev. 2008;28(3):451–7.

48. Osgood DW, Foster EM, Courtney ME. Vulnerable populations and the transition to adulthood. Futur Child. 2010;20:209–29.

49. Courtney ME, Dworsky A. Early outcomes for young adults transitioning from out-of-home care in the USA. Child Fam Soc Work. 2006;11:209–19.

50. Smith CA, Park A, Ireland TO, Elwyn L, Thornberry TP. Long-term outcomes of young adults exposed to maltreatment: the role of educational experi-ences in promoting resilience to crime and violence in early adulthood. J Interpers Violence. 2013;28:121–56.

51. Havlicek J, Courtney ME. Maltreatment histories of aging out foster youth: a comparison of official investigated reports and self-reports of maltreatment prior to and during out-of-home care. Child Abus Negl. 2016;52:110–22.

52. Loman LA. Families frequently encountered by child protection services: a Report on Chronic Child Abuse and Neglect. Missouri: St. Louis; 2006.

53. Darlington Y, Healy K, Feeney JA. Approaches to assessment and inter-vention across four types of child and family welfare services. Child Youth Serv Rev. 2010;32:356–64.

54. Domburgh, Van L, Vermeiren R, Doreleijers TAH. Screening and assess-ment. In: Loeber R, Slot NW, Laan, van der PH, Hoeve M, editors. Tomor-row's Crim. Dev. child Delinq. Eff. Interv. Aldershot: Ashgate; 2008. p. 165–78.

55. Montgomery P, Donkoh C, Underhill K. Independent living programs for young people leaving the care system: the state of the evidence. Child Youth Serv Rev. 2006;28:1435–48.

56. Kapp SA. Pathways to Prison: life histories of former clients of the child welfare and juvenile justice systems. J Soci Soc Welf. 2000;27:63–74.

57. International Research Triagle Institute. Adolescents involved with child welfare: a transition to adulthood. Washington D.C.: National Survey of Child and Adolescent Well-Being (NSCAW); 2008.

58. Fergusson DM, Lynskey MT. Physical punishment/maltreatment during childhood and adjustment in young adulthood. Child Abuse Negl. 1997;21:617–30.

59. Jonson-Reid M, Kohl PL, Drake B. Child and adult outcomes of chronic child maltreatment. Pediatrics. 2012;129:839–45.

60. Smith CA, Ireland TO, Thornberry TP. Adolescent maltreatment and its impact on young adult antisocial behavior. Child Abus Negl. 2005;29:1099–119.

61. Moffitt TE, Caspi A, Harrington H, Milne BJ. Males on the life-course-persistent and adolescence-limited antisocial pathways: follow-up at age 26 years. Dev Psychopathol. 2002;14:179–207.

62. Mun EY, Windle M, Schainker LM. A model-based cluster analysis approach to adolescent problem behaviors and young adult outcomes. Dev Psychopathol. 2008;20:291–318.

63. Maschi T, Hatcher SS, Schwalbe CS, Rosato NS. Mapping the social service pathways of youth to and through the juvenile justice system: a compre-hensive review. Child Youth Serv Rev. 2008;30:1376–85.

64. Barnes JC, Boutwell BB. On the relationship of past to future involvement in crime and delinquency: a behavior genetic analysis. J Crim Justice. 2012;40:94–102.

65. Garland A, Aarons GA, Brown SA, Wood PA, Hough RL. Diagnostic profiles associated with use of mental health and substance abuse services among high-risk youths. Psychiatr Serv. 2003;54:562–4.

66. Corrales T, Waterford M, Goodwin-Smith I, Wood L, Yourell T, Ho C. Childhood adversity, sense of belonging and psychosocial outcomes in emerging adulthood: a test of mediated pathways. Child Youth Serv Rev. 2016;63:110–9.

67. Spies H, Tan S, Davelaar M. De Jeugd Maar Geen Toekomst? Naar Een Effectieve Aanpak Van Sociale Uitsluiting. Amsterdam: SWP; 2016.

68. Fassaert T, Lauriks S, Van De Weerd S, Theunissen J, Kikkert M, Dekker J, et al. Psychometric properties of the Dutch version of the self-sufficiency matrix (SSM-D). Community Ment Health J. 2014;50:583–90.

69. Fassaert T, Lauriks S, Van De Weerd S, De Wit M, Buster M. Ontwikkeling en betrouwbaarheid van de Zelfredzaamheid-Matrix. Tijdschr voor Gezond-heidswetenschappen. 2013;91:169–77.

70. Bannink R, Broeren S, Heydelberg J, van't Klooster E, Raat H. Psychometric properties of self-sufficiency assessment tools in adolescents in voca-tional education. BMC Psychol. 2015;33:10.

71. Culhane DP, Gross KS, Parker WD, Poppe B, Sykes E. Accountability, cost-effectiveness, and program performance: progress since 1998. Retrieved from http://repository.upenn.edu/spp_papers/114.

72. Luijks MJ, Bevaart F, Zijlmans J, van Duin L, Marhe R, Doreleijers TA, et al. A multimodal day treatment program for multi-problem young adults: Study protocol of a randomized controlled trial in clinical practice. Trials. 2017;18:1–15.

73. Het Kwaliteitskader van de Raad voor de Kinderbescherming. Utrecht; 2013.

74. McHugh ML. Interrater reliabilty: the kappa statistic. Biochem Medica. 2012;22:276–82.

75. Landis JR, Koch GG. The measurement of observer agreement for cat-egorical data. Biometrics. 1977;33:159–74.

76. Keij I. Standaarddefinitie allochtonen. Index: Cent Bur voor Stat; 2000.

77. Achenbach TM, Rescorla LA. Manual for the ASEBA adult forms and profiles. Burlington: ASEBA; 2003.

78. Vanheusden K, van der Ende J, Mulder CL, van Lenthe FJ, Verhulst FC, Mackenbach JP. The use of mental health services among young adults

with emotional and behavioural problems: equal use for equal needs? Soc Psychiatry Psychiatr Epidemiol. 2008;43:808–15.

79. van der Laan AM, Blom M. WODC-Monitor Zelfgerapporteerde Jeugd-criminaliteit—Meting 2005. Den Haag: WODC Memorandum; 2006.

80. van der Laan AM, Blom M, Kleemans ER. Exploring long-term and short-term risk factors for serious delinquency. Eur J Criminol. 2009;6:419–38.

81. Bosma A, Asscher J, Van der Laan P, Stams J. Procesevaluatie Tools4U. Amsterdam: Kohnstamm Instituut; 2011.

82. Collins LM, Lanza ST. Latent Class and Latent Transition Analysis. Balding DJ, Cressie NAC, Fitzmaurice GM, Johnstone IM, Molenberghs G, Scott DW, et al., editors. New Jersey: Wiley; 2010.

83. Lanza ST, Collins LM, Lemmon DR, Schafer JL. PROC LCA: a SAS procedure for latent class analysis. Struct Equ Model Multidiscip J. 2007;14:671–94.

84. Celeux G, Soromenho G. An entropy criterion for assessing the number of clusters in a mixture model. J Classif. 1996;13:195–212.

85. Field A. Discovering statistics using SPSS. 3rd ed. chennai: Sage Publications; 2009.

86. Raad voor de Kinderbescherming. 2016: ongeveer 35.000 kinderen in aanraking met de RvdK. 2017 https://www.kinderbescherming.nl/actueel/nieuws/2017/04/18/2016-ongeveer-35.000-kinderen-in-aanraking-met-de-rvdk Accessed 2017 Jun 30.

87. Nederlands Jeugdinstituut. Studie cijfers kindermishandeling. 2016. http://www.nji.nl/Kindermishandeling-Probleemschets-Cijfers.

88. LeBlanc ML, Bouthillier C. A developmental test of the general deviance syndrome with adjudicated girls and boys using hierarchical confirmatory factor analysis. Crim Behav Ment Heal. 2003;13:81–105.

89. Henry KL, Huizinga DH. School-related risk and protective factors associated with truancy among urban youth placed at risk. J Prim Prev. 2007;28:505–19.

90. McCluskey CP, Bynum TS, Patchin JW. Reducing chronic absenteeism: an assessment of an early truancy initiative. Crime Delinq. 2004;50:214–34.

91. Jessor R, Jessor SL. Problem behavior and psychosocial development: A longitudinal study of youth. San Diego: Academic Press; 1977.

92. Shonkoff JP, Fisher PA. Rethinking evidence-based practice and two-generation programs to create the future of early childhood policy. Dev Psychopathol. 2013;25:1635–53.

93. Myers JEB. A short history of child protection in America. Fam Law Q. 2008;42:449–63.

94. HM Government. Working together to safeguard children. 2015. https://www.gov.uk/government/publications/working-together-to-safeguard-children--2.

95. Berg T, Vink C. Jeugdzorg in Europa—Lessen over strategieën en zorgsystemen uit Engeland, Duitsland. Utrecht: Noorwegen en Zweden; 2009.

9

Global burden of mental disorders among children aged 5–14 years

Marie Laure Baranne*[iD] and Bruno Falissard

Abstract

Background: The global burden of disease (GBD) study provides information about fatal and non-fatal health outcomes around the world.

Methods: The objective of this work is to describe the burden of mental disorders among children aged 5–14 years in each of the six regions of the World Health Organisation. Data come from the GBD 2015 study. Outcomes: disability-adjusted life-years (DALYs) are the main indicator of GBD studies and are built from years of life lost (YLLs) and years of life lived with disability (YLDs).

Results: Mental disorders are among the leading causes of YLDs and of DALYs in Europe and the Americas. Because of the importance of infectious diseases, mental disorders appear marginal in Africa for YLLs although they play an important role in YLDs there. Because the epidemiological transition that has taken place in Europe and the Americas (i.e., a switch from acute and infectious conditions to chronic and mental health issues) is likely to happen sooner or later across the entire planet, mental health problems in youth are likely to become one of the main public health challenges of the twenty-first century.

Conclusion: These results should improve health care if policy-makers use them to develop health policies to meet the real needs of populations (especially children) today.

Keywords: Mental health, Children, Burden of disease

Background

Determination of the health problems that most often or most severely affect specific populations is necessary to optimise health services and prioritise health policies. Until recently, the indicators most frequently chosen to understand population needs were mortality, life expectancy, and their causes and risk factors. As advances in medical knowledge have increased life expectancy in most of the world's regions, the dichotomy between fatal vs non-fatal effects has become much less relevant [1]. In 1992, the World Health Organisation (WHO) asked C. Murray and his collaborators to develop a more comprehensive indicator that would reflect not only the mortality but also the level of disability due to particular diseases. The Lancet published four articles applying this

perspective in 1997, all based on the concept of the global burden of disease (GBD) [2]. They assessed GBD through a new indicator called the DALY, for disability-adjusted life years [3]. Since then, studies of DALYs and GBD, because they provide a comprehensive picture of population needs, have become essential part of the public health literature. Technically, DALYs are estimated from mortality and disability data. Disability is estimated from the prevalence of a given disease, its average duration, and a subjective appreciation of its day-to-day impact (often obtained through revealed preference surveys in the general population) [2]. The first set of GBD studies did not clearly identify psychiatric disorders, which were grouped with neurologic disorders. The situation was even worse for most child and adolescent psychiatric disorders, which have been seriously considered only since 2010 [4].

Although some papers have already presented the results of the most recent GBD studies of young people,

*Correspondence: marie-laure.baranne@etu.parisdescartes.fr
CESP, INSERM U1018, Université Paris-Saclay, Université Paris-Sud, UVSQ, APHP, Paris, France

most of their analyses were conducted at the level of the planet and thus masked the huge specificities that exist between regions [5]. For this reason, these analyses were unable to interpret the global weight of mental disorders adequately in the paediatric population.

The objective of the present paper is to describe and analyse the global burden of mental disorders among children aged 5–14 years throughout the world from the latest data available (GBD 2015), with a focus on each WHO region and an explicit summary of the relative importance of mortality and disability in each.

Methods

For GBD 2015, diseases were defined according to the International Classification of Diseases, 10th revision (ICD-10), and organised in a hierarchical classification [6, 7]. The first level of this classification comprises three main disease groups: communicable diseases (group 1), non-communicable diseases (group 2), and injuries (group 3). These three groups are divided in 21 categories. The communicable disease categories include, for example, infectious and parasitic diseases and neonatal conditions. Categories of non-communicable diseases include mental disorders, as well as malignant neoplasms and endocrine, blood, and immune disorders. Injuries regroup intentional and non-intentional injuries. The third level of classification is closer to the usual ICD-10 categories. Mental disorders, for instance, are divided into 13 subcategories: major depressive disorders, dysthymia, bipolar disorders, schizophrenia, alcohol use disorders, drug use disorders, anxiety disorders, eating disorders, autism spectrum disorders (reported in the GBD database as Autism and Asperger syndrome), conduct disorders, attention-deficit/hyperactivity disorder (ADHD), idiopathic intellectual disability, and other mental and behavioural disorders.

The aggregate data from the 2015 GBD study are freely available [7]. This dataset provides DALYs for the six WHO regions—Africa (AFR), the Americas region (AMR), South-East Asia (SEAR), Europe (EUR), the Eastern Mediterranean region (EMR), and the West Pacific region (WPR)—for each sex and for seven age groups: <28 days, 1–59 months, 5–14, 15–29, 30–49, 50–69 years, and 70 and older [6].

Formally, DALYs are the sum of years of life lost (YLLs) and years lost due to disability (YLDs) for disorder (d), age (a), sex (s), and year (t).

$$\text{DALY (d, a, s, t)} = \text{YLL (d, a, s, t)} + \text{YLD (d, a, s, t)}.$$

YLLs and YLDs are estimated as follows:

$$\text{YLL} = \text{N(d, s, a, t)} \times \text{L(s, a)},$$

where: N(d, s, a, t) is the number of deaths due to disorder (d) for a given age (a) and sex (s) in year (t). L(s, a) is a function specifying the number of YLLs for a person of sex (s) dying at age (a).

The equation for YLDs is:

$$\text{YLD} = \text{P(d, s, a, t)} \times \text{DW(d, s, a)} \times \text{L(d, s, a, t)},$$

where: P(d, s, a, t) = prevalence of the disorder of interest (d) at age (a) and sex (s); DW(d, s, a) = disability weight for the disorder of interest (d) at age (a) and sex (s); L(d, s, a, t) = average duration of the case until remission or death (years).

In the GBD 2015 study, disability weights were obtained from two international surveys in the general populations of nine countries in 2011 and 2013: Bangladesh, Indonesia, Peru, Tanzania, the USA, Hungary, Italy, the Netherlands and Sweden [8, 9]. Two approaches were used: face-to face interviews and online surveys. The method relied on the revealed preference paradigm. More precisely, respondents were asked to determine the healthier of two situations in a series of questions. Concerning ADHD, for example, one question was:

"Who do you think is healthier overall (in terms of having fewer physical or mental limitations on what the person can do in life), the first or the second person:"

- Person 1: "ADHD: the person is hyperactive and has difficulty concentrating, remembering things, and completing tasks."
- Person 2: "Partially controlled asthma: The person has wheezing and coughing once a week, which causes some difficulty with daily activities."

The duration of each disability L(d, s, a, t) until remission or death was estimated by experts on the basis of a literature review.

The GBD 2015 study differed in some aspects from the previous studies [7]:

- Age weighting is now uniform across the lifespan; earlier versions had assigned less weight to years of healthy life lost at extreme ages [10].
- YLDs are now based on prevalence estimates, although the earlier GBD studies used disease incidence preferentially.
- YLDs are now adjusted for independent comorbidities.
- Disease weights and prevalence estimation have been revised and updated.

At classification level two, where mental disorders appear as a broad category, we extracted the five main categories of disorders causing loss of DALYs in each of the six WHO regions, for children and adolescents aged from 5 to 14 years of each sex. At level 3 (the level of specific disorders), we considered the 20 disorders that explain the greatest losses of DALYs.

Then we standardised DALYs by the size of the population aged 5–14 years:

DALY1000 = Number of DALYs/Total relevant (youth) population in the region.

We also estimated the relative trends of the DALY1000 between 2000 and 2015 in each region.

$$[(\text{DALY1000 in 2015} - \text{DALY1000 in 2000})$$
$$/(\text{DALY1000 in 2000})] * 100$$

To evaluate the relative weight of death and disability in the burden of mental disorders, we explored the relative proportion of YLLs and YLDs. We also compared YLDs caused by mental disorders with all causes of YLDs in group 2 (non-communicable diseases).

Results
The WHO regions are presented in Fig. 1.

Burden of mental disorders in 2000 and in 2015 in children aged 5–14 years
In the Americas and Europe, mental disorders in 2000 ranked third among the causes of DALYs (Fig. 2). By 2015, they had reached second place (Fig. 3).

In 2000, mental disorders were the fourth leading cause of DALYs in South-East Asia, the Eastern Mediterranean, and the Western Pacific. In 2015, their rank remained stable in South-East Asia, fell to fifth place in the Eastern Mediterranean (likely because of wars in this region, which increased the number of deaths due to injuries), and reached third place in the Western Pacific.

In Africa, mental disorders were not in the top five causes of losses of DALYs in either 2000 or 2015. Infectious diseases were the most prevalent cause of DALYs among children of this region. In Europe, from 2000 to 2015, the impact of infectious diseases on DALYs decreased, while that of mental disorders increased. The same was true in the Western Pacific and South-East Asia and to a lesser extent in the Americas. Only in the Eastern Mediterranean did this situation differ.

In addition to this period effect, there is also an income effect: the continent with the highest gross domestic product has globally fewer problems with infectious diseases and more problems with mental disorders. This is especially true in Western Europe, where infectious diseases are no longer in the top 5 DALY causes, but mental

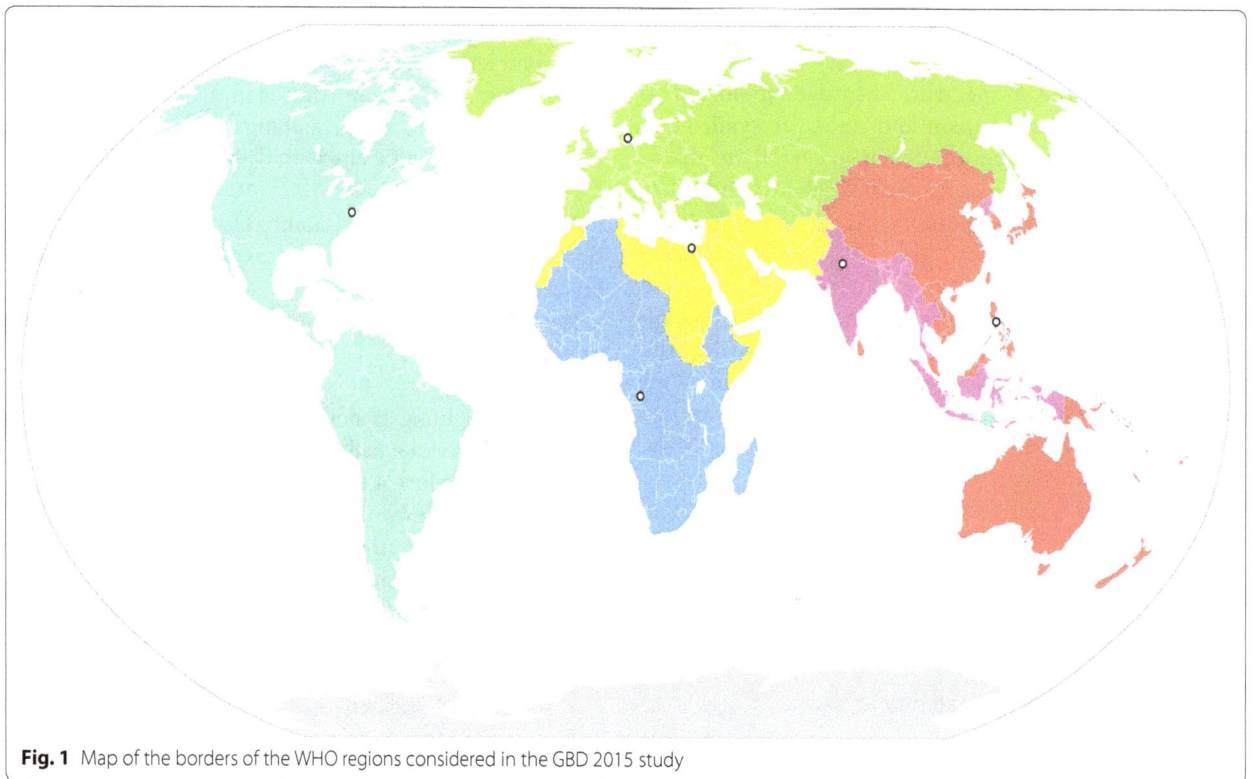

Fig. 1 Map of the borders of the WHO regions considered in the GBD 2015 study

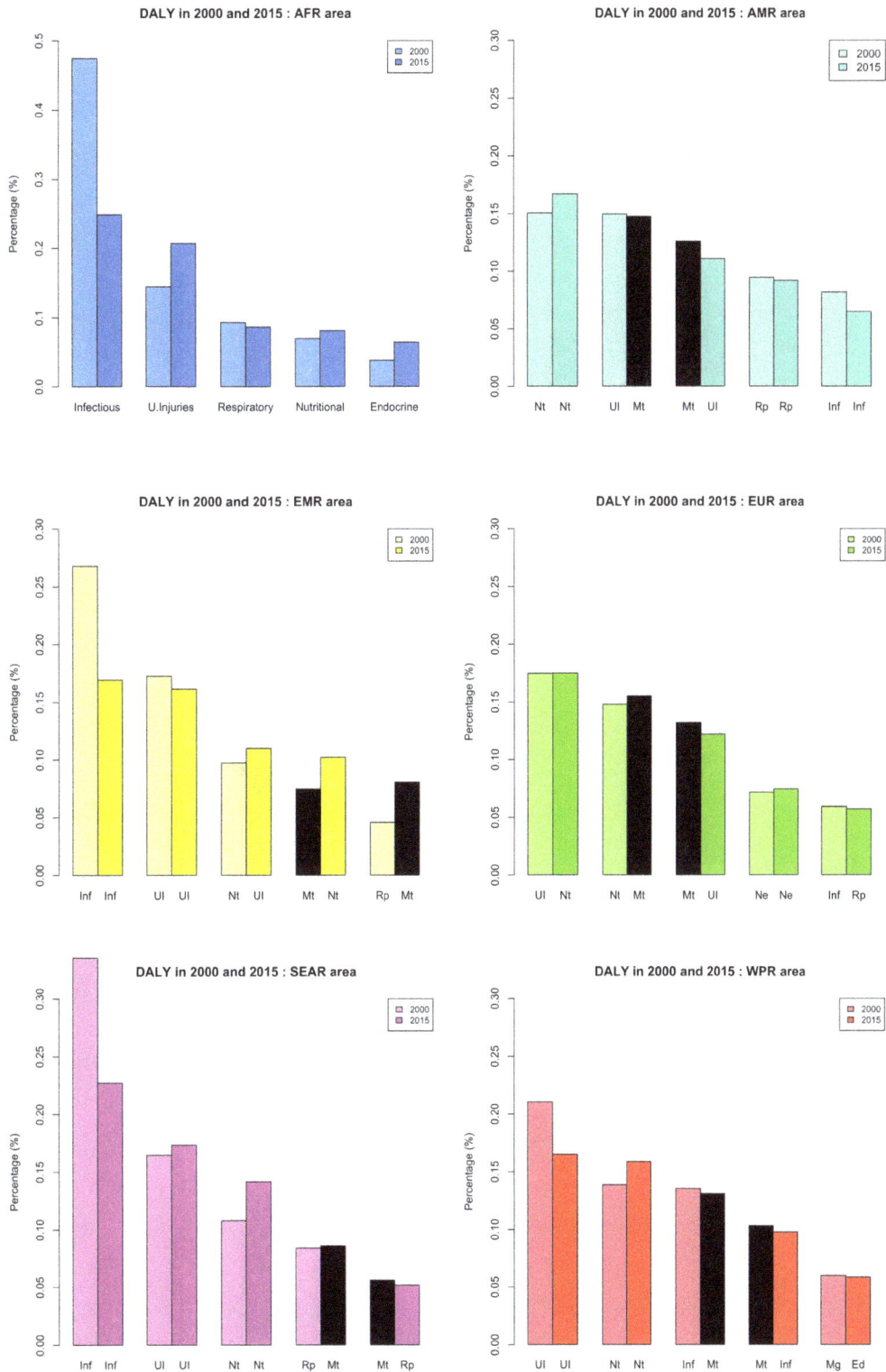

Fig. 2 The five leading level-2 causes of DALY1000 in each WHO region for the 5–14-year age group in 2000 and in 2015. *Nt* nutritional disorders, *UI* unintentional injuries, *Mt* mental and substance use disorders, *Rp* respiratory diseases, *Inf* infectious and parasitic diseases, *Nt* nutritional disease, *Ne* neurologic disorders, *Sk* skin diseases, *Ed* endocrine, blood, immune disorders, *Mg* malignant neoplasms

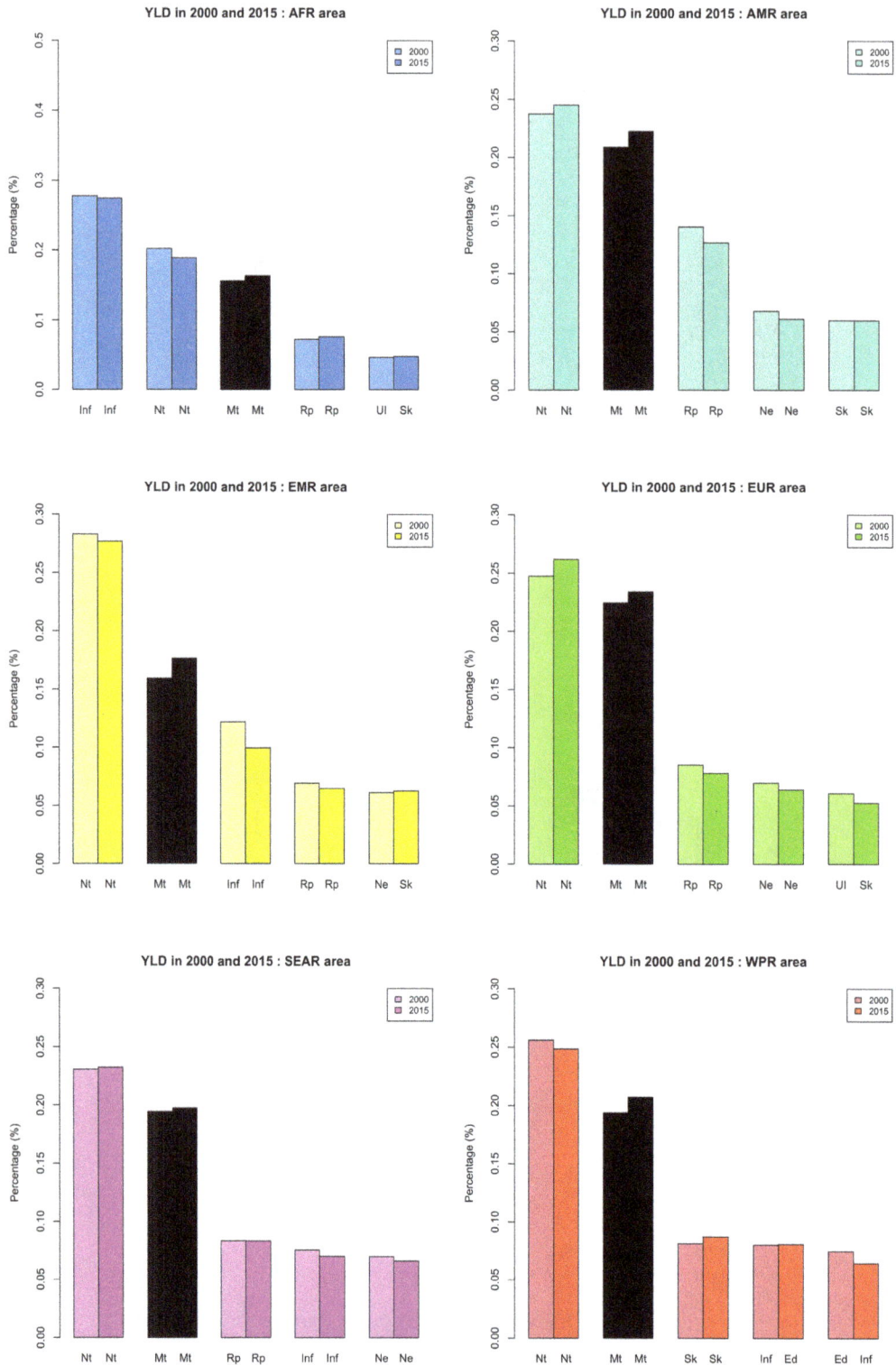

Fig. 3 The five leading level-2 causes of YLDs per 1000 inhabitants in each WHO region for the 5–14-year age group in 2000 and 2015. *Nt* nutritional disorders, *Ul* unintentional injuries, *Mt* mental and substance use disorders, *Rp* respiratory diseases, *Inf* infectious and parasitic diseases, *Nt* nutritional disease, *Ne* neurologic disorders, *Sk* skin diseases, *Ed* endocrine, blood, immune disorders, *Mg* malignant neoplasms

disorders are in the first place. This phenomenon is called an epidemiological transition, which we will consider in more detail in the discussion. The epidemiologic transition concerns all age groups of a population. Our results show clearly that it is especially relevant in the 5–14 age group.

Mental disorders have an important impact on the YLDs in Africa (Fig. 3). This point is important because the organisation of health care systems depends strongly on the profile of patients with important disabilities.

Trends of the normalised burden of mental disorders from 2000 to 2015

Because the burden of disease evaluated from DALYs depends on the population size, it is also interesting to look at a standardised estimate of the DALY, the DALY1000 described in the methods section. The course of this indicator was stable in most regions during the study period. As Table 1 shows, two regions had a relative variation in the DALY1000 between 2000 and 2015 that reached 5%: Europe and the Americas. Surprisingly, these variations moved in opposite directions. In Europe, the DALY1000 associated with mental disorders decreased by 5.3%. The simultaneous increase in the relative weight of mental disorders implies that the global health of children and adolescents aged from 5 to 14 improved substantially. In the Americas, the DALY1000 associated with mental disorders increased by 4%.

Principal mental disorders (level 3 of analysis) that affect losses of DALYs (Additional file 1: Table S1 and Additional file 2: Table S2)

We focus here on the 20 diseases (considered fairly broadly) that caused the most DALYs. Except for Africa (which has no mental disorder in its top 20), most regions typically had four mental disorders in the top 20 in both 2000 and 2015: conduct disorders and anxiety disorders were respectively first and second among mental disorders, while major depressive disorders and

autism-Asperger syndrome alternated between ranking third or fourth, depending on continent and period, although one or the other was occasionally surpassed by idiopathic intellectual disability.

Among boys, the most common mental disorders in the top 20 causes of losses of DALYs in 2015 were conduct disorders (in all regions), autism-Asperger syndrome, and anxiety disorders. Among girls they were anxiety disorders, conduct disorders, and major depressive disorder.

Relative importance of YLLs and YLDs

As expected, in the 5–14-year age group, the importance of YLLs due to mental disorders was marginal. YLDs are clearly the main component of these DALYs.

Discussion

Without data about DALYS, YLLs, and YLDs, it is difficult to determine health priorities rationally. When people hear the words leukaemia, stroke, Alzheimer, or schizophrenia, they experience feelings, emotions, and often compassion, but according to a metric that is not necessarily fair. For example, most consider that Hodgkin disease is clearly much more severe than anorexia nervosa, although the prognosis for survival is the same for both [11, 12]. Mental disorders, which are still considered mysterious in most societies because they are supposed to affect the mind more than the body, are often neglected and even denied by populations. Policy-makers are thus often tempted to cut spending in this domain. This is even truer for child and adolescent psychiatry, where some pathologies, such as conduct disorders, are considered deviance rather than a health problem that requires compassion and care. For a long time, public health professionals did not significantly help repair this injustice; their quantitative work was limited to mortality statistics, while many important child and adolescent psychiatric disorders, such as autistic spectrum disorder or anxiety disorders, have only a marginal impact

Table 1 Trends over time of DALYs caused by mental disorders from 2000 to 2015 in children aged 5–14 years

Region	Age (years)	Population (thousands) 2015	Population (thousands) 2000	DALY (000 s) in 2000	DALY (000 s) in 2015	DALY change 2000–2015 (%)	DALY1000 in 2015	DALY1000 in 2000	DALY1000 change 2000–2015 (%)
AFR	5–14	259,866.6	179,060.3	1,863,516	2,676,614	43.6	10.30	10.41	− 1.0
AMR	5–14	153,998.0	155,225.3	1,664,443	1,717,707	3.2	11.15	10.72	4.0
SEAR	5–14	364,810.6	348,134.3	3,429,175	3,689,155	7.6	10.11	9.85	2.7
EUR	5–14	105,064.9	120,968.3	1,378,652	1,133,424	− 17.8	10.79	11.40	− 5.3
EMR	5–14	134,825.1	120,066.3	1,404,740	1,553,569	10.6	11.52	11.70	− 1.5
WPR	5–14	221,655.7	312,317.4	2,967,064	2,139,505	− 27.9	9.65	9.50	1.6

on mortality, although their effect on daily life can be extreme.

The development and recording of DALYs and YLDs are thus an important breakthrough in the context of global health. We now have data covering several years for DALYs and YLDs due to mental disorders for 5–14-year-olds in the different regions of the globe. This paper focuses on this crucial statistic.

The impact of mental disorders on the burden of disease among children aged 5–14 years appears to be very strong in the Americas and in Europe. In other regions, mental disorders also play a notable role that will surely increase in the future, as they undergo the "epidemiological transition". Omran describes this concept as "focus[ing] on the complex change in patterns of health and disease and on the interactions between these patterns and their demographic, economic and sociologic determinants and consequences" [13]. Europe and the Americas are the two regions where the epidemiological transition was first observed, because of their high level of development. This transition begins with a decrease in mortality from infectious and epidemic diseases and then the modification of the health problems encountered by populations, which because they are living longer, face new and different health challenges [13]. An epidemiological transition results in the regression of communicable diseases and injuries, at the same time as non-communicable diseases, such as mental disorders but also degenerative disorders and cancers, tend to grow in importance. These changes have already taken place in Europe and the Americas. This trend is also notable but less advanced in the Western Pacific and South-East Asia regions. In the Eastern Mediterranean, the rank of mental disorders among 5–14 years has declined over the study period, while intentional injuries are now in the top five. This finding is most likely due to recent war in this region. This hypothesis is buttressed by the major increase between 2000 and 2015 of "Collective violence and legal intervention" as a cause of DALYs. In Africa, where infectious diseases remain common and lethal, mental disorders appear to play a lesser role. Nevertheless, the level 3 classification of diseases, which is more precise, showed the appearance of conduct disorders among 5–14 year-old boys in 2015. This may reflect the first sign of an epidemiological transition.

When we focus on the YLDs, which give an overview of the morbid impact of diseases, we see that even in emerging regions, the burden of mental disorders is already high and constant over time.

Furthermore, the many comorbidities make it difficult to disentangle the specific role of disease categories. For example, unintentional injuries play an important role in disability in many regions, but several mental disorders,

such as conduct disorders and attention-deficit/hyperactivity disorders, are associated with higher rates of injuries [4]. This highlights the difficulties in assessing the actual prevalence of mental disorders in less developed areas. Populations with less access to health and psychiatric care are diagnosed less often, and the consequences of their disorders are not considered to be health-related. In 2011, Gore et al. analysed the burden of disease in the 10–24 age group from earlier GBD date and showed the predominant place of mental disorders [14]. Even though these diseases were aggregated with neurologic disorders, the authors were able to show the importance of specific psychiatric disorders and discussed the difficulties in assessing them, as well as their low priority for researchers, especially in low- and middle-income countries.

This work obviously has some limitations. The calculation of DALYs requires the estimation of many parameters that are known only approximately, at best. Mortality statistics are likely to be accurate because most countries have a system for registering deaths [15]. DALYs are assessed from three parameters (prevalence, disability weight, and average duration of the case until remission or death) evaluated from multiple points of view (epidemiological surveys, opinion surveys, and expert knowledge). These multiple sources of information present many possible sources of error that magnify the uncertainty of the DALY estimates [16]. The individualisation of child psychiatric disorders is a breakthrough but also a challenge. Estimating its prevalence is difficult; it requires, among other things, a good health care system.

Furthermore, disease weighting is likely to be the trickiest part of these estimations. Respondents had to choose between two heath situations explained in simplistic terms. For example, the description of ADHD does not come close to an accurate description of the reality experienced by patients and their families in their daily lives: "is hyperactive and has difficulty concentrating, remembering things, and completing tasks" [7]. This presentation ignores the impact of ADHD on social exclusion, stigmatisation, school difficulties, accidents, etc. The consequence is a quite debatable relative ranking [17]. For example, ADHD has a disease weight of 0.045, whereas symptomatic benign prostatic hypertrophy (the lay description of which is: "feels the urge to urinate frequently, but when passing urine, it comes out slowly and is sometimes painful") has a disease weight of 0.067. Disease weighting is a powerful approach toward capturing the population's point of view of health situations. It is limited, however, by the fact that it collects abstract and subjective representations of people who have never dealt with or perhaps even seen the disorder, as opposed to the real experience of patients and their families. Another important limitation comes from the definition of burden of disease, which does not include the impact of disorders on caregivers [18, 19]. In many ways, mental disorders cannot be considered standard diseases, especially among children. Psychiatric diseases in a population aged 5–14 years must be considered systemic. That is, they affect a community, most often a family, which must be considered as a whole [20].

This paper is intended as an urgent signal of alarm to national and international public health institutions and policy-makers. The world is experiencing an epidemiologic transition. The relative burden of disease of mental disorders among children aged 5–14 years is increasing and will accelerate even more in the near future. This change and the problems accompanying it will require specific responses. Psychiatric diseases in children must be considered specifically. Planning a vaccination program or an antibiotic prescription is very different from organising a global policy for mental health and psychiatric care. It requires a long-term perspective, specially trained professionals, and careful preparation in view of the numerous obstacles that must be anticipated, including local representations of psychiatric diseases, the time necessary for effectiveness, and the extensive resources, financial and human, that will be required. This is a major challenge.

Conclusions

The recognition of mental disorders in children and their consequences has improved, thanks, in particular, to very macroscopic studies such as the Global burden of disease study. Our description shows two major trends: the rates of mental disorders per inhabitant have remained stable over time and at the same time the epidemiological transition has placed them among the main causes of disease burden in this age group. These results ought to lead to improved health care if policy-makers use them to develop health policies to meet the real needs of populations today. Prevention, diagnosis, treatment and family support should be organised according to these findings.

Abbreviations
ADHD: attention deficit and hyperactivity disorders; AFR: African region; AMR: Americas; DALY: disability-adjusted life-years; EMR: Eastern Mediterranean region; EUR: European region; GBD: Global burden of disease; SEAR: South East Asian region; WHO: World Health Organisation; WPR: West Pacific region; YLDs: years of life lived with disability; YLDs: years of life lost.

Authors' contributions
MLB analysed the available data and wrote the article based on the results obtained. BF directed this work, offered advice, and reviewed the article. The version has been reviewed by a professional native-English-speaking editor and translator. Both authors read and approved the final manuscript.

Acknowledgements
Not applicable.

Competing interests
Not applicable.

Funding
Not applicable.

References
1. WHO | Global health estimates. WHO. http://www.who.int/healthinfo/global_burden_disease/en/. Accessed 11 Sept 2017.
2. Murray CJ, Lopez AD. Mortality by cause for eight regions of the world: global burden of disease study. Lancet. 1997;349(9061):1269–76.
3. Murray CJ. Quantifying the burden of disease: the technical basis for disability-adjusted life years. Bull World Health Organ. 1994;72(3):429–45.
4. Erskine HE, Ferrari AJ, Polanczyk GV, Moffitt TE, Murray CJL, Vos T, et al. The global burden of conduct disorder and attention-deficit/hyperactivity disorder in 2010. J Child Psychol Psychiatry. 2014;55(4):328–36.
5. Global Burden of Disease Pediatrics Collaboration, Kyu HH, Pinho C, Wagner JA, Brown JC, Bertozzi-Villa A, et al. Global and national burden of diseases and injuries among children and adolescents between 1990 and 2013: findings from the global burden of disease 2013 study. JAMA Pediatr. 2016;170(3):267–87.
6. WHO | International classification of diseases. WHO. http://www.who.int/classifications/icd/en/. Accessed 11 Sept 2017.
7. WHO | Health statistics and information systems. Estimates for 2000 and 2015. Disease burden. WHO. http://www.who.int/healthinfo/global_burden_disease/estimates/en/index2.html. Accessed 11 Sept 2018.
8. Salomon JA, Vos T, Hogan DR, Gagnon M, Naghavi M, Mokdad A, et al. Common values in assessing health outcomes from disease and injury: disability weights measurement study for the global burden of disease study 2010. Lancet. 2012;380(9859):2129–43.
9. Salomon JA, Haagsma JA, Davis A, de Noordhout CM, Polinder S, Havelaar AH, et al. Disability weights for the global burden of disease 2013 study. Lancet Glob Health. 2015;3(11):e712–23.
10. Health I of M (US) C on SM of P, Field MJ, Gold MR. Ethical issues in the development of summary measures of population health status. National Academies Press; 1998. https://www.ncbi.nlm.nih.gov/books/NBK230306/. Accessed 26 Jan 2018.
11. Huas C, Caille A, Godart N, Foulon C, Pham-Scottez A, Divac S, et al. Factors predictive of 10-year mortality in severe anorexia nervosa patients. Acta Psychiatr Scand. 2011;123(1):62–70.
12. Castellino SM, Geiger AM, Mertens AC, Leisenring WM, Tooze JA, Goodman P, et al. Morbidity and mortality in long-term survivors of Hodgkin lymphoma: a report from the childhood cancer survivor study. Blood. 2011;117(6):1806–16.
13. Omran AR. The epidemiologic transition: a theory of the epidemiology of population change. 1971. Milbank Q. 2005;83(4):731–57.
14. Gore FM, Bloem PJN, Patton GC, Ferguson J, Joseph V, Coffey C, et al. Global burden of disease in young people aged 10–24 years: a systematic analysis. Lancet. 2011;377(9783):2093–102.
15. WHO | Almost half of all deaths now have a recorded cause, WHO data show. WHO. http://www.who.int/mediacentre/news/releases/2017/half-deaths-recorded/en/. Accessed 11 Sep 2017.
16. Murray CJ, Salomon JA, Mathers C. A critical examination of summary measures of population health. Bull World Health Organ. 2000;78:981–94.
17. Nord E. Disability weights in the Global Burden of Disease 2010: unclear meaning and overstatement of international agreement. Health Policy. 2013;111(1):99–104.
18. Karp DA, Tanarugsachock V. Mental illness, caregiving, and emotion management. Qual Health Res. 2000;10(1):6–25.
19. Dixon LB, Lucksted A, Medoff DR, Burland J, Stewart B, Lehman AF, et al. Outcomes of a randomized study of a peer-taught family-to-family education program for mental illness. Psychiatr Serv. 2011;62(6):591–7.

10

Serious juvenile offenders: classification into subgroups based on static and dynamic charateristics

Sanne L. Hillege[1,2]*, Eddy F. J. M. Brand[3], Eva A. Mulder[2,4], Robert R. J. M. Vermeiren[1,4] and Lieke van Domburgh[1,2]

Abstract

Background: The population in juvenile justice institutions is heterogeneous, as juveniles display a large variety of individual, psychological and social problems. This variety of risk factors and personal characteristics complicates treatment planning. Insight into subgroups and specific profiles of problems in serious juvenile offenders is helpful in identifying important treatment indicators for each subgroup of serious juvenile offenders.

Methods: To identify subgroups with combined offender characteristics, cluster-analyses were performed on data of 2010 adolescents from all juvenile justice institutions in the Netherlands. The study included a wide spectrum of static and dynamic offender characteristics and was a replication of a previous study, in order to replicate and validate the identified subgroups. To identify the subgroups that are most useful in clinical practice, different numbers of subgroup-solutions were presented to clinicians.

Results: Combining both good statistical fit and clinical relevance resulted in seven subgroups. Most subgroups resemble the subgroups found in the previous study and one extra subgroups was identified. Subgroups were named after their own identifying characteristics: (1) sexual problems, (2) antisocial identity and mental health problems, (3) lack of empathy and conscience, (4) flat profile, (5) family problems, (6) substance use problems, and (7) sexual, cognitive and social problems.

Conclusions: Subgroups of offenders as identified seem rather stable. Therefore risk factor scores can help to identify characteristics of serious juvenile offenders, which can be used in clinical practice to adjust treatment to the specific risk and needs of each subgroup.

Keywords: Serious juvenile offenders, Risk factors, Cluster-analysis, Subgroups

Background

The population of serious juvenile offenders in Juvenile Justice Institutions (JJIs) is heterogeneous in its background, mental health issues, offending behavior and attitude towards treatment [1, 2]. Serious juvenile offenders often display problems in several life areas that all impact daily functioning and show risk factors on different domains. Therefore, the potential number of different combinations of risk factors in individuals is substantial. So far, many studies on characteristics of serious juvenile offenders are based on the population as a whole and do not take the heterogeneity within this population into consideration. However, given their heterogeneity, findings based on overall group statistics cannot automatically be used in individual clinical treatment planning and therefore leaves a gap between science and practice [3]. Identifying subgroups of serious juvenile offenders in the larger population may help to find more specific treatment indicators for more homogeneous subgroups of individuals. This is a step towards the development of individualized treatment for these juveniles.

*Correspondence: s.hillege@vumc.nl
[1] Department of Child and Adolescent Psychiatry, VU University Medical Center, Duivendrecht, P.O. Box 303, Amsterdam 1115 ZG, The Netherlands
Full list of author information is available at the end of the article

The main objectives of treatment of serious juvenile offenders in JJIs are to reduce criminal recidivism, to prevent further harm to society, and to create a positive future on different domains for the individual. Well-known theoretical frameworks such as the Risk Needs and Responsivity model (RNR) [4] and the Good Lives Model (GLM) [5] state that treatment works best when tailored to specific individual characteristics. Based on the RNR model, the intensity of treatment has to be adjusted to the level of *risk* and interventions should aim at the *needs* related to criminogenic factors. According to the *responsivity* principle, interventions should also match the offenders personal characteristics, such as learning style and motivation. Several studies demonstrate that the number of risk factors are more predictive of reoffending behavior, than one particular risk factor [6]. Hence, information about characteristics related to these three elements is needed in order to work on reducing recidivism. However, within forensic psychiatry, clinicians not only focus on recidivism reduction, but also on treating individuals with mental health problems. Therefore clinicians constantly have to find a balance between protecting the society against 'offenders' and providing care for 'patients' [7]. Forensic practitioners have therefore previously been described as 'double agents' using different objectives when developing treatment plans [8]. Since recent studies demonstrate high prevalence rates of chronic and comorbid mental health problems [2, 9–11], cognitive impairment [12], and trauma [13] in incarcerated adolescents, these offender characteristics should be integrated in treatment as well. This in order to provide good care and to create optimal circumstances for treatment and development for the individual serious juvenile offender. Thus, problems that are not directly linked to criminal behavior or recidivism, need to be taken into account during individualized treatment planning as well.

In everyday practice, it is challenging to integrate these different models, and to design individual treatment trajectories considering all possible risk factors and offender characteristics for each of the serious juvenile offenders in care. To support clinicians in this process, it will help to identify subgroups with a common pattern of risk factors within the group of serious juvenile offenders. If clinicians are able to choose interventions matching the specific needs of a subgroup a juvenile belongs to, a next step will be taken towards individualized treatment. Thus, knowledge is needed on which subgroups can be recognized based on clustering of risk factors and which risk factors point towards treatment indicators within these subgroups. Classification of a larger population into subgroups also enables clinicians to learn from previous experiences and to study treatment interventions for specific subgroups of serious juvenile offenders.

For decades, the population of serious juvenile offenders has been studied and classifications of this heterogeneous group have been developed [12, 14, 15]. So far, most studies on subgroups of serious juvenile offenders have used offending behavior [16, 17] or the severity, nature, and chronicity of the careers of the offenders [6] to distinguish subgroups. Characteristics of the serious juvenile offenders that are considered important for treatment according to the above mentioned models, such as motivation for treatment, cognitive skills and attitude in the institution together with mental health issues, are not included in these studies on typologies of serious juvenile offenders. Studies that did focus on mental health issues in serious juvenile offenders [1, 18–20], or on gender [21, 22] mainly focused on specific subgroups of offenders without making comparisons *between* subgroups of serious juvenile offenders. In addition, these studies focused on relatively small populations, which makes it impossible to identify clear subgroups and provide clinicians with valuable information. As a result, data on the uniqueness of offender characteristics, other than offense characteristics, for specific subgroups of offenders, is lacking. To overcome these limitations, Mulder, Brand, Bullens, and van Marle identified subgroups of offenders based on a wide variety of risk factors in a nation-wide sample of incarcerated youth [23]. This study of Mulder and colleagues identified subgroups based on data driven research which provided certain fit values, combined with the face value after the consultation of experts in the forensic field. Six subgroups with different risk profiles were found, named: (1) antisocial identity, (2) frequent offenders, (3) flat profile, (4) sexual problems and weak social identity, (5) sexual problems, and (6) problematic family background [23]. Since the identification of subgroups by algorithms is an exploratory heuristics process that can create as well as reveal structure, replication is critical to establish validity [24]. Besides replication, the clinical value of the subgroups would improve when more insight is provided about differences and resemblances in risk factors between the identified subgroups on an item level, as this could inform clinical intervention strategies. Therefore, the present study aims to replicate the previous study by Mulder and colleagues and to study the subgroup characteristics on item level.

Using cluster-analyses, the present study identifies subgroups within a nationwide population of serious juvenile offenders from JJIs. We are interested in the identification of subgroups in the total JJI population, including male and females. A sample twice as large as the original sample was used with information on offender characteristics, including a wide variety of static and dynamic risk factors and mental health problems. In order to identify the solution with the highest clinical relevance, different subgroup solutions and their risk profiles were discussed with clinicians. Finally, the present study takes the identification of the subgroups one step further by taking a more detailed look at the differences between subgroups on item level of the different risk factors. These analyses result in combinations of distinguishing offender characteristics per subgroup, that enables clinicians to tailor treatment to individual needs according to the principles of prevailing theories on offender treatment and create optimal treatment circumstances per individual.

Methods
Subjects
The subjects of this study were adolescents aged 12–22 years and sentenced with a mandatory treatment order in a JJI in the Netherlands between January 1994 and December 2013. This mandatory treatment order (PIJ, Placement in Juvenile Justice Institution) [25] is the most severe measure in the Netherlands and is intended for adolescents between the age of 12 and 22 who committed a severe crime and have a mental disorder or deficient (emotional or cognitive) development [26]. The mandatory treatment order initially lasts 2 years, but can be extended to 4 or 6 years in case of insufficient development concerning risk factors and reintegration.

The total sample included 2010 adolescents and represented the most serious offenders in the Netherlands. The majority (95%, n = 1911) was male and only 5% (n = 99) was female and both genders were included since the interest of the present study was on the total population of serious juvenile offenders in the JJIs. The background and characteristics (age by start treatment order, IQ, and origin of offenses) of both genders did not differ significantly, therefore both genders were included in the current study. The mean age at the start of the treatment order was 17.0 years (SD 1.46), 4.6% was 14 years or younger, and only 1.4% was older than 20 at the start of the treatment order. The offenses leading to the mandatory treatment order were violent offense (58.7%), sexual offenses (25.6%), and (repeating) property offenses (15.7%). In line with policy of the Dutch Ministry of Safety and Justice, no information about ethnicity was collected. The study of Mulder and colleagues [23] included 1107 adolescents, which are also included in the current sample.

Instruments
Juvenile Forensic Profile (JFP)
We used a list of 70 items specially constructed for forensic research based on file information, the Juvenile Forensic Profile (JFP) [27]. This list of items was developed in 2003 and 2004 and contains items similar to items in internationally and nationally validated instruments for

risk assessment together with instruments for measuring problem behavior, including the Child Behaviour Check List [28], the Structured Assessment of Violence Risk in Youth [29], the Psychopathy Check List: Youth Version [30], the Juvenile-Sex Offender Assessment Protocol [31], and the HCR-20 Violence Risk Assessment Scheme [32]. The JFP is related to the adult version of the Forensic Profile list, the FP40 [33]. Both instruments are often used to study the Dutch forensic population. The 70 items are divided into seven domains: 'History of criminal behavior', 'Family and environment', 'Offense related risk factors and substance abuse', 'Psychological factors', 'Psychopathology', 'Social behavior/interpersonal relationships' and 'Behavior during stay in the institution'.

The items are scored on a three point scale with $0 =$ no problems, $1 =$ some problems, and $2 =$ severe problems. Previous studies have demonstrated that the JFP is a solid instrument based on file information, with acceptable inter-rater reliability ($r = .73$; $\kappa = .61$), strong convergent validity with the SAVRY [34], adequate predictive validity [35], adequate face validity and clinical value [36] and overall satisfactory psychometrics qualities [27]. Studies on domain scores across gender in the adult population demonstrated no differences [37].

Procedure
The JFP-list was scored after 1 year of treatment, since necessary (historical) information is available at that moment and to be able to include (dynamic) risk factors during treatment, such as motivation and attitude towards treatment. All files (n = 2010) were read and scored anonymous with the JFP-list by (psychology or criminology) master-students in their last year before graduation. The students were trained for 3 weeks before scoring the instrument individually. This training included a test of the quality of scoring in order to check the files were read and scored as intended.

Statistics
During the statistical analyses of this study, sequential steps were made in clustering individuals into subgroups. These steps were based on Everitt [38] and have been previously used in the forensic field [39]. All statistics were calculated with SPSS, IBM, version 24.0.

First, descriptives were calculated. Second, we performed a Principal Axis Factor analysis (PAF) to cluster the 70 items of the JFP-list into dimensions of related items, in order to be able to work with a usable number of variables during cluster-analysis. This reduction in variables was needed as to prevent the effect that is known as the 'Curse of dimensionality' [40, 41]. This effect may occur as a large number of variables increases the risk that the variables are less dissimilar and specific aspects covered by these variables can be overrepresented in the clustering solution [42]. Third, cluster analyses were performed. For the present study, a two-step method of cluster analyses was used which starts with hierarchical cluster-analysis, followed by an iterative cluster-analysis to form the subgroups. During hierarchical cluster-analysis 4.5% of 2010 the outliers were removed using the Mahalanobis distance (> 25.0) and Cooke's distance (> .0050). The information of the hierarchical cluster analysis was used as starting point. In the consecutive steps, the iterative clustering, all case are appointed to a cluster, thus no outliers were removed. Euclidean distance [43, 44], was used together with z-scores ranged 0–1 in order to standardize the distance between subjects. Fourth, Ward's method, also known as the 'Minimum sum of squares' [45], was used to set the distance between clusters, merging at the point that leads to minimum increase in total within-cluster variance. A clinical useful aspect of Ward's method is that this leads to subgroups with more equal sizes than when other cluster methods are used [46]. Different fit indexes (D-index; Hartigan; Scott; Friedman) were measured for the different cluster solutions. All these measures have an index pointing towards the optimal number of clusters [47, 48]. All cluster solutions are nested, which means that in each consecutive step one cluster is split into two clusters.

Next, we presented the different subgroup-solutions resulting from the cluster-analyses at six clinicians working in JJIs during a group session in order to test the clinical validity of the subgroups. These clinicians were considered experts in their field and included psychiatrist, psychotherapists and psychologists with extensive experience in the treatment of serious juvenile offenders in the JJI or in outpatient settings. Cluster solutions for 5 to 8 clusters were presented, in order to end up with as few clusters as possible to be able to understand them and be practical, but also having enough clusters to identify the subtle differences between clusters [42]. Additional benefit of this step is that the relatively subjective step of choosing the number of clusters is taken away from the researcher [49].

Based on clinical relevance and statistical measures, we choose the optimal cluster solution. During a post hoc comparison with ANOVA's that focused on the differences between subgroups on factor level and mean item scores the uniqueness of the subgroups were checked.

Finally, we studied the 70 item scores on the different risk factors from the final subgroup solution, in order to find indicators for tailored treatment per subgroup. Posthoc analyses using ANOVA's were used, in order to find distinguishing (elevated) item scores between subgroups.

Results

Factor analyses

The PAF analyses of the 70 items of the FPJ-list resulted in nine factors, named *Antisocial behavior, Sexual problems, Family background, Mental health problems, Substance use, Conscience and Empathy, Cognitive and social skills, Social network* and *Offenses*. Table 1 demonstrates the 70-items of the JFP-list and the factors they belong to, based on the PAF analyses. Compared to the nine factor solution of Mulder and colleagues, 94.5% out of the 70 items fell under the same factor in this study (see Additional file 1).

Cluster-analyses

We used the results of factor analyses as input for the cluster-analyses to identify subgroups with comparable scores over the nine factors. Based on individual scores of 2010 adolescents on these nine factors, cluster-analyses identified four cluster solutions with adequate fit measures, which were presented to clinical experts. Table 2 gives an overview of the four identified subgroups and their fit indexes. Based on these statistics the solution with six clusters, demonstrates the best fit.

The consultation of the clinical experts resulted in a cluster solution of seven subgroups of serious juvenile offenders, since this solution dived the subgroup of juveniles with sexual problems into two subgroups and therefore connected best with clinical practice. The clusters were named after the offender characteristics that differentiated the subgroups from each other: (1) sexual problems, (2) antisocial identity and mental health problems, (3) lack of empathy and conscience, (4) flat profile, (5) family problems, (6) substance use problems, and (7) sexual, cognitive and social problems. Each of the seven subgroups contained between 7 % (n = 141) to 21.1% (n = 424) of the serious juvenile offenders and the females were fairly equally divided over the seven subgroups, with the exception of the sexual problems subgroups (see Additional file 2). The final 7-cluster solution and the mean scores on the factors per cluster are shown in Table 3. The subgroups are listed in order in which the hierarchical cluster-analyses detected the seven subgroups and can be described as follows:

Subgroup 1: sexual problems

Compared to the other groups, juveniles in this subgroup display predominately problems with sexuality, such as problematic (pedo)sexual behavior or committing a sexual offense. They also display mental health issues such as peer rejection. This subgroup represents 7% of the sample.

Table 1 Results of the PAF analyses with items from JFP-list per factor and their loadings

	N = 2010
Factor 1: antisocial behavior during treatment	
Antisocial behavior in institution	.717
Negative coping	.701
Lack of cooperation with treatment	.673
Incidents, aggression in institution	.592
Treatment motivation	.583
Lack of positive coping	.511
Lack of commitment to school/work	.504
Negative attitude in the institution	.415
Lack of contact, trust, openness	–
Factor 2: sexual problems	
Sexual offense	.931
Problematic sexual behavior	.913
Pedosexual behavior	.616
Past offense, searching for a victim	.477
Threat to be involved in prostitution (–)	.381
Involvement in criminal environment (–)	.368
Sadism	.325
Victim of sexual abuse	.316
Truancy (–)	
Factor 3: family background	
Witnessing violence in the family	.647
Lack of consistency of parents/parental control	.605
Presence/accessibility by parents	.584
Problematic family situation	.577
Substance abuse by parents	.552
Criminal behavior of family	.446
Physical/emotional abuse	.445
Psychopathology in parents	.352
Factor 4: mental health problems	
Psychotic symptoms	.542
Offense following psychosis/medication stop	.405
Depression (past year)	.387
Anxiety	.355
Peer rejection	.346
Autism spectrum disorder	.287
Poor selfcare	–
Factor 5: substance use	
Substance use preceding/during the offense	.859
Drugs abuse	.722
Alcohol abuse	.629
Factor 6: conscience and empathy	
Lack of conscience	.618
Lack of empathy	.618
Lack of problem apprehension	.590
Personality traits cluster B	.292
Factor 7: cognitive and social skills	
Low academic achievement	.542
Low IQ	–.469

Table 1 continued

	N = 2010
Low social skills	.361
Self-esteem	.350
Self-reliance	.323
Neurobiological disorder	.249
Suggestibility	–
Previous contact with mental health care services	–
Factor 8: social network	
Network, low quantity	.369
Network, lack of emotional support	.332
Impulse regulation in the past	.316
Cooperative behavior, problems with authorities	.229
ADHD	.219
Coping, avoidance (–)	.218
Lack of social activities	–
Factor 9: offenses	
High number of past offenses	.732
Violent criminal behavior	.501
Young age first conviction	.473
Young age of onset problem behavior	.394

Subgroup 2: antisocial identity and mental health problems

This group consists of juveniles characterized by antisocial behavior and mental health problems. The prevalence of substance use problems in this subgroup is high, compared to the other subgroups. This subgroup represents 10.8% of the sample.

Subgroup 3: lack of empathy and conscience

The juveniles in this subgroup are quite similar to the ones in subgroup 2, but without the mental health and substance use problems. Additionally, these juveniles display a development towards personality disorders in the direction of antisocial, narcissistic of borderline personality disorder. This subgroup represents 19.6% of the sample.

Subgroup 4: flat profile

On all domains the scores of these juveniles are relatively average compared to the other subgroups. However, compared to the general population, the problems of these adolescents are still considerable. Juveniles from this profile show the most problems around their social network. This subgroup represents 21.1% of the sample.

Subgroup 5: family problems

Compared to the other groups, juveniles in this subgroup mainly experience family problems, such as inconsistent parenting, abuse and witnessing violence in the family. Additionally, these juveniles also have mental health

Table 2 Descriptions of the subgroups from the 5-, 6-, 7- and 8-cluster solutions and their fit measures

	5	6	7	8	Number of optimal clusters
D-index	2.33	2.25	2.23	2.22	6
Hartigan	125.52	35.20	30.92	63.44	6
Scott	2615.53	3478.60	3851.44	4015.40	6
Friedman	2.04	2.81	3.11	3.35	6
Cluster description	Sexual problems	Sexual problems	Sexual problems	Sexual problems	
			Sexual, social and cognitive problems	Sexual, social and cognitive problems	
	Antisocial behavior and multi problems	Antisocial behavior and multi problems	Antisocial behavior and multi problems	Antisocial behavior and multi problems	
		Problems around empathy and conscience	Problems around empathy and conscience	Problems around empathy and conscience	
	Group with mild problems around network	Group with mild problems around network	Group with mild problems around network	Group with mild problems around network	
	Family background problems	Family background problems	Family background problems	Family background problems	
	Substance use problems	Substance use problems	Substance use problems	Substance use problems	
				Substance use and network problems	

problems as well as substance abuse problems. This subgroup represents 14.3% of the sample.

Subgroup 6: substance use problems

These juveniles mainly demonstrate problems with substance abuse, often preceding their offending behavior. They also experience problems in their social network. This subgroup represents 16.8% of the sample.

Subgroup 7: sexual, cognitive and social problems

This group consists of juveniles who display problems with sexuality in combination with a lack of social and cognitive skills. Additionally, they display mental health problems. These adolescents have suffered peer rejection and autism spectrum disorders. This subgroup represents 10.4% of the sample.

ANOVA's resulted in strong significant ($p < .0005$) differences between the seven subgroups on all nine factors, as demonstrated in Table 3. The cluster solution scores from the 2010 study can be found in Additional file 3.

Figure 1 provides a graphical overview of the seven subgroups and their scores on the items belonging to the different factors.

Item scores from different subgroups

For each of the nine factors, item scores were compared between the seven subgroups. Since all items are scored on a three point scale (0, 1 or 2), scores in the direction of 2 indicate severe problems. All item scores differed significantly between subgroups ($p < .0005$). The item scores

from the different factors and the differences between subgroups will be discussed (see Additional file 4 for numerical values and Additional file 5 for the graphical images).

Regarding the first factor, *Antisocial behavior*, the "Antisocial identity and mental health problems" subgroup (.91–1.31) displayed the highest mean scores on items from this factor, followed by the "Lack of empathy and conscience" subgroup (.91–1.29). These two subgroups had particular high mean scores on the items: 'negative coping', 'lack of positive coping', and 'lack of motivation for treatment'. Juveniles from the "Sexual problems" subgroup had the lowest mean scores (.15–.65) on items from this factor.

Turning to the second factor, *Sexual problems*, the highest scores were found in the "Sexual, cognitive and social problems" subgroup (.37–1.75) and the "Sexual problems" subgroup (.15–1.62). High scores were found at the items 'problematic sexual behavior', 'pedosexual behavior', and 'sexual offense'. Mean scores on the items 'threat to be involved in prostitution' and 'involvement in criminal environment' were higher among juveniles from the other five subgroups.

On the third factor, *Family background*, the "Family problems" subgroup (.95–1.77) was the highest scoring subgroup, followed by the "Antisocial identity and mental health problems" subgroup (.66–1.59). These two subgroups displayed the highest scores on the items 'lack of consistency of parents/parental control', 'presence/accessibility of parents', and 'physical/emotional abuse'. In

Table 3 Mean factor scores per cluster solution (range 0–2) and differences between subgroups on the factors

Nine factor scores	Cluster 1: n = 141	Cluster 2: n = 218	Cluster 3: n = 394	Cluster 4: n = 424	Cluster 5: n = 287	Cluster 6: n = 337	Cluster 7: n = 209	F (df = 6,1894)	Sign.
Antisocial behavior during treatment	− .802	.995	.878	− .628	− .429	− .169	− .013	287.81	$p < .005$
Sexual problems	1.613	− .032	− .393	− .441	− .277	− .451	1.691	823.10	$p < .005$
Family background	− .705	.449	.075	− .549	1.016	− .274	.031	125.43	$p < .005$
Mental health problems	.288	1.177	− .397	− .492	.287	− .316	.440	74.99	$p < .005$
Substance use	− 1.087	.851	− .101	− .413	.094	.986	− .845	249.19	$p < .005$
Conscience and empathy	− .868	.536	.789	− .183	− .606	− .233	.113	177.32	$p < .005$
Cognitive and social skills	− .353	.569	− .073	− .361	− .205	.015	.775	60.72	$p < .005$
Social network	− .240	− .440	− .016	.279	− .237	.372	− .192	29.73	$p < .005$
Offenses	− .586	.035	.280	− .403	− .268	.369	.416	41.19	$p < .005$

Cluster 1: sexual problems, cluster 2: antisocial identity and mental health problems, cluster 3: lack of empathy and conscience, cluster 4: flat profile, 5: family problems, cluster 6: substance use problems, and cluster 7: sexual, cognitive and social problems

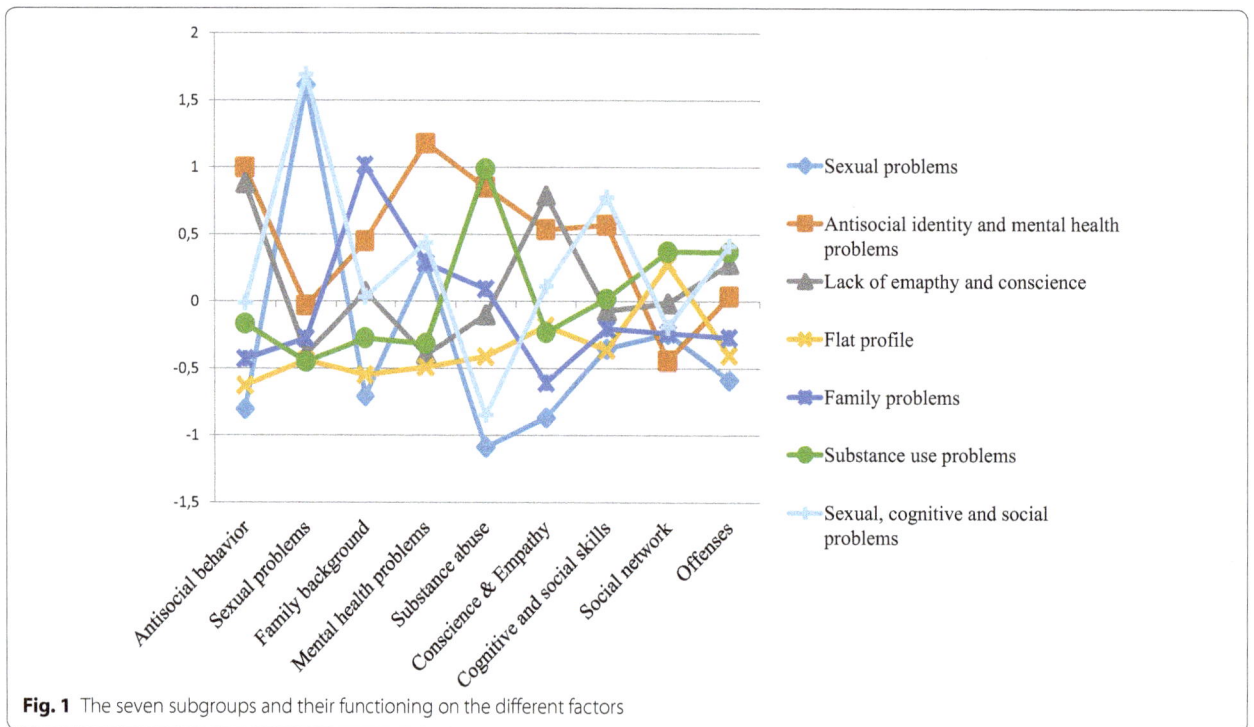

Fig. 1 The seven subgroups and their functioning on the different factors

contrast, juveniles from the "Sexual problems" subgroup (.17–.82) had the lowest mean scores on the items from this factor.

Regarding the fourth factor, *Mental health problems*, the "Antisocial identity and mental health problems" subgroup had the highest scores in relation to the other subgroups. The items; 'peer rejection' (1.04), 'psychotic symptoms' (.78), and 'depression' (.59) stood out for their high scores. The "Sexual, cognitive and social problems" subgroup and "Sexual problems" subgroup demonstrated the highest scores, compared to the other subgroups, especially for the items 'peer rejection' (1.24 and 1.03), and 'autism spectrum disorder' (.82 and .66).

Regarding the fifth factor, *Substance abuse*, the "Substance use problems" subgroup (.82–1.55) had the highest scores, followed by the "Antisocial identity and mental health problems" subgroup (.78–1.59). The "Sexual, cognitive and social problems" subgroup (.07–.27) and the "Sexual problems" subgroup (.08–.22) had the lowest scores on items from this factor.

The sixth factor, *Conscience and Empathy*, showed high overall item scores in all seven subgroups. The "Lack of empathy and conscience" subgroup (1.76–1.86) and "Antisocial identity and mental health problems" subgroup (1.61–1.72) had the highest scores on this factor. Items 'lack of problem apprehension' and 'personality traits Cluster B' demonstrate the highest scores in this factor. The "Sexual problems" subgroup (.80–1.36) had the lowest mean item scores on this factor.

The seventh factor, *Cognitive and social skills*, demonstrated the highest scores for the "Sexual, cognitive and social problems" subgroup (.47–1.58) and "Antisocial identity and mental health problems" subgroup (.26–1.36). All subgroups had the highest mean item score on the item 'self-esteem'.

Regarding the eighth factor, mean item scores on factor *Social network* were highest in the "Antisocial identity and mental health problems" subgroup (.63–1.69), especially on the item 'cooperative behavior, problems with authority'. The "Sexual problems" subgroup had the lowest item scores on this factor (.28–.91).

Finally, item scores on the ninth factor *Offenses* demonstrated quite similar scores for all subgroups. The "Substance use" subgroup (.40–1.64) and "Lack of empathy and conscience" subgroup had the relatively highest items scores on these factor (.34–1.61).

Discussion

Present study aimed to identify subgroups of serious juvenile offenders in JJIs based on specific sets of offender characteristics that can serve as an important starting point for tailored treatment. Cluster-analyses in a sample of 2010 serious juvenile offenders and checks of cluster solutions by clinicians resulted in seven subgroups of serious juvenile offenders: (1) a sexual problems subgroup, (2) an antisocial identity and mental health problems subgroup (3) a lack of empathy and conscience subgroup, (4) a flat profile subgroup, (5) a family

problems subgroup, (6) a substance use problems subgroup, and (7) a sexual, cognitive and social problems subgroup.

The present study is a replication of the previous study by Mulder and colleagues [23] and thereby a validation of the earlier described subgroups. Factor analyses on the 70 items of the JFP-list of risk factors demonstrated almost the same nine factors in the present as the previous study on a sample twice as large. This implies that the risk factors of the JFP-list are consistently divided over nine factors. Results of the present study further indicate towards a good replication of the identification of robust subgroups of serious juvenile offenders. The original study identified six subgroups, whereas the present study identified seven subgroups. The present six subgroups were supplemented with a subgroup of juveniles marked by substance use.

Although the other subgroups are more or less identical between the studies of 2010 and 2017, the subgroup of offenders with substance use problems is remarkable. This especially because it was not the last cluster that originated from a larger subgroup during the hierarchical cluster-analyses, which could imply that it is a subgroup of a subgroup. Furthermore, this subgroup is fairly large (16.8%). These results suggest that over the years problematic alcohol and drugs use in Dutch serious juvenile offenders increased to the extent that it influences delinquent behavior. Statistics from the Trimbos Instituut, the Dutch institute for mental health and substance use, show, however, a decrease in the use of alcohol, soft-drugs and hard-drugs since 2003 in the total population of Dutch adolescents [50]. Research that focused specifically on the population in the JJI in the Netherlands has shown different substance use behavior, since the problematic use of alcohol and the use of substances during criminal behavior has increased between the years 1995 and 2010 [51]. The specific subgroup of serious juvenile offenders with substance use problems was also acknowledged by the clinicians as a separate group in their existence and need for a specific approach during treatment, which will be discussed hereafter.

Including female adolescents and adolescents from a large age-span in the current sample, provided the opportunity to find out whether these groups form a separate subgroup based on their offender characteristics. This was not the case, since the female, younger and older adolescents were distributed over the subgroups that were found. However, the present sample includes only a small percentage of females or older adolescents and therefore can present findings not be generalized to these groups of serious juvenile offenders. Thereby, prevalent theories on the development of criminal behavior

[14, 52] discuss the differences between boys and girls that are also seen in clinical practice. Further research into these subgroups, with larger samples is needed in order to be able to say anything conclusive about female or older serious juvenile offenders.

Since the present study is based on a large sample and identified almost the same subgroups as the previous study, based on solid performed cluster-analyses that are also validated with clinical experts, we feel confident to adopt these seven subgroups and take a closer look at the characteristics of the juveniles per subgroup. It is not possible to develop a set protocol for the treatment of serious juvenile offenders per subgroup. However, insight can be given in treatment ingredients towards specific offender characteristics and tailored treatment. The interventions suggested are not new, but they can be seen as suggestions to support clinicians tailoring treatment depending on subgroup characteristics and in this way focus on the most important factors for the specific individual in treatment. Next, the unique offender characteristics per subgroup will be described to be able to point towards treatment indicators per subgroup, but not before we pay attention to the following issue. Although present subgroups are the result of extended analyses in a large sample of serious juvenile offenders and of high clinical relevance, it is important to interpret current results with some caution. As always when making classifications, different nuances can be found in offender characteristics. Not all serious juvenile offenders who cluster into a subgroup are exactly the same, although they do share distinguishing characteristics that could be relevant for treatment and treatment outcome. Since young offenders are still developing, subgroups also need to be put in a developmental perspective.

A large part of the serious juvenile offenders belong to the "Lack of empathy and conscience" subgroup. As this profile is quite common, all clinical practitioners in juvenile justice institutions should be equipped with adequate intervention techniques to promote the development of empathy and conscience. This is in line with clinical practice as most correctional programs are working on increasing empathy. However, studies on the effect of these interventions are still scarce. Specific interventions based on cognitive behavioral therapy (CBT) that work on critical and moral reasoning, social skills and empathy have shown promising results [53] and could therefore be suitable for treatment of offenders from this subgroup. This subgroup further displays high risks to develop personality disorders (antisocial, borderline, narcissistic), negative coping styles and orientation towards a criminal environment. Suitable interventions to work on these criminogenic factors are based on CBT and schema focused therapy with training in social skills and problem

solving or focus in the system of the juvenile like Multi Systemic Therapy (MST) [54].

Another subgroup identified in this study was the subgroup "Substance use problems". This indicates that it is essential to pay special attention to these problems, all the more because previous studies have demonstrated high prevalence rates (60%) of substance use problems in detained adolescents [2, 55, 56]. It has been stated that substance abuse and delinquent behavior could have a different etiology and are linked with different psychological and social processes. Interventions focused on reducing substance abuse and those focused on reducing reoffending behavior should therefore aim at different processes and mechanisms [57]. Promising interventions for substance abuse problems for serious juvenile offenders are cognitive behavioral therapy and Multi-Dimensional Family therapy (MDFT) [58].

The subgroup "Antisocial identity and mental health problems" contains serious juvenile offenders with a clear antisocial identity. Negative coping style, lack of motivation for treatment and a negative attitude have a particular high prevalence in these juveniles. Although it is important for every juvenile from every subgroup to address motivation, juveniles from the subgroup "Antisocial identity" seem to have specific problems concerning their attitude towards treatment and motivation for change, compared to other subgroups. Therefore it seems important to focus on motivating and engaging with the adolescent first, in order to be able to work on underlying problems at a later stage. In order to develop motivation for treatment, the juvenile needs to be provided with the optimal balance of autonomy, competence and relatedness [59]. Motivation for treatment is found to be a crucial factor for engaging juveniles in the process of change in treatment trajectories [60] and reducing the risk of reoffending [61].

Further, the results reveal two separate subgroups of offenders that demonstrate sexual problems (sexual problems and sexual, cognitive and social problems). The presence of committing a sexual offense, however, does not mean that all these juveniles are identified as a member of one of these two subgroups. Around a third of the sexual offenders from the current sample (167 from 467) was divided over the other five subgroups, with the largest part in the "Lack of empathy and conscience" subgroup. This is in line with previous studies that describe differences within the group of juvenile sex offenders and suggest differentiation in treatment approaches [17, 18, 62]. According to the clinicians participating in a discussion group with focus on the different subgroup solutions, the juveniles with cognitive, social and sexual problems need a different approach than the juveniles only displaying sexual problems, since the first group is more vulnerable and has different needs with respect to reintegration. It has been stated that the (sexual deviant) behavior of these juvenile is more visible and less sophisticated [60] and therefore needs more practical corrections, whereas the other group of sexual offenders has developmental needs on more cognitive and moral level. Further investigation of the differences in item scores between sexual offenders that are included in the different subgroups could provide data driven starting points for treatment.

Further, a distinct subgroup was identified as the "Family problem" subgroup, including lack of consistency in parenting, presence/accessibility of parents and criminal behavior of the parent. Although these are static risk factors and might not be present at the time of incarceration, they may still influence family interactions. It could be important to identify juveniles with these specific characteristics and start family oriented intervention at an early stage of treatment. For example, MST [63], Functional Family Therapy (FFT) [64] and MDFT [65] have shown promising results on family factors as well as other offender characteristics [66, 67].

A strength of this study is that results lead to subgroups with specific characteristics that are of great practical value when creating tailored treatment in JJIs. Clinicians know, based on these results, which offender characteristics are distinguishing between the population of serious juvenile offenders, need focus during treatment and might point towards missing information that is necessary to develop a suitable treatment trajectory. The use of fit values for the cluster-solutions in combination with the face value of the clinicians, strengthens our findings and overcomes limitations of the identification of subgroups in other studies when the choice of the optimal subgroup solution is often made by the researcher [49]. The large sample on which this study is performed makes the results relevant for a large population of serious juvenile offenders. Thereby, the identification of seven subgroups with distinguishing offender characteristics makes it possible to perform future research on the effects of treatment interventions for different groups of serious juvenile offenders. Currently, evaluation studies of treatment interventions in incarcerated adolescents use a relatively heterogeneous population, while the evaluation of more homogeneous groups as presented in the subgroups in this study could reveal a more realistic outcome of treatment. This makes it possible to not only study *what works?*, but also *what works for whom?* The next step in research should be focused on the experience of the clinician working with juveniles from these different clusters to gain information about best practice interventions, since the identification of the subgroups was data-driven and not theory-driven. This information

should be transferred to the clinical field in order to be of great value for clinicians as well as the juveniles. Together with information on future delinquent behavior of juveniles from the seven subgroups this provides practical information on the characteristics that could be targeted to maximize treatment effect in each subgroup.

Notwithstanding the strengths of this study, some limitations must be mentioned. The present study focused on file information of characteristics of Dutch serious juvenile offenders placed in JJIs and therefore focused on a specific group of young offenders. The fact that file based information is used may have led to missed information that was not present in the files, for instance on protective factors or trauma. Moreover, the list that is used to collect the data focused on risk factors and, thereby, overlooks the value of protective elements in a juveniles life. Thereby, the interrater reliability and other psychometric characteristics of the JFP-list for the total current sample were not measured, only for a part of the sample. Present results and the use of the JFP-list to identify subgroups of serious juvenile offender would be stronger if these measures of the total sample could be provided and is the focus of future research. The strength of the large sample in current study can also be regarded as a limitation, because the sample includes a small percentage of girls (4.9%), younger (< 14 years, 4.6%) and older adolescents (> 20 years 3.5%). We were interested in the total population of serious juvenile offenders with a mandatory treatment order and therefore included all juveniles in the sample. When preferring a more homogeneous set of data, these theoretical outliers that appear in daily practice, should be excluded. Present study can be considered an exploration of serious juvenile offenders, as the sample consists of the total population of serious juvenile offenders under a mandatory treatment order in Dutch JJI's, where also some female offenders and older juveniles reside. Future research based on these specific 'subgroups' of serious juvenile offenders is necessary in order to be able to generalize current result to female, younger or older serious juvenile offenders. The results of present study are based on risk factors and offender characteristics of serious juvenile offenders that can be measured in other countries as well and are known factors in international literature. Therefore, the main focus of current results are internationally generalizable: The group of serious juvenile offenders is heterogeneous and there are specific groups (with sexual problems, substance use problems, family problems, antisocial behavior, conscience and empathy problems) with specific needs. Nevertheless, in most Western countries are serious juvenile offenders placed in different facilities and the population of juveniles in JJI's differs across countries. Future research is necessary to be able to study the international generalizability of our results.

Conclusions

Present study identified seven subgroups of serious juvenile offenders with distinguishing offender characteristics. Because these subgroups all have their own specific combination of offender characteristics and risk factors, they provide information for clinical practice to apply this knowledge to daily practice and tailored treatment to the needs and possibilities of each specific subgroup. Clinicians should identify specific offender characteristics in order to find suitable intervention strategies for the individual juvenile in the JJI.

Additional files

Additional file 1. Results of the PAF analyses with items from JFP-list per factor and their loadings from 2017 and 2010.

Additional file 2. Division of female, younger and older serious juvenile offenders over the total sample (N = 2010).

Additional file 3. Mean factor scores per cluster solution (range 0–2) on the factors in 2010.

Additional file 4. Mean scores on factor items per subgroups (range 0–2) and the differences between subgroups in 2017.

Additional file 5. Item functioning of the seven subgroups on the factor Antisocial behavior. Item functioning of the seven subgroups on the factor Sexual problems. Item functioning of the seven subgroups on the factor Family background. Item functioning of the seven subgroups on the factor Mental health problems. Item functioning of the seven subgroups on the factor Substance use. Item functioning of the seven subgroups on the factor Conscience and empathy. Item functioning of the seven subgroups on the factor Cognitive and social skills. Item functioning of the seven subgroups on the factor Social network. Item functioning of the seven subgroups on the factor Offenses.

Authors' contributions
SH and EB contributed to the conceptualization as well as design of this study. EB supervised the data collection. SH, EB, and EM were involved in the analysis and interpretation of data. All authors were involved in drafting and revising the manuscript. All authors read and approved the final manuscript.

Author details
[1] Department of Child and Adolescent Psychiatry, VU University Medical Center, Duivendrecht, P.O. Box 303, Amsterdam 1115 ZG, The Netherlands. [2] Intermetzo-Pluryn, Nijmegen, The Netherlands. [3] Department of Justice, National Agency of Correctional Institutions, The Hague, The Netherlands. [4] Curium-LUMC, Leiden University Medical Center, Leiden, The Netherlands.

Acknowledgements
The authors would like to acknowledge ZonMw for funding this project, as well as the Department of Safety and Justice in the Netherlands for this cooperation.

Competing interests
The authors declare that they have no competing interests.

Funding
All authors, except EB, are affiliated with the Academic Workplace Forensic Care for Youth, funded by The Netherlands Organization for Health Research and Development (ZonMw, The Hague; Grant Number 159010002). These funding sources had no involvement in the study design, in the collection, analysis and interpretation of data, in the writing of the report, and in the decision to submit the article for publication.

References
1. Espelage DL, Cauffman E, Broidy L, Piquero AR, Mazerolle P, Steiner H. A cluster-analytic investigation of MMPI profiles of serious male and female juvenile offenders. J Am Acad Child Adolesc Psychiatry. 2003;42(7):770–7.
2. Teplin LA, Abram KA, McClelland GN, Dulcan MK, Mericle AA. Psychiatric disorders in youth in juvenile detention. Arch Gen Psychiatry. 2002;59:1133–43.
3. Lutz W, Lambert MJ, Harmon C, Tschitsaz A, Schürch E, Stulzl N. The probability of treatment success, failure and duration: what can be learned from empirical data to support decision making in clinical practice? Clin Psychol Psychother. 2006;13:223–32.
4. Andrews DA, Bonta J. The psychology of criminal conduct. Abingdon: Routledge; 2010.
5. Ward T, Brown M. The good lives model and conceptual issues in offender rehabilitation. Psychol Crime Law. 2004;10(3):243–57.
6. Cox SM, Kochol P, Hedlund J. The exploration of risk and protective score differences across juvenile offending career types and their effects on recidivism. Youth Violence Juv Justice. 2016. https://doi.org/10.1177/1541204016678439.
7. Barnao M, Ward T, Robertson P. The good lives model: a new paradigm for forensic mental health. Psychiatry Psychol Law. 2015. https://doi.org/10.1080/13218719.2015.1054923.
8. Blackburn R. "What works" with mentally disordered offenders. Psychol Crime Law. 2004;10:297–308.
9. Colins O, Vermeiren R, Vreugdenhil C, van den Brink W, Doreleijers T, Broekaert E. Psychiatric disorders in detained male adolescents: a systematic literature review. Can J Psychiatry. 2010;55(4):255–63.
10. Fazel S, Doll H, Långström N. Mental disorders among adolescents in juvenile detention and correctional facilities: a systematic review and meta-regression analysis of 25 surveys. J Am Acad Child Adolesc Psychiatry. 2008;47(9):1010–9.
11. Vermeiren R, Jespers I, Moffitt T. Mental health problems in juvenile justice populations. Child Adolesc Psychiatr Clin N Am. 2006;15:333–51.
12. Loeber R, Menting B, Lynam DR, Moffitt TE, Stouthamer-Loeber M, Stallings R, Farrington DP, Pardini D. Findings from the Pittsburgh Youth Study: cognitive impulsivity and intelligence as predictors of the age–crime curve. J Am Acad Child Adolesc Psychiatry. 2017;51(11):1136–49.
13. Abram KM, Teplin LA, Charles DR, Longworth SL, McClelland GM, Dulcan MK. Posttraumatic stress disorder and trauma in youth in juvenile detention. Arch Gen Psychiatry. 2004;61(4):403–10.
14. Moffitt TE. Adolescence-limited and life-course-persistent antisocial behavior: a developmental taxonomy. Psychol Rev. 1993;100:674–701.
15. Smiley WC. Classification and delinquency: a review. Behav Disord. 1977;2(4):184–200.
16. Hendriks J, Bijleveld CCJH. Juvenile sexual delinquents: contrasting child abusers with peer abusers. Crim Behav Ment Health. 2004;14(4):238–50.
17. Hunter JA, Figueredo AJ, Malamuth NM, Becker JV. Juvenile sex offenders: toward the development of a typology. Sex Abuse. 2003;15(1):27–48.
18. Potter CC, Jenson JM. Cluster profiles of multiple problem youth mental health problem symptoms, substance use, and delinquent conduct. Crim Justice Behav. 2003;30(2):230–50.
19. Stefurak T, Calhoun GB, Glaser BA. Personality typologies of male juvenile offenders using a cluster-analysis of the Millon Adolescent Clinical Inventory introduction. Int J Offender Ther Comp Criminol. 2004;48(1):96–110.
20. Vaughn MG, Freedenthal S, Jenson JM, Howard MO. Psychiatric symptoms and substance use among juvenile offenders: a latent profile investigation. Crim Justice Behav. 2007;34(10):1296–312.

21. Odgers CL, Moretti MM, Burnette ML, Chauhan P, Waite D, Reppucci ND. A latent variable modeling approach to identifying subtypes of serious and violent female juvenile offenders. Aggress Behav. 2007;33(4):339–52.

22. Stefurak T, Calhoun GB. Subtypes of female juvenile offenders: a cluster-analysis of the Millon Adolescent Clinical Inventory. Int J Law Psychiatry. 2007;30(2):95–111.

23. Mulder EA, Brand EFJM, Bullens RAR, van Marle H. Toward a classification of juvenile offenders: subgroups of serious juvenile offenders and severity of recidivism. Int J Offender Ther Comp Criminol. 2010. https://doi.org/10.1177/0306624X10387518.

24. Breckenridge JN. Validating cluster-analysis: consistent replication and symmetry. Multivar Behav Res. 2000;35(2):261–85.

25. Lodewijks HP, Doreleijers TA, de Ruiter C, Borum R. Predictive validity of the Structured Assessment of Violence Risk in Youth (SAVRY) during residential treatment. Int J Law Psychiatry. 2008;31(3):263–71.

26. Kwakman N. Het wetsvoorstel adolescentenstrafrecht. In Casu. 2013;20(4):41–3.

27. Brand EFJM, van Heerde WK, Handleiding Forensisch Profiel Justitiële Jeugdigen (FPJ-lijst). The Hague: Department of Safety and Justice, National Agency of Correctional Institutions; 2004/2010.

28. Achenbach TM. Manual for the child behavior checklist/4–18 and 1991 child profile. Burlington: University of Vermont, Department of Psychiatry; 1991.

29. Borum R. Manual for the Structured Assessment of Violence Risk in Youth (SAVRY). Odessa: Psychological Assessment Resources; 2006.

30. Forth AE, Hare R. The Hare PCL: youth version. Toronto: Multi-Health Systems; 2003.

31. Prentky R, Righthand S. Juvenile sex offender assessment protocol-II (J-SOAP-II) manual. Washington: Department of Justice, Office of Juvenile Justice and Delinquency Prevention; 2003.

32. Webster CD, Douglas KS, Eaves D, Hart SD. HCR-20: Assessing Risk for Violence (Version 2). Burnaby: Simon Fraser University; 1997.

33. Brand EFJM, van Emmerik JL. Handboek Forensisch Psychiatrische Profielen: Handleiding FP40. The Hague: Department of Safety and Justice, National Agency of Correctional Institutions; 2001.

34. Skeem JL, Mulvey EP, Appelbaum P, Grisso T, Silver E, Clark Robbins P. Identifying subtypes of civil psychiatric patients at high risk for violence. Crim Justice Behav. 2004;31(4):392–437.

35. Brand EFJM. Onderzoeksrapport PIJ-Dossiers 2003-C: Predictieve validiteit van de FPJ lijst. The Hague: Department of Safety and Justice, National Agency of Correctional Institutions; 2005.

36. van Heerde WK, Mulder EA. Research Study PIJ-Files 2003-B. Klinische evaluatie van de FPJ-Lijst & SAVRY in Eikenstein en FORA. The Hague: Department of Safety and Justice, National Agency of Correctional Institutions; 2005.

37. Brand EFJM, van Emmerik JL. FP40 Handleiding Forensische Profiel Lijsten. The Hague: Department of Safety and Justice, National Agency of Correctional Institutions/FPC Oostvaarderskliniek; 2006.

38. Everitt BS. Cluster-analysis. London: Heinemann; 1974. p. 1994.

39. van Heerde WK, Brand EFJM, van 't Hof GICM, Mulder EA. Inter-rater reliability and convergent validity of the juvenile forensic profile. The Hague: Department of Safety and Justice, National Agency of Correctional Institutions; 2004.

40. Fielding AH. Cluster and classification techniques for the biosciences. Cambridge: Cambridge University Press; 2007.

41. Frieman JH. On bias, variance, 0/1—loss, and the curse-of-dimensionality. Data Min Knowl Discov. 1997;1:55–77.

42. Mooi E, Sarstedt M. A concise guide to market research. Berlin: Springer; 2011. p. 237–84.

43. Aldenderfer MS, Blashfield RK. Cluster-analysis. Sage University paper series on quantitative applications in the social sciences 07-044. Beverly Hills: Sage Publications; 1984 (**tDAR ID: 111467**).

44. Hair JF, Black WC. Cluster-analysis. In: Grimm LG, Yarnold PR, editors. Reading and understanding more multivariate statistics. Washington: American Psychological Association; 2000. p. 147–205.

45. Ward T. Hierarchical grouping to optimize an objective function. J Am Stat Assoc. 1963;58(301):236–44.

46. Everitt BS, Landau S, Leese M, Stahl D. Hierarchical clustering. Cluster-analysis. 5th ed. West Sussex: Wiley; 2012. p. 71–110.

47. Charrad M, Ghazzali N, Boiteau V, Niknafs A, Charrad MM. NbClust: an R package for determining the relevant number of clusters in a data set. J Stat Softw. 2014;61:1–36.

48. Team, RC. R: a language and environment for statistical computing (Version 3.1. 2). Vienna: R Foundation for Statistical Computing; 2012. http://www.R-project.org.

49. Everitt BS, Landau S, Leese M, Stahl D. Hierarchical clustering. Cluster-analysis. 5th ed. West Sussex: Wiley; 2012. p. 126–30.

50. Verdurmen J, Monshouwer K, Dorsselaer SV, Lokman S, Vermeulen-Smit E, Vollebergh W. Jeugd en riskant gedrag 2011. Kerngegevens uit het peilstationsonderzoek scholieren. Utrecht: Trimbos-instituut; 2012.

51. Brand EFJM, a'Campo AMG, van den Hurk AA. 15 jaar PIJers in beeld: Kenmerken en veranderingen van jeugdigen die de PIJ-maatregel opgelegd kregen in de periode 1995–2010. The Hague: Department of Safety and Justice, National Agency of Correctional Institutions; 2013.

52. Loeber R. Development and risk factors of juvenile antisocial behavior and delinquency. Clin Psychol Rev. 1990;10(1):1–41.

53. Ross R, Ross R. Thinking straight: the reasoning and rehabilitation program for delinquency prevention and offender rehabilitation. Ottawa: Air Training and Publications; 1995.

54. Bateman AW, Gunderson J, Mulder R. Treatment of personality disorder. Lancet. 2015;385(9969):735–43.

55. Abrantes AM, Hoffmann NG, Anton R. Prevalence of co-occurring disorders among juveniles committed to detention centers. Int J Offender Ther Comp Criminol. 2005;49(2):179–93.

56. Vermeiren R. Psychopathology and delinquency in adolescents: a descriptive and developmental perspective. Clin Psychol Rev. 2003;23(2):277–318.

57. Prendergast ML, Pearson FS, Podus D, Hamilton ZK, Greenwell L. The Andrews' principles of risk, needs, and responsivity as applied in drug treatment programs: meta-analysis of crime and drug use outcomes. J Exp Criminol. 2013;9(3):275–300.

58. Taxman FS, Perdoni ML, Caudy M. The plight of providing appropriate substance abuse treatment services to offenders: modeling the gaps in service delivery. Vict Offenders. 2013;8(1):70–93.

59. Deci EL, Ryan RM. The" what" and" why" of goal pursuits: human needs and the self-determination of behavior. Psychol Inq. 2000;11(4):227–68.

60. Salekin RT, Lee Z, Schrum Dillard CL, Kubak FA. Child psychopathy and protective factors: IQ and motivation to change. Psychol Public Policy Law. 2010;16(2):158–76.

61. Mulder EA, Brand EFJM, Bullens RAR, van Marle HJC. Profiling juvenile offenders in juvenile institutions: change in risk factors in their population. Int J Forensic Ment Health. 2012;9(2):93–100.

62. Hackett S, Masson H, Balfe M, Phillips J. Individual, family and abuse characteristics of 700 British child and adolescent sexual abusers. Child Abuse Rev. 2013;22(4):232–45.

63. Henggeler SW, Schoenwald SK, Borduin CM, Rowland MD, Cunningham PB. Multisystemic treatment of antisocial behavior in children and adolescents. New York: Guilford; 1998.

64. Alexander JF, Parsons BVV. Functional family therapy: principles and procedures. Carmel: Brooks & Cole; 1982.

65. Liddle HA, Hogue A. Multidimensional family therapy for adolescent substance abuse. In: Wagner EF, Waldron HB, editors. Innovations in adolescent substance abuse interventions. Kidlington: Elsevier; 2001. p. 229–61.

66. Baldwin SA, Christian S, Berkeljon A, Shadish WR. The effects of family therapies for adolescent delinquency and substance abuse: a meta-analysis. J Marital Fam Ther. 2012;38(1):281–304.

67. van der Stouwe T, Asscher JJ, Stams GJJM, Deković M, van der Laan PH. The effectiveness of multisystemic therapy (MST): a meta-analysis. Clin Psychol Rev. 2014;34(6):468–81.

11

Photo-elicitation with adolescents in qualitative research: an example of its use in exploring family interactions in adolescent psychiatry

J. Sibeoni[1,2]*, E. Costa-Drolon[1,2], L. Poulmarc'h[1], S. Colin[1], M. Valentin[1], J. Pradère[1] and A. Revah-Levy[1,2]

Abstract

Background: Photo-elicitation is a method used increasingly often in qualitative health research, and its positive effect on the research process is well established today. Photo-elicitation appears to facilitate verbalization and insight and to improve relationships between the researcher and participants, thereby enriching the quality of the data collected. Nonetheless, it is barely used at all in the field of adolescent psychiatry. With the aim of exploring the potential of these methods for research with adolescents receiving psychiatric care, we conducted a qualitative photo-elicitation data collection study with this population, asking them about family interactions around food.

Methods: The data were collected from 15 adolescents and 17 parents during semi-structured interviews in which a photo taken by the adolescent served as the focus of discussion. Data were explored through inductive thematic analysis.

Results: Photo-elicitation played a threefold role in this study: (1) it induced the teens' interest, thought, and pleasure, (2) it played a mediating function during the interviews, and (3) it enabled family interactions to be viewed from the adolescent's perspective. Three themes concerning family interactions were found: (1) parent–child relationship patterns, (2) the functioning of the family group, and (3) the adolescent's individual relation with food, that is, the issue of the adolescent's autonomy.

Conclusions: Photo-elicitation proved to be an innovative technique in qualitative research in the area of adolescent psychiatry, one that enriched the data and enabled the emergence of new themes in this field, related in particular to the process by which adolescents develop autonomy.

Keywords: Photo-elicitation, Adolescence, Family functioning, Qualitative methods, Methodology

Background

Visual narrative research methods are used increasingly often in the field of qualitative health research. Derived from work in visual anthropology, photo-elicitation involves the use of photographs as support during a research interview [1]. Currently, the participants themselves most often take these pictures. The positive effects of photo-elicitation on the research process have been widely described in qualitative literature studying adults. It appears to improve the quality of the data collected [2] by promoting active cognitive involvement and better participation in the research [3]. The principle of photo-elicitation *empowers* participants, by putting them in a more active position and thereby giving them the opportunity to influence the research process more strongly [4]. Photo-elicitation may also facilitate the construction of a bond between participants and researchers [5] and may promote verbalization of thoughts and emotions [6].

*Correspondence: jordansib@hotmail.com
[1] Service Universitaire de Psychiatrie de l'Adolescent, Argenteuil Hospital Centre, Argenteuil, France
Full list of author information is available at the end of the article

In recent years, qualitative health research has also been developing among adolescents. The qualitative approach makes it possible to consider adolescents as active participants in research, to recognize their right and autonomy of thought and to give them a voice [7]. Qualitative research within this population nonetheless raises specific questions, in terms of both ethics [8] and methodology [9], including the use of visual methods [10]. Qualitative research with adolescents in the general population requires consideration of the developmental aspects of this life stage, both cognitive and affective, and of the anxiety inherent in the situation, the imbalance in the researcher–adolescent relationship, the adolescents' lack of involvement for the research, and the adolescents' difficulties—common at this age—in expressing themselves and especially their emotions verbally [9]. These points are even more salient when the adolescent presents a psychiatric disorder. The methodological literature describes adolescents with psychiatric disorders to be "doubly vulnerable persons" [11], with "multi-faceted vulnerability" [12], and qualitative research in this population is considered a methodological challenge. Moreover, certain psychiatric symptoms, either cognitive or affective, may directly affect the interview. It is therefore difficult to obtain a detailed and deep narrative of experience from this group population. Accordingly, many qualitative studies exploring psychiatric issues of adolescents involve interviews with parents, caregivers, or physicians. At the same time, mental health professionals in general and those working with adolescents in the mental health field in particular endeavor to take into account the needs of the patients and take their subjective health status into consideration [13].

The literature already includes several qualitative studies of adolescents that used photo-elicitation [14, 15]. Nonetheless, photo-elicitation has not been used in research in the field of adolescent mental health, with the exception of a qualitative study of the school experience of adolescents with autistic spectrum disorders [16]. In an earlier study, we used photo-elicitation to explore the role of food in the family relationships of obese adolescents [17]. The question of food and the family meal appeared relevant for exploring these adolescents' family interactions, consistent with the data in numerous studies that have demonstrated the important role of food in family interactions among adolescents. On the one hand, research has shown that factors such as parental dietary preferences, family meal structure, and single parenthood can influence body mass index (BMI) in childhood and especially adolescence [18]. On the other hand, many authors have described the important part food plays in family interactions, as seen both in the consideration of the act of nurturing [19] and in the issues of power and control that arise between parents and adolescents around food [20].

We have focused for several years on the crossed perspectives of care in adolescent medicine and psychiatry—the views of teens, their parents, and the professionals providing them with care [17, 21, 22]. In our study using photo-elicitation with obese adolescents and their parents, we obtained an elaborate narrative about food and family interactions from both the groups. In line with this study, we used the same design among adolescents receiving psychiatric care to examine whether this visual method of photo-elicitation is an effective tool for exploring family interactions with adolescents receiving care for psychiatric disorders unassociated with food and with their parents. Furthermore, exploring family interactions among adolescents receiving psychiatric care is an important issue in the practice of adolescent psychiatry. Regardless of the disorders presented, this exploration most often provides new insights that illuminate both evaluation and treatment perspectives.

Methods

Table 1 presents the overall study design in detail. This exploratory multicenter study used a qualitative methodology: sampling was purposive [23]; Adolescents were asked to take a photograph of a family meal that would subsequently be discussed in two individual interviews a week later, first with the adolescent, and then separately with one or both parents; data saturation was achieved according to the principle of theoretical sufficiency [24]; and a five stage thematic analysis was used to explore the data [25] (Table 2). This study complied with the COREQ guidelines [26].

The study included 15 adolescents, 10 girls (F) and 5 boys (M). Table 3 summarizes their characteristics. A total of 17 parents were also interviewed giving data from a total of 32 participants. All the adolescents recruited agreed to participate. Nonetheless, some parents refused to be interviewed; some explained that food was a subject too personal and private to be shared or, on the contrary, that the subject was neither interesting nor relevant. Numerous fathers shared the latter opinion and chose not to participate. In the families in which the parents were separated, the parents not having primary custody did not want to or could not participate.

Results

We present first the results of the role of photo-elicitation in the research process and then the results about the family interactions around food. Extracts of the transcripts have been selected to exemplify the themes described and transcribed in English for the sole purpose of this article. All personal information

Table 1 Study design

Qualitative approach	Phenomenology
Research paradigm	Constructivism
Setting	Study developed in a research group seeking to develop the use of qualitative research in adolescent psychiatry
Ethical issues	The relevant French Institutional Committee of the Paris North University Hospital Group approved this study All patients and their parents provided written *consent* before inclusion
Sampling strategy	Purposive sampling strategy: selective and deliberate
	Researchers first contacted clinicians at recruitment sites (Argenteuil and Remiremont Hospitals) where recruitment was planned and explained the study design and objectives to them in detail
	Clinicians identified potential participants—adolescents and parents—whom they considered most likely to provide useful information
	Clinicians mentioned the study to potential participants and gave them an information sheet about it
	Researchers met each interested teen and his/her parents
	To describe the study
	To collect social and demographic data
	To obtain their written consent
Inclusion/exclusion criteria	Adolescents between 12 and 18 years at the time of the interview
	Adolescents and parents must speak French fluently
	Adolescents must not have an eating disorder (i.e., anorexia nervosa, bulimia, avoidant/restrictive food intake disorder, or another unspecified eating disorder) or a weight-related disorder such as obesity
	Adolescents could have food-related symptoms and their effects on the family relationships would be part of our field of exploration
	Adolescents must not present acute or severe psychiatric disorders—schizophrenia, bipolar disorder, or autistic spectrum disorders—(the focus of this study was not the adolescents' psychopathology but rather the relevance of photo-elicitation in research in adolescent psychiatry)
	Families must not have major dysfunctional patterns, such as neglect or abuse
	Adolescents must be able to talk about their experience of family relationships around food and the family meal
	Adolescents must have been receiving care for at least 6 months
Participants	Adolescents receiving psychiatric care in an outpatient setting and one or both of their parents
	All saw their psychiatrist at least once a month
	All had chronic mental disorders that had begun during adolescence (depression, anxiety, social phobia, personality disorder). This diagnosis was made by each patient's referring psychiatrist, according to DSM 5 criteria
	None had a somatic disease
Data saturation	Data saturation according to the principle of theoretical sufficiency:
	When new participants were not adding anything significant to the database
	When the themes obtained offered a sufficient explanatory framework in view of the data collected
	Two further individual interviews were conducted with no new themes emerging, to ensure full data saturation
Data collection period	From April 2015 to November 2015
Data collection methods	Individual in-depth interviews using photo-elicitation:
	At the end of the preliminary interview, the adolescent was given a digital camera. They could refuse and use their own equipment (smartphone) if they preferred
	Instructions: *"You must take a photograph of the table after a family meal. The table should not yet have been cleared. No person should appear in the picture, so everyone at the table must have gotten up. You can take as many pictures as you want, but you will have to choose just one that you will talk about with the researcher at the interview"*
	We chose to ask for a photo after the family meal to encourage a narrative of the entire meal
	For ethical reasons, no person could appear in the photographs
	Individual interviews a week after:
	Of the adolescent and immediately after of the parent(s)
	The selected photograph was displayed on a computer screen during both interviews
	The interviewer began by asking the adolescent for a description of the family meal from which the photograph resulted
	At any point during the interview, the interviewer and the participant could go back to the photograph

Table 1 continued

	Individual in-depth interviews:
	Unstructured, open-ended approach
	One introductory prompt: "can you tell us about this family meal?"
	To get rich and detailed personal data from each participant
	To enter the interviewees' psychological and social world
	To remain open and attentive to any unknown issues that they might introduce
	All interviews were:
	Audio-recorded with participants' permission
	Transcribed word for word, including nonverbal aspects (pauses, laughter, etc.)
	Anonymized
Interviewers	The same researcher (JS), an adolescent psychiatrist, conducted all the interviews
Duration of the interviews	From 60 to 90 min
Data analysis	Thematic analysis:
	To identify, analyze and report themes within data
	To identify the similarities and the differences in the participants' narratives
	To discern recurrent patterns and to integrate new elements that emerged from the analysis
	In a data-driven analysis with inductive approach = coding the data without any reference to theoretical notions or researcher's preconceptions
Criteria to ensure validity	Analysis conducted independently by the three researchers (JS, EC, LP)
	To verify that the themes identified were an exact reflection of the data
	Research group monthly meetings:
	To discuss the results
	To be supervised by a researcher more distant from the material (ARL)
	To resolve disagreements on the inclusion or exclusion of a theme (discussion continued until a consensus was reached)

Table 2 Process of inductive thematic analysis

	Activities	Rationale
Stage 1	Repeatedly read each transcript, as a whole	Obtain a global picture of the interview and become familiar with the interviewee's verbal style
Stage 2	Code the transcript by making notes corresponding to the fundamental units of meanings	Make descriptive notes using the participant's own words
Stage 3	Make conceptual notes through processes of condensation, abstraction, and comparison of the initial notes	Categorize initial notes and reach a higher level of abstraction
Stage 4	Identify initial themes Provide text quotes that illustrate the main ideas of each theme	Themes are labels that summarize the essence of a number of related conceptual notes
Stage 5	Identify recurrent themes across transcripts and produce a coherent ordered table of the themes, gathered into domains of experience	Move from the particular to the shared across multiple experiences. Recurrent themes reflect a shared understanding of the phenomena among all participants

has been removed, to protect the confidentiality of the participants.

The role of photo-elicitation

We observed that using photo-elicitation added specific, original input to this project with adolescents on the issue of family. First of all, they were invested in the task given to them and showed creativity, thought, and also feelings of pleasure in taking the photograph. Next, this picture did indeed serve a mediating function during the interview, both for the participants and the interviewer. Finally the task assigned to the adolescent, to take this picture, was itself the object of family interactions.

Take a picture: participate in this study with pleasure and engagement

The teens' act in taking the picture by itself facilitated their commitment to the study. Better, they were all invested in the task assigned to them. All reported thinking about the production of the photograph. Some

Table 3 Adolescents' characteristics

	Gender	Age	Body mass index (kg/m²)	Psychiatric diagnosis	Adjunctive treatment	Duration of treatment in months	Parental situation	Parents interviewed
F1	Girl	18	19,6	Depression	Sertraline 100 mg/day	22	Divorced	Mother
F2	Girl	17	23	Anxiety disorder	Individual psychotherapy	8	Divorced	Mother
F3	Girl	16	21	Borderline personality disorder	Individual psychotherapy, day hospital	18	Divorced	Mother
F4	Girl	14	18.4	Anxiety disorder	Fluoxetine 20 mg/day	8	Married	Father
F5	Girl	13	21	General anxiety disorder	Individual psychotherapy	14	Married	Parents
F6	Girl	16	22.3	Panic disorder	Individual psychotherapy	12	Divorced	Mother
F7	Girl	17	21.5	Borderline personality disorder	Individual psychotherapy	6	Married	Parents
F8	Girl	15	19.6	Depression	Individual psychotherapy, fluoxetine 20 mg/day	11	Married	Father
F9	Girl	16	18.3	Depression	Individual psychotherapy	16	Divorced	Mother
F10	Girl	14	20.6	Panic disorder	Sertraline 100 mg/day	7	Divorced	Mother
M1	Boy	13	22.7	Depression	Fluoxetine 20 mg/day, day hospital	24	Divorced	Mother
M2	Boy	16	19.1	Borderline personality disorder	Individual psychotherapy	15	Divorced	Mother
M3	Boy	17	18.7	Depression	Fluoxetine 40 mg/day, day hospital	24	Divorced	Mother
M4	Boy	15	21	Depression	Individual psychotherapy	16	Married	Father
M5	Boy	16	19.6	Borderline personality disorder	Individual psychotherapy, day hospital	15	Divorced	Mother

mentioned a desire to show the most or the best, others described esthetic concerns about the questions of light, color, or symmetry of the objects on the table, and especially about the shot selected.

> F1: "I chose that one because it's beautiful, because I did it really well."

Taking the photo and then choosing it required a thoughtful effort that included anticipating and imagining the conversations of the research interview.

> M4: "Finally I opted for seeing everything that I usually see, so that we can do the best examination of the picture."

The adolescents sought with their pictures to reflect their experience as closely as possible. They were thus able to impose their point of view on the scene and directly influence the research process.

> F8: "I chose this picture because it is exactly what I see from my seat, it's taken exactly as if it were my eyes."

Beyond their investment in the study, the teens also enjoyed performing this task. Taking only one photograph did not suffice to express the enthusiasm for this project.

> M2: "Why were we limited to a single picture? Me, I took lots of them, with a zoom, from above (...) do you want to see them?"

Parents also explicitly mentioned the child's pleasure and investment.

> Mother of F1: "We were taken aback the day that she said, 'don't clear the table, I have to take a picture.' I don't know if her stepfather was more astonished by the story of the photo or by her attitude, how she took it to heart."

The photographic image: a support for the narrative

During the interviews with the adolescents, the photo was at the center of the verbal exchanges. The presence of the photo as the basis for the conversation made it possible to disinhibit the adolescent-researcher relationship.

> F5: "I would never have imagined you could say so much about a photo!"

The teens leaned on the photo to verbalize their memories and their emotional experiences.

> M5: "Do you see this fruit basket at the center? eh, I made it in school, for Mother's Day, when I was in kindergarten."

The researcher also used the picture to facilitate conversation and to approach a new subject.

Interviewer: Whose plate is that, with the no-fat yogurt?

F2: "Ah that's my mother's, they are her yogurts and no one else can touch them!"

Finally, the photograph embodied the teen's point of view during the interviews with the parents.

Mother of F3 (about Fig. 1): "I was wondering why she chose to keep that one; she took others, better ... at least, in my opinion."

Access to family interactions through the object that was photographed

The taking of the picture The task assigned to the teen often led to conversations in the families and became a family task. That is, the entire family felt concerned and gave advice, either at the teen's request, or spontaneously.

M2: "I think my little brother also wanted to take pictures; so I asked for his advice and he was so happy. He had the idea of taking pictures of our two plates to show the difference, but my mother said it would be better to be able to see the whole table."

Sometimes parents had exercised a right of oversight or censorship, illustrating the issues of control and asymmetry in the adolescent-parent relationship.

M1: "Isn't my dog's head in this picture? Ah no! But at the beginning I had kept it but my mother must have deleted it when she was checking."

Taking the picture also gave some adolescents the opportunity to assert themselves within the family as the person to whom this task was assigned.

F4: "...it was me! They were there, but I am the one who chose and who took the pictures."

View of the family visible in the still-life photograph The image most often let us see a view of the family and of the family functioning—a view proposed by the adolescents, either by the choice of a specific meal to photograph or by the specific shot. Some teens chose to photograph the only meal where the entire family was together, thus noting the rarity of these moments and the lack of family communication and cohesion.

F1: "A meal where we are all together because on Monday my mother has English and I have dance in the evening (...) Tuesday we are all together."

Other adolescents on the contrary stressed a particular relationship in adapting the instructions and choosing a meal where only some family members were present .

F4 (Fig. 2): " Breakfast with brother and sister... it's an important moment for us, when the two of us are really together."

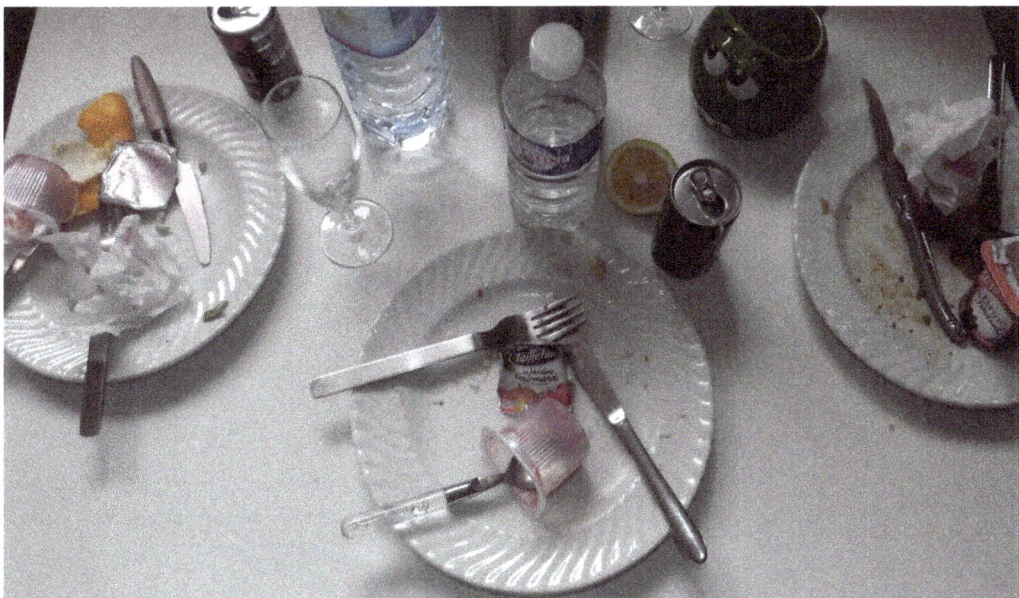

Fig. 1 F3's photograph

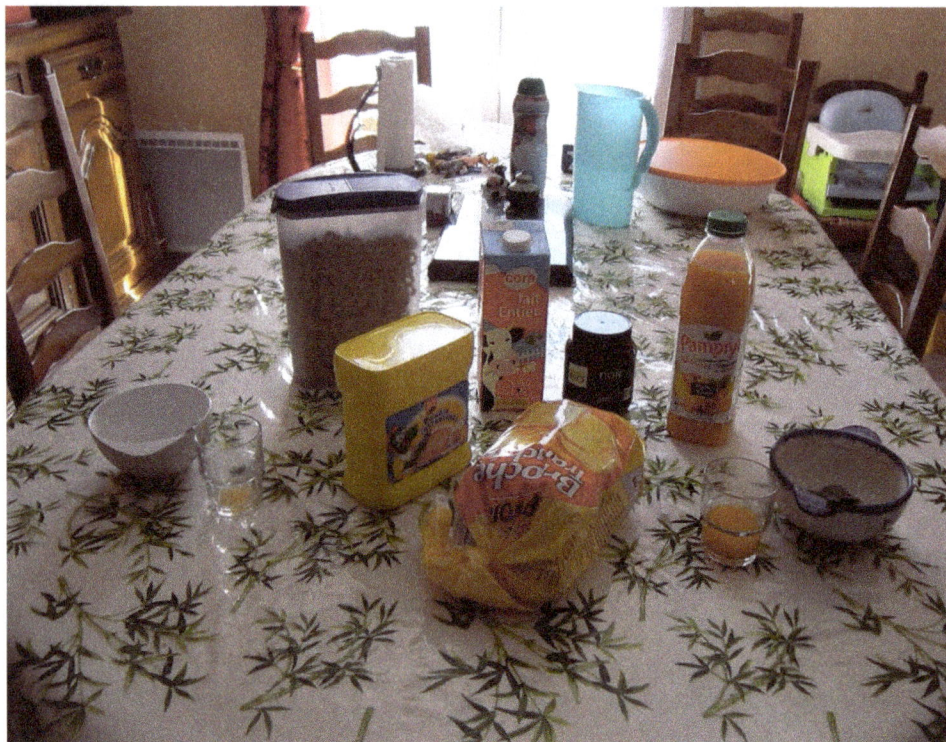

Fig. 2 F4's photograph

Finally, some adolescents choose a particular shot to illustrate the family history. The view of the photograph taken by F3 (Fig. 1) gives the impression of a horizontal slice. She presents a view from above of a table with three plates, but shot such that the viewer cannot tell how the table continues and whether or not there is a fourth plate outside the field of view. She used this project to illustrate her distress about the separation of her parents, a recurrent topic during the interview.

> F3: *"I don't know why I kept this picture. It's true that the framing is bad, you could say it's cut (...) But this table doesn't hold four people. When my father still lived with us, we didn't eat there anyway, we ate in the living room."*

Exploration of family interactions around meals and food

The analysis of the interviews allowed us to identify three themes concerning family interactions around food. The first concerns parent–child relationship patterns, the second the functioning of the family group, and the third the adolescent's individual relation to food and therefore the process of separation from the family.

Parent–child relationship patterns

Express both difference from and resemblance to others by food   We first found in these adolescents a desire to differentiate themselves from their parents through what they eat, but also to confirm that they belonged to their family and claimed its heritage. They signaled this continuity explicitly by appropriating the parental discourse about food.

> M4: *"In fact, it works like that, I have to taste everything each time. My mother repeated it incessantly and now it's like her voice is in my head."*

The differentiation could be observed through the adolescent's new tastes, most often accompanied by attraction to a cuisine different from that of the family. This issue of difference and resemblance was clearly illustrated by the adolescents' acts of cooking. Some reproduced family recipes, other compromised with a variant of a basic family dish, while others invented completely different recipes to demonstrate their individual relation to food.

> M1: *"I began to invent recipes, just for me. Once I made a mixture of pears and potatoes in the blender."*

Food: expressing love within the parent–child relationship   Food was a way of expressing love within the family. Mothers made this discourse explicit.

> *Mother of F9: "there's love in it, it's nothing but love (…) because they know I sacrificed to make it…"*

Adolescents also considered food as a way of expressing love.

> *F5: "I don't really like boiled beef (…) I make myself eat a little, because I know it makes her happy when I do."*

Functioning of the family group

Family cohesion and a relational game   The family group experienced authentic cohesion around the family meal. These moments were special because they were together and sharing. Food was actually secondary and was sometimes only a pretext for getting together.

> *F10: "Sometimes the meal is over but we stay there, we sit, and we talk."*

Family cohesion during meals was especially the foundation of a relational game within the family, a flexible game that allowed the expression and sharing of all sorts of emotions.

> *Father of F7: "That can be two minutes of screaming and two minutes later we are all going to laugh."*

Everything was part of the game. The teens refused to be at the table with their parents and played at not eating but nonetheless ended up eating. The parents were perfectly aware of this.

> *Mother of F6: "There was a phase when she didn't eat, at least, not in front of me, but there was this strange phenomenon of food that disappeared from the refrigerator."*

The teens also played with parental control around food. They could break the rules, but it was still part of the game.

> *M2: "In fact, I have packages of chips hidden in my room (…) my mother yells at me but at the same time she laughs because she did the same thing when she was my age."*

Transmission and family history   Food also served a function in the transmission of family history.

> *Father of F4: "We are epicureans, when we get together for these occasions, and we have to transmit that to the children."*

This implied first of all transmission of the family history, based on ways of cooking things, special recipes that were transmitted from generation to generation and carried with them the culture of the family.

> *Mother of F5: "There was also Grandma Alice's apple charlotte, there's something special when I cook these recipes."*

Food also gave access to the current family situation: reorganizations of family life were illustrated by changes in food or diet.

> *M1: "My father never let us have onions or butter. Now for example, we can make onion tarts often."*

For the adolescents, parental separation furnished two parallel histories, and food could serve as a witness to both and thus confirm the separation.

> *F9: "My father is kind of random, my mother very straightforward. My mother is steak, salad, yogurt, and an apple; my father is an omelet and chips and then merguez mixed with anything."*

An individual relation to food

This theme was unexpected in our exploration of family interactions around food, but we found that adolescents asserted their own individual relations to food. It did not involve simply claiming their own tastes in food but also deciding when, where, and with whom to have meals. The adolescents showed that they wanted to choose and make decisions about food based on their own experience.

> *F7: "I think that my parents never made me eat something, so I always said, I don't like it. But now I try, I verify if I really don't like it….. and sometimes I like it and sometimes I don't.*

They showed a desire to cook for themselves even if they remained attached to the family cuisine.

> *Mother of F6: "In fact, she is totally 'I can make it but I'd prefer if you do it."*

In fact, the transmission of culinary practices was a progressive movement toward autonomy, preparing the teen for a future life outside the family home. These practices were thus transmitted in several ways, from a passive *watch it being done* to *I'm making it all by myself.*

> *F4: "First, I watched my mum and then she showed me and after that she let me do it, but stayed behind me. After that, she just watched and now I do it alone."*

The individual relation with food was also found in the adolescents' interactions with their peer groups.

F4: "With my friends, we talk a lot about food, we organize 'crepe parties' just for us, and it's great."

Finally, the parents too asserted their own individual relation with food. They had their own tastes and desires in food and refused to sacrifice them.

Mother of F3: "Yes, I cook brussels sprouts, I cook them for me; it would bother me to think that I deprive myself of something I like because of my daughters' tastes… after all, the fridge is big enough."

Discussion

The main objective of this study was to examine the value and feasibility of using photo-elicitation in research in adolescent psychiatry via an exploration of the role of food in family relationships.

Photo-elicitation appeared to be feasible in adolescent psychiatry research and helpful for interviewing teens with diverse psychiatric disorders. There are three aspects especially important to point out here.

First, taking the photo promoted the adolescents' involvement in the project and generated a positive feeling toward it. Some authors suggest that modern vocabulary and contemporary modes of expression are useful in research interviews with adolescents [8]. The use of the photo-elicitation tool fits into this approach. Photography is a favored mode of expression for youth, occupying an important place in their daily lives, in particular in their social networks. Here, 11 adolescents spontaneously refused to use the cameras we planned to give them and preferred to use their own smartphones. This idea also appears in the study by Yi-Frazier et al. [15], they asked teens with diabetes to use Instagram—a social network whose primary medium is photographs—as a form of photo-elicitation for their study.

Second, most adolescents are quite skilled at photography, and this gives them the opportunity to better express their point of view [9]. Accordingly, as Mack et al. [8] wrote, *"Research will be a positive experience for adolescents when they know that their input is important and valued".* We consider that in this study, the teens were fully able to influence the research process because, although we initially sought to focus on the family interactions around food, our most original result concerns the adolescents' individual relations with food. Our study fits within the constructivist paradigm, and the visual method helped to co-construct the results [27]. Our methodological choice to use photo-elicitation— and probably also our instructions—empowered the adolescents, by asking them to perform an action they were skilled at and comfortable with, to reveal their own vision. We placed them in the position of author. This

position enabled the emergence of a theme focused on the issue of the adolescent's empowerment in the construction of his or her own self.

A last point about the photograph is that the teens experienced and expressed pleasure in taking the picture, choosing it, showing it, and talking about it. Sutton et al. [28] argued that the presence of pleasure increases the success of study recruitment. We note that all the adolescents who were asked to participate in this research project agreed to do so. In her review of the literature about qualitative research with children and adolescents, Kirk [9] concluded that it is important to use child-friendly techniques so that the participants can have fun during the data collection.

Tested in our study, photo-elicitation was a tool that enabled us to obtain rich narratives of experiences that led to innovative results. Two of the themes in our results (parent–child relationship patterns and the functioning of the family group) have also been found in studies of obese adolescents [17, 29]. The literature describes the cohesive function of the family meal [18], like that of food, as a vector of transmission of the family history and culture [30]. These dimensions are above all cultural and are related to family structure in Western countries. The third theme, which shows adolescents' individual relation to food, is an original result of our study. That is, the adolescents insisted on their taste in food and their own attitudes towards it. They consider themselves the authors of their food-related actions and choices. This result can be linked to the issue of identity construction in adolescence, especially through the idea of *self-concept* [31]; this notion underlines the importance of the definition individuals give to themselves, how they perceive themselves. This idea of *self-concept* in adolescence has been developed in the recent literature, both in a cognitive, neurobiological dimension [32] and in an environmental perspective [33]. The adolescent's *self-concept* is constructed from multiple dynamics: his or her individual society, peer group, and family [34]. Food may be an accessible marker of this potential identity construction. These links between identity construction and food have already been described in sociology in relation to the general population of adolescents [35, 36]. From a methodological perspective, this result also shows that photo-elicitation can be used to identify and explore dynamic examples of self-concept and identity construction.

To the best of our knowledge, no study in the field of adolescent psychiatry has described the importance of this individual relation with food in a population of adolescents with a variety of psychiatric disorders. This particular context raises a question: is this preoccupation of adolescents about their food-related desires and choices linked to the adolescent process of identity construction, or is it a marker of treatment that may have promoted the adolescent's autonomy? The development of the adolescent's *self-concept* may be considered, in the latter case, as a treatment effect, resulting from the various kinds of care he or she has received.

Implications for adolescent mental health research

As we mentioned above, qualitative research among adolescents with psychiatric disorders is considered as a methodological challenge. It is already clear from the literature that photo-elicitation is a methodologically relevant choice with adolescents, with many advantages: greater control over the visual and verbal discourse, easier relationship between researcher and adolescent, greater influence on the research process [10, 37, 38]. Yet, its potential interest with adolescents with psychiatric disorders has not previously been explored. Our results highlight the positive aspects of using this tool with this specific population as well as its methodological relevance in qualitative research among them.

Limitations

One limitation is inherent to photo-elicitation as a tool and its generalizability. Its use may be restricted to teens able to take pictures, although we found no teens in our sample who were unable to do so and it is limited to teens with reasonably good vision.

Two other limitations concern the results of the analysis of the content of the patients' experience. The first is the difficulty in determining whether results are specific to our population of adolescents receiving psychiatric care or if, instead, they might be true for all adolescents. Certainly, the advantages of using photo-elicitation with this age group and its use as a vehicle for discussing family functioning seem clear and are not specific to our study population. To verify these assertions, however, would require an identical qualitative study in the general population of adolescents, and then a quantitative research design with matched comparison groups from the general population. The second limitation involves the diagnostic heterogeneity of the members of our sample: 6 with depression (3F:3M), 4 with borderline personality disorder (2F:2M), 2 with anxiety disorder (2F:0M), 2 with panic disorder (2F:0M), and 1 with generalized anxiety (1F:0M). We thus cannot prejudge the relevance of our results in particular clinical situations.

Conclusions

This qualitative study used the tool of photo-elicitation to explore the family interactions around food in adolescents receiving psychiatric care.

From the methodological perspective, our results simultaneously illustrate the value of developing qualitative research in adolescent psychiatry and the need to adapt this research to this specific population by using innovative and original techniques that enable teens with psychiatric disorders to express their subjective experience.

Abbreviation
BMI: body mass index.

Authors' contributions
Conceived and designed the study: JS, ARL. Collected the data: JS, LP. Analyzed the data: JS, EC, LP, ARL. Contributed reagents/materials/analysis tools: JS, EC, LP, MV, SC, JP. Wrote the paper: JS, EC, ARL. All authors read and approved the final manuscript.

Author details
[1] Service Universitaire de Psychiatrie de l'Adolescent, Argenteuil Hospital Centre, Argenteuil, France. [2] ECSTRA Team, UMR-1153, Inserm, Paris Diderot University, Sorbonne Paris Cite, Paris, France.

Acknowledgements
The authors thank the participants of this study, and JA Cahn for the translation.

Competing interests
The authors declare that they have no competing interests.

Funding
None.

References
1. Harper D. Talking about pictures: a case for photo elicitation. Vis Stud. 2002;17(1):13–26.
2. Pain H. A literature review to evaluate the choice and use of visual methods. Int J Qual Methods. 2012;11(4):303–19.
3. Guillemin M, Drew S. Questions of process in participant-generated visual methodologies. Vis Stud. 2010;25(2):175–88.
4. Oliffe JL, Bottorff JL. Further than the eye can see? Photo elicitation and research with men. Qual Health Res. 2007;17(6):850–8.
5. Rhodes T, Fitzgerald J. Visual data in addictions research: seeing comes before words? Addict Res Theory. 2006;14(4):349–63.
6. Daniels D. Using visual methods to bring people to the center. Global Issues and Adult Education: perspectives from Latin America, Southern Africa and the United States. Jossey Bass; 2006.
7. Grover S. Why won't they listen to us? On giving power and voice to children participating in social research. Childhood. 2004;11(1):81–93.
8. Mack R, Giarelli E, Bernhardt BA. The adolescent research participant: strategies for productive and ethical interviewing. J Pediatr Nurs. 2009;24(6):448–57.
9. Kirk S. Methodological and ethical issues in conducting qualitative research with children and young people: a literature review. Int J Nurs Stud. 2007;44(7):1250–60.
10. Darbyshire P. Multiple methods in qualitative research with children: more insight or just more? Qual Res. 2005;5(4):417–36.
11. Moore L, Miller M. Initiating research with doubly vulnerable populations. J Adv Nurs. 1999;30(5):1034–40.

12. Liamputtong P. Researching the vulnerable. London: Sage; 2007.

13. Deroche K, Lahman M. Methodological considerations for conducting qualitative interviews with youth receiving mental health services. forum qualitative sozialforschung/forum. Qual Soc Res. 2008;9(3):17–35. doi:10.17169/fqs-9.3.1016.

14. Johnson CM, Sharkey JR, McIntosh AW, Dean WR. "I'm the Momma": using photo-elicitation to understand matrilineal influence on family food choice. BMC Women's Health. 2010;10:21.

15. Yi-Frazier JP, Cochrane K, Mitrovich C, Pascual M, Buscaino E, Eaton L, Malik F. Using instagram as a modified application of photovoice for storytelling and sharing in adolescents with type 1 diabetes. Qual Health Res. 2015;25(10):1372–82.

16. Hill L. Some of it I haven't told anybody else': using photo elicitation to explore the experiences of secondary school education from the perspective of young people with a diagnosis of autistic spectrum disorder. Educ Child Psychol. 2014;31(1):79–89.

17. Lachal J, Speranza M, Taïeb O, Falissard B, Lefèvre H, Moro MR, Revah-Levy A, Qualigramh. Qualitative research using photo-elicitation to explore the role of food in family relationships among obese adolescents. Appetite. 2012;58(3):1099–105.

18. Berge JM, Jin S, Hannan P, Neumark-Sztainer D. Structural and interpersonal characteristics of family meals: associations with adolescent body mass index and dietary patterns. J Acad Nutr Diet. 2013;113(6):816–22.

19. Wong OL. Meaning of food in childhood obesity: an exploratory study in a Chinese family context. Soc Work Health Care. 2010;49(4):362–77.

20. Bassett R, Chapman GE, Beagan BL. Autonomy and control: the co-construction of adolescent food choice. Appetite. 2008;50(2–3):325–32.

21. Sibeoni J, Orri M, Valentin M, Podlipski MA, Colin S, Pradere J, Revah-Levy A. Metasynthesis of the views about treatment of Anorexia Nervosa in adolescents: perspectives of adolescents, parents, and professionals. PLoS ONE. 2017;12(1):e0169493.

22. Sibeoni J, Orri M, Campredon S, Revah-Levy A. The efficacy of care as perceived by adolescents presenting anxiety-based school refusal. Soins Pediatr Pueric. 2017;38(295):43–7.

23. Patton MQ. Qualitative research & evaluation methods. 3rd ed. Thousand Oaks: SAGE Publications, Inc; 2001.

24. Dey I. Grounding grounded theory: guidelines for qualitative inquiry. San Diego: Academic Press; 1999.

25. Braun V, Clarke V, Terry G. Thematic analysis. In: Rohleder P, Lyons AC, editors. Qualitative research in clinical and health psychology, vol. 7. Basingstoke: Palgrave Macmillan; 2014.

26. Tong A, Sainsbury P, Craig J. Consolidated criteria for reporting qualitative research (COREQ): a 32-item checklist for interviews and focus groups. Int J Qual Health Care. 2007;19(6):349–57.

27. Merriam SB, Tisdell EJ. Qualitative research: a guide to design and implementation. Wiley; 2015.

28. Sutton LB, Erlen JA, Glad JM, Siminoff LA. Recruiting vulnerable populations for research: revisiting the ethical issues. J Prof Nurs. 2003;19(2):106–12.

29. de Almeida Mota Ramalho J, Lachal J, Ferro Bucher-Maluschke JSN, Moro M-R, Revah-Levy A. A qualitative study of the role of food in family relationships: insight into the families of Brazilian obese adolescents using photo elicitation. Appetite. 2016;96(1):539–45.

30. Bowen R, Devine C. "Watching a person who knows how to cook, you'll learn a lot" linked lives, cultural transmission, and the food choices of Puerto Rican girls. Appetite. 2011;56(2):290–8.

31. O'Dea J. Self-concept, self-esteem and body weight in adolescent females: a three-year longitudinal study. J Health Psychol. 2006;11(4):599–611.

32. Sebastian C, Burnett S, Blakemore SJ. Development of the self-concept during adolescence. Trends in Cognit Sci. 2008;12(11):441–6.

33. Tarrant M, MacKenzie L, Hewitt L. Friendship group identification, multidimensional self-concept, and experience of developmental tasks in adolescence. J Adolesc. 2006;29(4):627–40.

34. Ybrandt H. The relation between self-concept and social functioning in adolescence. J Adolesc. 2008;31(1):1–16.

35. Fox NJ, Ward KJ. You are what you eat? Vegetarianism, health and identity. Soc Sci Med. 2008; 66(12): e2585–e2595.

36. Stead M, McDermott L, MacKintosh AM, Adamson A. Why healthy eating is bad for young people's health: identity, belonging and food. Soc Sci Med. 2011;72(7):1131–9.

37. Didkowsky N, Ungar M, Liebenberg L. Using visual methods to capture embedded processes of resilience for youth across cultures and contexts. J Can Acad Child Adolesc Psychiatry. 2010;19(1):12–8.

38. Drew SE, Duncan RE, Sawyer SM. Visual storytelling: a beneficial but challenging method for health research with young people. Qual Health Res. 2010;20(12):1677–88.

Attributions and private theories of mental illness among young adults seeking psychiatric treatment in Nairobi: an interpretive phenomenological analysis

Judy Wanjiru Mbuthia[1], Manasi Kumar[1,2]* , Fredrik Falkenström[3], Mary Wangari Kuria[1] and Caleb Joseph Othieno[1]

Abstract

Background: Mental illness affects every segment of population including young adults. The beliefs held by young patients regarding the causes of mental illness impact their treatment-seeking behaviour. It is pertinent to know the commonly held attributions around mental illness so as to effectively provide psychological care, especially in a resource constrained context such as Kenya. This helps in targeting services around issues such as stigma and extending youth-friendly services.

Methods: Guided by the private theories interview (PTI-P) and attributional framework, individual semi-structured interviews were carried out with ten young adults of ages 18–25 years about their mental health condition for which they were undergoing treatment. Each interview took 30–45 min. We mapped four attributions (locus of control, stability, controllability and stigma) on PTI-P questions. Data was transcribed verbatim to produce transcripts coded using interpretive phenomenological analysis. These codes were then broken down into categories that could be used to understand various attributions.

Results: We found PTI-P to be a useful tool and it elicited three key themes: (a) psychosocial triggers of distress (with themes of negative thoughts, emotions around mental health stigma and negative childhood experiences, parents' separation or divorce, death of a loved one etc.), (b) biological conditions and psychopathologies limiting intervention, and (c) preferences and views on treatment. Mapping these themes on our attributional framework, PTI-P themes presented as causal attributions explaining stigma, locus of control dimensions and stability. External factors were mainly ascribed to be the cause of unstable and uncontrollable attributions including persistent negative emotions and thoughts further exacerbating psychological distress. Nine out of the ten participants expressed the need for more intense and supportive therapy.

Conclusion: Our study has provided some experiential evidence in understanding how stigma, internal vs external locus of control, stability vs instability attributions play a role in shaping attitudes young people have towards their mental health. Our study points to psychosocial challenges such as stigma, poverty and lack of social support that continue to undermine mental well-being of Kenyan youth. These factors need to be considered when addressing mental health needs of young people in Kenya.

Keywords: Youth in psychiatric facilities, Attributions of mental illness, Locus of control, Private theories interview, Stigma

*Correspondence: m.kumar@ucl.ac.uk
[1] Department of Psychiatry, College of Health Sciences, University of Nairobi, P.O.Box 19676, Nairobi 00202, Kenya
Full list of author information is available at the end of the article

Background

Mental illness affects every segment of the population. Mental health issues among the youth can negatively impact the national development of a country. More so, the beliefs held by the community about the causes of mental illness are likely to impact individual treatment-seeking behavior [1–4]. Available literature from developing countries show that acceptance of help with mental health issues and engagement with services can be affected by various factors such as belief in evil spirits and stigmatization of mental health problems [2, 4–7]. Young people's attitudes towards peers with mental illnesses has been studied and the findings suggest that young people differentiate between perceptions of how dangerous and fear provoking the individuals might be [8]. However, no research has explored young peoples' beliefs and attributions associated with their illnesses. Cultural components such as social attitudes, peer group rules, religious beliefs, family morals, and other socio-cultural factors strongly contribute to the behavior and attributions towards mental illness held by the youth [9]. Data on years lived with disability (YLD) demonstrate that, in Kenya, the burden of mental health is significant and access to specialist care is limited [10, 11]. The gaps in meeting mental health needs and providing services for young adults are worrying, given increasingly high levels of depression and incidents of suicide by young adults in Kenya [12–14].

Young adults' attributions of mental illness are not well-researched; hence, we know very little about their patterns of help-seeking behavior or their commonly used description of distress. Our study is an exploratory step towards understanding young adults' expression of distress, their attributions associated with mental illness, and factors that prevent or contribute to management of mental disorders. By gathering mental illness-related attributions held by the young adults, we made it possible to extrapolate aspects of their psychotherapy care which need further strengthening. Exploring the beliefs young people hold about their illness and pathways to cure are important steps to facilitating early access to mental health services and improving psychological wellbeing. This includes alerting the practitioners about possible barriers that hinder positive psychotherapy outcome. Through this research we gained a critical knowledge piece that will provide insight into barriers young adults encounter in seeking mental health services. To achieve this, we used two theoretical lenses to review subjective appraisal from young adults: attributional framework and the private theories interview.

The private theories interview patient version (PTI-P)

The private theories interview [15] is an interview that was developed in the context of psychotherapy research, and is used to study psychotherapy patients' subjective beliefs about their problems, their causes, and any ideas they may have about what would be needed for them to feel better. We used the patient version of the interview (PTI-P). We superimposed this interview on an attribution model developed by Weiner [16]. We used these two frames to capture the interviewee's attempts to give meaning to their interpersonal, psychic, and somatic distress, while including these experiences in the patient's private context of meaning. The PTI-P is a semi-structured, brief qualitative interview, which can be used to understand participants' personal assumptions of treatment, mental health or illness qualitatively. We adopted the PTI-P, developed by [17], as it is with minimal changes. The attribution-focused questions were superimposed on the PTI-P, by adding extra probes to questions in the PTI-P. See Table 2 for the newly designed attribution-focused questions.

The attributional framework

Depression, anxiety, and stress are commonly associated with negative thinking and attributions. We outlined our attribution framework from the original attributional framework done by Bernard Weiner [18]. Attribution refers to the assessments of the cause of an action or behavior [19]. It also refers to the internal (thinking) and external (talking) process of interpreting and understanding what is behind our own and others' behaviors. Attribution theory explains an occurrence and determines the cause of the happening or behavior. It starts with the idea that individuals are driven to understand the causes of the happenings or behavior and that this desire allegedly grows out of individuals' wish to understand, foresee, and control the environment [20–22]. The attributions are known to be of different types. According to Weiner et al. [23], there are three dimensions of causal attributions which include the following.

Locus of control (internal vs. external)

A person's belief that the events which occur in life are either a result of personal control and efforts or an outside force like luck or fate is referred to as locus of control (LoC). *Controllable* vs. *uncontrollable attribution:* Weiner's controllability dimension concerns a situation that is regarded as controllable if the individual is personally able to guide, influence, or prevent it. It is the extent to which the individual has control over the cause, as perceived by observers. Försterling [24] used "drunkenness" as an example to describe the controllability of causes, suggesting that "drunkenness" is perceived as a controllable cause. Causes that can neither be influenced nor guided such as a physical handicap, for example blindness, are regarded as being uncontrollable [24]. The external locus of control are often thought to be relatively uncontrollable and associated with perceived social stress that young adults might encounter [25].

Stability of causal attribution (stable vs. instability)

Stability is the time-based nature of causes [16]. Some causes remain stable over time while others increase or decrease. Causal attributions, when viewed as stable and unchanging as opposed to unstable and fluctuating, are directly related to a person's expectancy of successful results [24] implying that the stability attribution makes the person less inclined to believe that his/her problems will improve. As the mental illness deteriorates in an individual, it perpetuates an irrational outcome and damages self-governing functions. This could be explained by the knowledge that mental-behavioral or internal stigmas are normally considered unstable or reversible, while physically based stigmas are perceived as stable, or irreversible [26]. Stability and instability of attributions refer to how fixed or how flexible the mental schemas associated with these can be. Unstable attributions may help with the motivation to work in treatment, whereas stable attributions may lead to hopelessness and not seeking treatment. The more stable an attribution is, the harder it is to change it [16]. Inferences on the stability and instability of an attribution depends on how controllable or uncontrollable one experiences an event or an individual attribute to be; it is also contingent on whether one views the event or attribute it from an internal or external locus of control.

Attribution of stigma (internalized vs. externalized)

Stigma is defined as a social scratch that leads to questioning of associates of a group, such as people with mental illness [27]. According to Rüsch et al. [28], the negative properties of stigma among individuals with mental illness lessen self-esteem and health care seeking behavior, and increase discrimination. The tendency towards self-stigma has been documented in Sub-Saharan African patients and along this are also religious and supernatural attributions given to mental health conditions in the form of punishments [29]. Experiences of stigma catalysed by self-stigma revolve around experiences of devaluation, exclusion, and disadvantage [30]. Moreso, mental illness stigma is one factor that hinders seeking care by distressed people, hence undermining the service system [31]. The individuals are not only troubled by the external mental illness stigma but also by the self-stigma, leading to low self-esteem and self-efficacy [32].

Methods

Setting

The study took place at the Kenyatta National Hospital's Youth clinic. The clinic runs every weekday from 7.30 am to 5.00 pm, and roughly ten new patients are registered each week and around fifteen more new patients are added during school holiday periods. It is overseen by resident psychiatrists, psychiatric nurses, and psychotherapists including clinical psychology interns. The services are free to all youth regardless of type of diagnosis, and the clinic also provides outreach services for HIV testing and counselling (HTS). This setting was chosen because it serves nationwide referrals and walk-in patients who are predominantly fluent in either English or Kiswahili. Most clients are referred from various schools, colleges, and universities, and it is also a clinic for walk-in cases and emergencies.

Participants

Our participants were between ages 18 and 25 years. 18 years is the legal age for an adult in Kenya [12], while 25 is the age limit for patients attending the youth clinic (Table 1).

Sampling

In this exploratory study, we purposely selected young adults who were seeking psychiatric treatment at the clinic, were willing to give consent, and had fluency in Kiswahili or English (the two official languages spoken in Kenya). Assessments from the psychiatrists and clinical psychologists were used to determine the severity of the patients' mental illness. Two patients who were eligible for the study were excluded because both had severe psychosis in addition to limited fluency in English and Kiswahili. None of the participants we approached for the study declined to give consent and participate.

Ethical approval and considerations

We received approval from the Kenyatta National Hospital and University of Nairobi Ethical Review Committee (no. KNH/UoN P105/02/2015). The participants were informed verbally and also provided with a written document about the purpose of study. In addition, consent to audio-record the interview was sought. Participants were informed that participation or refusal to take part in the study would not affect their current contact with the clinic. No rewards were given for participation.

Instruments

A brief socio-demographic questionnaire was used to capture key demographic information. These included the age of the participant, Kiswahili and English literacy levels, educational level, and gender of the participants. These were gathered to synthesize the information with their interviews. Data was gathered by use of semi-structured interviews with open-ended questions encouraging exploration of experiences within the conceptual

Table 1 The Socio-demographic information

Participant no.	Age	Gender	Level of education	Diagnosis
Patient 01	20	Male	University	Major depressive disorder
Patient 02	19	Male	High school	Substance induced psychosis
Patient 03	18	Female	College	Secondary enuresis
Patient 04	22	Female	University	Schizoaffective disorder
Patient 05	19	Female	High school	Depression
Patient 06	24	Female	University	Depression and epilepsy
Patient 07	20	Female	High school	Conduct disorder
Patient 08	22	Male	College	Somatic disorder
Patient 09	19	Male	High school	Substance induced psychosis
Patient 10	20	Female	College	Post-traumatic stress disorder

Table 2 Private theories interview patients' version and attributions focused questionnaire guide

Private theories questions	Attributions focussed domains
What is it that leads you to seek treatment today?	Internal locus of control External locus of control
What are your thoughts about the psychological issues you are experiencing?	Controllability Uncontrollability
Tell me about some or other important experiences or events in your life that you associate with your difficulties and how these problems	Stability Instability
In relation to the problem (MI) how do you see yourself and others around you?	Experiencing stigma Not experiencing stigma
What do you desire that would ease your pain/distress?	Desired treatment plan or cure

framework used. The five questions from the *Private Theories Interview-Patient version* (PTI-P) were the primary interview questions. We developed an *Attributions Focused Question guide* that was embedded within the PTI questions as probes in such a way as to elicit attributions. The probes were designed to get the participants to elaborate on the 'how', 'why', and 'when' associated with the five private theories questions. The attribution-focused question guide was mapped onto these questions to create a subset of categories that explain the attributions used by participants in understanding their problems and thinking about how these could be resolved. Given that mental illness continues to be a highly stigmatizing condition in Kenya [33], we included stigma as a category of attributions to see how our participants navigate it.

Since the PTI-P was first developed in Sweden, we were concerned how well these questions would fit the needs of our Kenyan young participants. In order to enhance cultural sensitivity and adapt the questions to the Kenyan context, the question-guide was translated into Kiswahili. The first author, who is fluent in Kiswahili and English, translated with the help of an English-Kiswahili dictionary to ensure that the meaning of each word was retained. Two Kenyan trainee-psychologists also gave

suggestions on a few semantic adjustments. The adjustments were only linguistic in nature. Given that these were semi-structured questionnaires there was no need to formally validate the tools. Instead, we tested their cultural sensitivity in pilot interviews. We used interpretative phenomenological analysis (IPA) [34]—a qualitative technique to analyze our data. IPA was chosen because our goal was to magnify the subjective experiences, both tone and tenor expressed by our participants while interpreting their idioms of distress, attributional patterns, and highlighting their barriers to mental health care.

These questions resulted in the attribution framework as shown in Table 2 below and embody each locus, stability, and stigma probes mapped on PTI-P. The questions were the following:

1. What is the problem?
2. How did the problems arise?
3. How can the problems be remedied?
4. What has changed?
5. What is your view of others and yourself?

Each of these questions was paired with a domain from the attribution theory. AFQ provided a deepening and expanding of the PTI-P framework and the scope of the analyses. The domains adapted from Wieners attribution theory were locus of control (internal vs. external), controllability (controllable vs. uncontrollable) stability (stable or unstable), and stigma as an independent domain.

Data collection

Three pilot interviews were conducted at the youth clinic to test the conceptual framework and gauge participants' reaction to the interview questions. The first author was trained in qualitative interview techniques by her senior mentor MK and had regular supervision with all her mentors on using IPA as well as analyzing the data thematically. The participants in distress were encouraged to continue with psychotherapy, and a referral mechanism was built in the study if anyone had self-harming thoughts or was at a risk of harming themselves or others. Once these procedures were identified, individual interviews took place in the counselling room at the youth clinic before or after the participants' counselling session. English or Kiswahili language was used as per the participant's preference. The first author conducted the audio-recorded interviews with one interviewee at a time. The interview duration ranged from thirty to 40 min. Data collected was safely stored without any identifiers to ensure confidentiality of the participants.

Data analytic plan

The recorded material was transcribed from the audio recorder to a MS Word document. The first step was to ensure that all experiential material about PTI-P and Attribution Focused questions were adequately answered in the data. The second step was to break the data as per the IPA framework. This was done because of the following reasons: (i). IPA is consistent with research aims since it is committed to the *examination of how people make sense of their major life experiences* [35], (ii). It is a phenomenological approach *focusing on exploration of experiences in its own terms* instead of attempting to reduce it to predefined or overly abstract categories. This means *that it is interpretative in that the researcher tries to make sense of the participants' experiences*, and (iii). IPA is concerned with personal experiences and involves interpretation, with ample consideration of a given context.

IPA as a scientific principle

IPA is idiographic in nature. It is concerned with revealing something about the experience of each of the individuals involved and is able to give a detailed conclusion about the participant group. Our third and next step was to ensure that we used IPA as a method in the service of teasing out PTI information and how young adults make attributions regarding their own well-being. The approach is committed to detail in-depth analysis as well as to understand how a particular experiential event or relationship (phenomenon) has been understood from a particular context by different individuals or groups.

IPA as a specific method in this study

We used IPA in the following ways: by carrying out verbatim transcription of the semantic content of each interview based on audio recording and followed by reading and re-reading of the content, while searching for richer, detailed sections and for contradictions and inconsistencies. At the initial noting stage, the first author and her supervisors identified specific ways the participants spoke of an issue, described what mattered to the participants, and the meaning of these things. This identified each participant's emergent themes and the connections/interrelations of the themes for each of the ten participants. Mapping of themes was done to connect and fit the themes in relation to the research questions. With each step, every individual participant's core themes were tallied with other participants' and we ensured that the analysis maintained a strong interpretive focus. The core themes were later merged with the attribution dimension and the PTI-P framework to make sense of the bigger picture. At this point, our key question was which themes were being articulated by our participants and where did these fit-in vis-à-vis identified attributions. We present themes emanating out of IPA from the private theories interview in the results section and in our discussion section we reflect on how these themes map onto attributions framework as a whole.

Results

Our results are presented in a twofold process. We highlight the themes that were drawn from the PTI-P: psycho-social triggers, biological origins, and preference for combined treatment as a way of addressing stigma. Table 3 lists the core themes arranged from the most prominent to the least, as derived from frequency count among the 10 participants, while Table 2 indicates the connections between the attributions and core themes. These themes are reviewed here, starting with the psycho-social attributions.

Psychosocial triggers of distress

Our participants were concerned about various psychosocial triggers that adversely impacted their lives. Employing IPA, we identified a number of thoughts and experiences as being the prominent causes of our participants' worries and distress.

Table 3 Building the connections (attributions vs. core themes) (to be placed in page 30, before internal and external locus of control)

Interview questions	Attribution dimensions	Core themes
What is it that leads you to seek treatment today?	Internal locus of control or dispositional attributions: based on behaviour within the client	Negative emotions and thoughts misconduct behaviour Transitional challenges-from teen to adult life Poor performance in school Self-stigma and shame of disclosure
	External locus of control or situational attributions: Based on behaviour (from others) to the individual	Negative childhood Experiences Strained relationships with parents and other family members Rejection from others and stigma Lack of finances Decline in social life
What are your thoughts about the psychological issues you are experiencing?	Controllability: if the individual is personally able to guide, influence or prevent the situation	Negative emotions and Thoughts
	Un-controllability: if the individual is personally not able to guide, influence or prevent the situation	Negative childhood experiences Strained relationships with parents and other family members Rejection from others and stigma Lack of finances Decline in social life
Tell me about some (other) important experiences or events in your life that you associate with your difficulties and how the problems began.	Stability: unchanging causes	Death of loved ones
	Un-stable: changing/fluctuating causes	Negative emotions and thoughts
In relation to the psychological issues, what is your view on others and yourself?	Stigma from others and self	Self-stigma Stigma from others
What do you think is needed for your illness to be cured or might ease your pain?	Treatment preference	Need for therapy Need for medication

Negative thoughts and emotions

The participants shared in their interviews that negative thoughts and emotions were the core reasons for their illness and distress. Adverse experiences created a spiral of negative thoughts and emotions about themselves and the world around them. The PTI question 1 was most reflective of this spiral thinking that our participants struggled to get out.

"I had a disagreement with mum. She wants me to be like her and I cannot. She separated with my dad and now she wants me to go live with my uncle who is very tough. She is also planning to go for further studies abroad." 20-year old young man.

"[...] I had a tough childhood; my brother uses drugs and abuses me. I also lost my dad at a young age..." 22-year old female participant.

These vignettes point to grim interpersonal context that generate self-doubt and apathy in the participants.

Parental separation, unexpected death of a loved one, and protracted bereavement thereafter worsened the situation and the participants' mental health, as experienced by the young adults interviewed. Female participants echoed such experiences more than their male counterparts. Vignettes such as the following are testament to these early deprivations and adversities which they highlighted:

"My dad does not care. Since the illness started from childhood, he has never sent money for medication. He went and got another wife. He only sends money for food for me and my sister. But for my medication, he has never sent ... money. My mother who lives with me does not work. She is a house wife and depends on the small amount send my father..." 24-year old female participant diagnosed with epilepsy.

"[...] I used to love my father but when my sister was born, it's like he forgot about me. He only cared about her. I started talking to boys and eventually lost my virginity. I still feel bad about it..." 19-year old female participant.

"My mum died. I still don't know how to deal with that. She was the most important person in my life. Always cheering me... I was her only child. I have no dad. I felt lost and never gotten over this. I do not understand myself anymore." 25-year old female

participant.

At a fairly early age, the participants had to deal with situations that left them emotionally scarred. Seven of them had an early childhood experience that they attributed to be the cause of their mental illness that brought them to the hospital in the first place.

Adjustment and behavioral problems in school and college

This theme captured the participants' thoughts about the need to be accepted by peers, family, and teachers. It also demonstrated the difficulty one may have in finding a friend who would guide and influence in a positive way. As we learnt in our interviews that the participants were mostly connected with difficult conduct-related behaviors (externalizing tendencies) for which the youth were seeking support. These vignettes underscore these problems:

"My friend and I had a phone in school. During prep time, the teacher on duty caught us playing games. We have been suspended for 2 weeks and told to go back to our parents..." 19-year old female participant.

"I started taking alcohol after high school. I thought it was normal for those in university to take alcohol since now you are a grown-up and other people especially my friends were taking it. So I thought, why not join them? I hope to stop completely as it is the cause of Bell's palsy that I have now..." 21-year old male participant.

Familial challenges and lack of support in transitioning process

Most of our male participants expressed difficulties in overcoming life transitions and alluded to absence of support in navigating resultant challenges. Six participants described the challenges of transiting from one phase of life to another i.e. from childhood to demands and expectations of youth, while some struggled with fitting in their social milieu due to mental illness. The following vignette explained these challenges further:

"I repeated form IV then joined university where I am studying mass communication. In the first semester, I started having weird feelings and thoughts. I felt like I do not fit into the school culture. People were just having fun. Right left and center. Then I got myself in this group of girls who had money from their boyfriends and older men. I wish I did not join them. Somehow I lost my virginity....." 22-year female participant.

"I am not comfortable with my life. I have not achieved the things I have wanted to achieve. Just the way my life is going.....my career...Everything is moving slowly. Am in a stage where I want to do new things and find my own place in life" 24-year old male participant.

"Since I went to boarding school in class six my performance dropped and was always punished for it...." 20-year old male participant.

As a result of challenges in transitioning to new environments (e.g. day schooling to boarding), death of a loved one, and lack of finances or strained relationships with significant others, four of them described their poor academic performance as a cause of their psychological distress. Some maintained this to be the main cause of their mental illness while others thought if they had better upbringing or did not have to face difficulties in their childhood, they would have performed much better academically.

"I used to think a lot after failing my KCSE[1]. I was wondering what next? This is when I started having too much headache and a lot of fear." 22-year old female participant.

Strained relationships with parents and other family members

Four participants attributed a conflictual relationship with their caregiver as a leading cause of their psychological distress. Coming from unsupportive families, abusive parents or siblings, parent child discrimination or preferential treatment, parental divorce or marital conflicts were shared as being the primary trigger of their current psychological distress. A client reported to have hated the day her younger sister was born:

"Dad started neglecting me and it is like all the love I had for him ended. He still prefers my sister and I feel like she is more special than me. Maybe it is because she is named after mum to my dad." 19-year female participant.

A client reported to have had no connection with his mum due to lack of motherly affection and attention since he was very young:

"I grew up with my extended family since mum had travelled out of the country for further studies. When she came back, she was a stranger to me. We still do not have a relationship." 19-year old male participant.

---

[1] (KCSE) Kenya Certificate of Secondary Education: End of high school level examination.

The PTI question "Tell me about some (other) important experiences or events in your life that you associate
with your difficulties and how the problems began" was
the most relevant to this theme:

*"I stay with my mum and brother. We are not close
to each other and I am not free to talk to them since
they do not care about my opinion. I just keep quiet."*
20-year old male participant.

*"I am angry at my dad. Really very angry. He listens
to his relatives more than he listens to us. Like now I
wanted to go further my education in UK but a sister
to my dad said I should not go because I am epileptic. My dad agreed with her. He does not like supporting me. But one day I will prove them wrong. I
will work hard and show them that epileptic people
can do great in life."* 24-year old female participant.

Stigma and rejection from significant others and a tendency towards self-stigma

Five out of ten participants attributed discrimination and
stigma emanating from people around them as further
triggering their mental illness and distress. Rejection,
being teased, and feeling judged by relatives was common
among the five participants. Peer pressure was mostly
described by the participants with substance abuse.

The PTI question "In relation to the psychological
issues, what is your view on others and yourself?" is illustrated here:

*"When am alone, I feel great. But when am with my
mother [sic] I feel bad because my mum thinks am
unimportant."* 19 years old male participant.

*"My friends used to undermine me because my mum
was old, deaf and dumb. And we were very poor. I
had no friends when growing up. They hated me."*
25-year old female participant

The inability of a parent to care, address the participants' needs, or social problems negatively impacted the
psychological wellbeing of our participants. Four out of
the 10 participants interviewed shared their suffering
from low self-esteem because their families did not support them or had socioeconomic or psychological problems themselves. They feared disclosing their illness or
others knowing that they were seeking psychiatric help
as it would bring stigma. They attributed their distress to
rejection or discrimination.

*"I used to be an active child but am now introverted.
I do not want my friends to know that I came for
counselling. I also did not tell my mum........ Also,*

*when I feel like everyone knows am not a virgin. I
don't want to hang out with boys so that they do not
find out about this."* 19-year old female participant.

*"After being caught with bhang, people viewed me
as a peddler making me feel so bad and couldn't
face people after that incident. My self-esteem was
affected. Some friends deserted me."* 19-year old
male participant.

Biological conditions and psychopathologies limiting intervention

Three of our participants shared their struggle with
organic conditions such as Epilepsy, Bell's palsy, and Psychosis (under remission).

An Illustration from a participant with Epilepsy:

In response to PTI question "What are your thoughts
about the psychological issues you are experiencing?" this
is what a participant had to say:

*"I was diagnosed with epilepsy when I was a young
child. Growing up as an epileptic person is very challenging. People do not want to be associated with
you, my father does not care about me. Maybe he
thinks I am a burden, since he doesn't buy my medicine. Were it not for epilepsy, I would be so happy. I
have never been happy in my entire life. But I will
prove people wrong. I want to show them that I can
achieve my goals despite being epileptic."* 24-year old
female.

This led to experiences of anger and emotional discon-
tent in our participant. She went on to describe her pain
as being "too much to bear." She thought that her unhap-
piness was due to the fact that she has always been epileptic and having to face stigma from close relatives and
friends.

An Illustration from a participant with Bell's palsy:

In response to PTI question "What are your thoughts
about the psychological issues you are experiencing?"

*"I cannot feel one side of my mouth. It is not there.
I have gone for physiotherapy but still... so my dad
being a psychiatrist thought I counselling would
help solve the issue. But am fine. It is only this side
of the mouth that is bringing me down and I am not
myself."* 22-year old male

*An Illustration from a participant diagnosed with
Psychosis:*

In response to PTI question "What are your thoughts
about the psychological issues you are experiencing?"

*"......Then I started getting headaches. Too many
fears and thoughts. When I went to hospital, the doc-*

tor said I had psychosis. Yes I have tried to Google what that means. It is not easy to live with that and when you tell people they say you are 'chizzy' (means 'mad' in Kiswahili)." 22-year old female

From the quotes above, it is evident that in the mind of these patients there was a fear about their long term well-being and a feeling of stigmatization from other relatives that led the participants to be withdrawn.

Preferences and views on cure

Nine out of the ten participants interviewed reaffirmed the tremendous value of psychotherapy as the most effective mode of intervention. One of our participants had had psychotherapy earlier; this prompted him to initiate therapy when the need arose. The following treatment-related preferences stood out:

Affirmation of psychotherapy as the most appropriate and helpful intervention

Our participants wanted concrete ways to move on from their current situation by guidance and support from a professional. It shows how several participants wanted to engage in counselling and believed that they could learn and improve their life situations with the skills they would learn during treatment.

In response to PTI interview question, "What do you think is needed for your illness to be cured or might ease your pain?"

> "*My dad often takes us for counselling just to make sure all is well. Prayers are good but I prefer something tangible such as counselling.*" 22-year old male participant.

Others wanted to learn coping mechanisms—learning how to manage their feelings in a constructive way or focus on important things in their life.

> "*I believe I need to control myself with regards to my anger. The only person I cannot control is my dad. So I let him be. But I need to know how to stop over reacting when I get angry.*" 24-year old female participant.

Seven participants believed that their negative childhood experiences caused their problems and continued to affect them, and these needed to be managed in order to move on with life. In this regard, a 20-year old female participant, who lost her mum at a young age made the following remarks:

> "*I still do not know how to deal with her demise. I want to understand myself better and be more productive in life. I am growing old. I need to know how to deal with mum not being around.*"

She believed that working through her past experiences would lead to a more productive life and consequently enable her to be psychologically healthy. The participant stated that she needed the support from a professional in order to come to terms with her mum's death. These participants thought that positive coping mechanisms coming from interaction with a professional psychotherapist were important in reshaping their lives. Another 19-year old male participant who had been suspended from school said that peer pressure was a cause to his psychological and emotional pain:

> "*If I had listened to my inner voice that was telling me to avoid those guys, I would be so ok. I would be in school like other students. I will be attentive to my thoughts when asked to do something next time.*"

A 24-year old young woman participant considered going back to school so that she could be happy:

> "*If I get the scholarship to UK, I will be happy. I want to be a better person and be busy. Being busy has helped me a lot. Now I do not concentrate on dad not buying medicine. I also do some volunteering work and get paid. Being busy helps a lot. But when idle, I get to think a lot and get angry over small issues.*"

Being involved in activities that the participants enjoyed doing and being in tune with their own feelings and thoughts were related to having a positive mental health. In this regard, the treatment offered life skills and problem-solving strategies. Professional help was emphasized over other alternative means of coping by our young participants. Involvement in activities that did not yield positive impact brought in the need for counselling. For those with substance abuse problems, participating in support groups that could reverse negative peer influences was a viable solution to psychological challenges. One of the female participants had tried various solutions like going to church and talking to friends but that did not put an end to her distress or problems.

> "*I used to go to church and share with my girlfriends but I was not content. I also think peer counselling would also be good.*" 20-year old female.

> "*I tried alcohol, cigarettes and generally going out for social events to feel ok but the pain was too deep in me. Especially after losing my dad and the insults I get from my brother. But the drinks did not help....*" 19-year old female participant.

Other participants who had been in psychotherapy before shared that it had a life-changing positive impact. Another client preferred psychotherapy as opposed to talking to friends and relatives. Some participants were concerned about the side-effects of medication and preferred psychotherapy as it presented no such risk.

> *"I do not share my issues with other people. People are superficial and cannot be trusted. I prefer counselling. My friend had advised me to ask for anxiety drugs but I am not ready for medication..."* 22-year old male participant

We explored different strategies that participants had thought of and practiced to ease their pain. Those participants who had adjustment problems in school and got suspended on account of misconduct mentioned that they were more mindful of this and chose their friends carefully. Listening to parental advice, getting involved in extracurricular activities like sports, and making use of their talents were the strategies that the participants had put into consideration and practiced. They believed that this would not only make them better people, but also help them improve in school performance, time management, and forming bonds with people with whom they shared similar goals in life. Our participants alluded to the family therapy sessions that were organized to address interpersonal problems and so their challenges were relayed to their caregivers. One of our participant echoes this further:

> *"If possible, I will ask my mum to come with me in next session. May be if the counsellor told her that I cannot be like her she will understand and stop being too harsh on me and having so high expectations form me."* 9-year old male participant

Valuing psychopharmacological support in their overall treatment

While we found a lot of validation of the psychotherapeutic treatments our participants received, one male participant particularly emphasized his preference for medication as a form of treatment during the interview saying:

> *"I am not a people person at all. Am hoping to be given some stress medicine and I will be good. Talking to people feels strange especially for a man. Men do not share their personal information."* 20-year old male participant diagnosed with major depressive disorder.

Discussion

We used a bifocal theoretical approach to guide this inquiry on attributions and private theories of mental illness amongst young adults. Weiner's attributional model [16] guided our conceptual model as we looked

at four domains: locus of control (internal vs. external), controllability of events (controllable vs. uncontrollable), stability of life circumstances (stable or unstable). Stigma (self/internal vs. external) was added as an independent domain given that mental illness can be highly stigmatizing in the Kenyan cultural context. The attributions were studied within the PTI-P [23]. In this process, we have tried to demonstrate that the attributional framework can help expand patients' private theories/experiences about their problems and perceived solutions.

Internal and external locus of control

In the present study, participants with an internal locus of control were relatively more resourceful in controlling their own behaviors once they were introduced to psychotherapy. The participants with an external locus of control do not have a determined role in shaping their response or energies towards a specific experience [36]. This implies that such individuals do not develop a sense of responsibility in establishing their own coping mechanisms and behavioral pathways, and hence their behaviors are shaped more in relation to the perceptions and interpretations of other people [37]. Consequently, we suspect, such individuals take longer to identify how the change could be made. Several studies have pointed to the interrelationship between increased levels of general self-efficacy, problem-oriented coping strategy, and internal locus of control as protective factors in bolstering mental health [38] and external locus of control is a good predictor of low mental health [39]. In a British study, one of the factors which facilitated the UK military personnel with post-traumatic stress disorder to engage in help-seeking behaviors was the sense of internal locus of control [40]. A case in point is that feelings of anger, fear, and thoughts of being unwell or the need to deal with one's stressors are some of the internal/dispositional factors leading to treatment-seeking behavior. These participants were well in control of their feelings and thoughts. However, their psychological stressors had roots in some external, uncontrollable traumatic factors such as separation from parents, death of a loved one, and excessive stigmatization and discrimination from others. In Julian B. Rotter's [41] explanation of external locus of control, events or outcomes depend on factors managed by environmental powers such as destiny or fortune outside of individual's control [42]. The skills of problem-solving and positive thinking offered in therapy provided one mechanism to cope given these adverse circumstances in the lives of our participants. For instance, participants, who spoke of their childhood experiences or stigma from the public, viewed these challenges as stemming from an outward cause (external locus of control) rather than from within their own thoughts, feelings, or behaviors. Those who attributed psychological problems internally spoke more of their negative thoughts and feelings leading them to experience a psychological problem. It is likely that those with an external locus of control will experience greater challenges with problem-focused coping when stressed.

Further implications of internal locus of control

Bitterness and hatred are internal processes. Each participant had a need for letting go of these emotional struggles [18]. Putting into consideration that these are within a person's internal locus of control explains our *second conjecture that the internal locus of control might be positively associated with early positive engagement with one's treatment such that it facilitates emotional regulation* and re-channeled our participants' efforts in the face of external stressors. One of the participants, as quoted above, sought help on how to manage her anger. She shared that anger was the reason why she could not deal with daily life challenges but instead had outbursts that accelerated the problem.

Stigmatizing contexts and relationships

Stigma can lead to excessive feelings of contempt and anger that triggers hostile behavior and other externalizing symptoms [43]. Unlike physical disabilities, persons with mental illness are perceived to be in control of their disabilities and be responsible for causing them. Furthermore, people are less likely to pity persons with psychiatric illness, instead reacting to psychiatric disability with anger and believing that help is not deserved [44]. This sentiment was also echoed by our research participants. For example, one of the participants attributed her psychological distress to being stigmatized by both family members and friends because of her epilepsy. Her father neglected her by not buying her medication and failing to pay her school fees. Another young participant shared that she had not told any of her friends or relatives about her decision to visit the clinic. She did not want people to know that she was seeking psychological help to avoid being labelled a mentally ill person.

Discrimination can also appear in public opinion about how to treat people with mental illness. For example, one client reported withdrawing from family functions due to stigma and discrimination from his immediate family members and relatives. It is worth noting that the behavioral impact (or discrimination) that results from public stigma may take four forms: withholding help, avoidance, coercive treatment, and segregated institutions [45]. Research also suggests that, instead of being diminished by the stigma, many persons become righteously angry because of the bias that they experienced [46]. This kind

of reaction empowers people to change their roles in the mental health system, becoming more active participants in their treatment plan and often pushing for improvements in the quality of services [44]. It is due to these external attributions (stigma from others) that various participants we interviewed felt the need to seek therapy and were quite committed to it. Hence, it can be argued that the participants viewed this external attribution as an unstable attribution factor that could be changed through therapy. Thus this was a controllable attribution as well, since they thought that by being in therapy, they were at a higher position of controlling how they felt and even reacted towards stigma from others.

Self-stigma and its links with attribution of controllability

An alternative reaction to anger about stigma is to turn prejudice inwards as self-discrimination. Research suggests self-stigma and fear of rejection by others lead people to quit pursuing life opportunities for themselves [47]. Self-esteem suffers, as does confidence in one's future, as indicated by participants interviewed in this study. Some felt lost and wanted to find their place in society. An individual with mental illness may experience diminished self-esteem/self-efficacy, anger, or relative indifference depending on the parameters of the situation [48].

Cognitive theories of depression argue that beliefs of low self-worth and the tendency to attribute negative events to causes that are global (widespread rather than specific) and stable (will persist rather than change in the future) is associated with the development of depressed mood (Pearson et al. 2015). In our interviews, self-esteem was viewed as proportionally connected to the distress one experienced: the more the distress the poorer the self-esteem. One of our participants shared that she sought therapy to regain self-esteem and confidence. Therefore, self-stigma was an internal attribution that was viewed as a reason for seeking help since it was within the participants' ability to be in control.

In the present study, prominent bio-psychosocial explanations of mental illness were identified from our ten participants. Previous research shows that patients tend to have more than one causal explanation for their mental illness [33]; an observation that echoes in our study too. Our participants attributed their problems to more than one cause.

Studies carried out in high-income countries [49] about public views regarding causes of mental illnesses reported that people predominantly held beliefs on mental illness to be social factors such as stressful life events, traumatic experiences, family problems, and social disadvantage [49–52]. Research carried out by Muga and Jenkins [3], Ikwuka et al. [53], and Samouilhan and Seabi [54] show that in Western contexts people might hold more biological explanations for their mental illness and increasingly seek medicines for these biological causes. However, in our study we noticed that whilst some of our participants had conditions that have biological determinants, the interface with therapy and work on psychosocial stressors remained the articulated needs of our participants.

Studies by Thwaites et al. [55] in UK and by Adewuya and Makanjuola, [56] in South Eastern Nigeria found that their participants attributed mental illnesses more to external than internal causes. Lingman and Lydén [33] found that causes such as poverty and negative family upbringing were common risk factors amongst young adults who sought psychological help. Environmental and social attributions have been identified as commonly seen stressors and our participants expressed similar concerns. In Ghana, for instance, participants mentioned issues such as unhealthy living conditions, lack of social support, relationships problems, society pressures, loneliness, and failure in life as reasons for becoming mentally ill [57].

A large community survey done in Nigeria [58] found that as many as one-third of the respondents suggested that possession by evil spirits could be a cause of mental illness, which was not the case in this present study. We suspect that as our work involved young adults' under-30 years of age, the belief in spirit possession and traditional healing might not be as common as it might be in older people. More recent studies from Ethiopia showed inclusion of biological and psychosocial factors as explanations of mental disturbances in addition to the age-old spiritual and magical views [59]. Similarly a survey from a small town in Western Ethiopia reported psychosocial problems such as poverty, stress, and drug abuse as common explanations for mental illness in addition to explanations from religious/magical views such as God's will or an attack by the evil spirit [60]. Another finding from North-western Ethiopia was that psychosocial and supernatural retribution were predominant explanations of mental illness, but less common for physical illnesses [61]. Mamah et al. [62] carried out a study on Kenyan youths' perceptions about mental illness where they found that spiritual explanations were highly prevalent. However, in contrast to our study, the attribution to a spiritual cause was not alluded to, which is also similar to the findings by Ikwuka et al. [53]. This study was carried out at a public hospital based in the country capital and the participants interviewed had acquired a high school education with free access to the services offered at the hospital's youth clinic; these factors may have influenced findings. In addition, we did not specifically explore spiritual attribution further in our interviewing.

Meyer and Garcia-Roberts [63] reported that the participants in their study preferred 'sharing and talking through their distresses as a cathartic and helpful strategy.' In our study, nine participants had tried other mediums of support such as prayers, focusing on their unique talent, avoiding bad company, and taking note of parental advice. In some ways, there was a development of an internal locus of control before they sought help from the health services. It could also be that there was a feeling that none of this could be sustained without adequate motivation and support that a professional could lend. This was a theme echoed by several participants of our study.

In a study from Pakistan, nearly half of the respondents reported psychiatric consultation to be the single most important management step [64]. This shows that people living in non-western countries endorse modern western medical care for mental health problems in addition to other more indigenous methods. Our participants tended to be contemplative and open-minded in seeking professional medical and psychosocial help for their mental illness, for which they were also willing to try various remedies for cure. Their views tended to be dynamic and agreeable to change, such as doing away with unwanted behavior that was a result of peer pressure in school. This is similar to other findings from non-western countries [65]. However, in our study it was evident that the private theories of several participants were influenced by Western views of pathogenesis and cure for mental illness. The apparent existence of Western conceptions could be the result of the participants being, what Sunday and Ibadan [66] describes as 'transitional Africans'. Transitional Africans have received a Western education and, therefore, often incorporate both the African and Western values. We found this flexibility in thinking very heartening and felt that our participants understood their problems and appraised solutions in fairly multidimensional ways.

Conclusions

Most research about etiological beliefs have investigated peoples' beliefs about mental illness in general but there is virtually no scholarship on young peoples' private theories of their own mental illness in Kenya. We have provided subjective explanations of Kenyan youths' perceptions of their mental illness. Three key themes, psychosocial triggers of distress, biological conditions, and psychopathologies limiting interventions and subjective views on cure were private theories that we unpacked. When these private theories were mapped onto the attributional framework we imposed on the PTI-P we found that those who attributed their distress to an internal locus of control had a positive outlook towards therapy and behavior change. External factors were mainly ascribed to be the cause of negative emotions and thoughts leading to psychological illness. Stigma and self-stigma particularly were challenging attributions that needed socio-cultural awareness and youth empowerment work. Our limited data suggests that certain aspects of our participants' lives emanated from uncontrollable events that shaped their locus of control to be externalized. Mental health care of young adults could benefit from exploration of their personal beliefs and attributions about their illness and cure in order to provide the best-adapted treatment for them and consequently make the mental health care more attuned to their concerns and needs.

Limitations and next steps

We interviewed participants after they had a psychotherapy session with their therapist and diagnoses were already established by then. This might have influenced the clients' thoughts and perceptions on mental illness and cure. However, the designed interview guide was structured in such a way that the client's personal perceptions on these issues were explored, independent from therapist's thoughts. The study was carried out in an urban setting with young adults, hence cannot be entirely generalized to youth living in rural or remote setting who may experience unique challenges in addition to their illness or those living in more marginal conditions, however the clinic serves as a referral for clients from all over the country. The experiences of our participants would most likely generalize to some other participants in the population.

We strongly feel that focusing on addressing experiences of young people in phenomenological ways offer insights into their psychosocial and intrapsychic processes. Future research efforts should be directed towards using this approach to understand attributions of mental illness in young people in diverse contexts, and more research is needed from resource-scarce context to understand mental health service implementation challenges. We believe that mental health needs of young people is an area requiring further phenomenological grounded theory based research. Such exercises would build an edifice of theoretical constructs useful for understanding what mental health, mental illness, and psychotherapies mean for young people in Kenya. And the findings from such studies may have wider resonance in other parts of Africa, too.

Abbreviations
AFQ: Attributions Focused Question guide; ERC: Ethics Review Committee; HIV: human immunodeficiency virus; IPA: interpretative phenomenological analysis; KNH: Kenyatta National Hospital; LoC: locus of control; PTI-P: private theories interview-patient version; UK: United Kingdom; UoN: University of Nairobi; VCT: voluntary counselling and testing; YLD: years lived with disability.

Authors' contributions
JWM carried out the research as a fulfillment of the Masters of Science in clinical psychology at the University of Nairobi, department of psychiatry. MK was her primary mentor who helped with conceptualizing and analyzing the study, CO was the second mentor to JWM and helped with translation of the tool and proofreading the manuscript, FF was the third mentor who helped in conceptualizing and proofreading the manuscript, MWK helped in proof reading the manuscript. All authors read and approved the final manuscript.

Author details
[1] Department of Psychiatry, College of Health Sciences, University of Nairobi, P.O.Box 19676, Nairobi 00202, Kenya. [2] Research Department of Clinical Health and Educational Psychology, University College London, Gower Street, London WC1E 6BT, UK. [3] Department of Behavioural Sciences and Learning, Linköping University, Linköping, Sweden.

Acknowledgements
We thank all the participants who took part in the research interviews making this study possible and to the clinicians and staff members at the Youth Clinic run by the Department of Mental Health, Kenyatta National Hospital who facilitated data collection. Acknowledgements are also due to the direct and indirect support of the three grants mentioned above.

Competing interests
The authors declare that they have no competing interests.

Funding
JWM received seed funding from NIMH funded Partnership for Mental Health Development in Sub-Saharan Africa (PaMD), CJO is a Co-I on the PaMD project and MK was awarded PRIME-K seed award as part of NIH funded MEPI/PRIME-K AWARD NUMBER 1R24TW008889.

References
1. Boldero J, Fallon B. Adolescent help-seeking: what do they get help for and from whom? J Adolesc. 1995;18:193–209. https://doi.org/10.1006/jado.1995.1013.
2. Jenkins R, Othieno C, Okeyo S, Aruwa J, Wallcraft J, Jenkins B. Exploring the perspectives and experiences of health workers at primary health facilities in Kenya following training. Int J Ment Health Syst. 2013;7(1):6. https://doi.org/10.1186/1752-4458-7-6.
3. Muga FA, Jenkins R. Public perceptions, explanatory models and service utilisation regarding mental illness and mental health care in Kenya. Soc Psychiatry Psychiatr Epidemiol. 2008;43(6):469–76. https://doi.org/10.1007/s00127-008-0334-0.
4. Musyimi CW, Mutiso VN, Nandoya ES, Ndetei DM. Forming a joint dialogue among faith healers, traditional healers and formal health workers in mental health in a Kenyan setting: towards common grounds.

J Ethnobiol Ethnomed. 2016;12(1):4. https://doi.org/10.1186/s1300 2-015-0075-6.

5. Helman CG. Culture, Health and Illness. Boca Raton: CRC Press; 2007. https://doi.org/10.1016/B978-0-7236-1991-8.50008-5.

6. Ndetei DM, Khasakhala LI, Mutiso V, Mbwayo AW. Knowledge, attitude and practice (KAP) of mental illness among staff in general medical facilities in Kenya: practice and policy implications. Afr J Psychiatry. 2011;14:225–35. https://doi.org/10.4314/ajpsy.v14i3.6.

7. Vaughn L, Jacquez F, Baker R. Cultural health attributions, beliefs, and practices: effects on healthcare and medical education. Open Med Educ J. 2009;2:64–74. https://doi.org/10.2174/1876519X00902010064.

8. O'Driscoll C, Heary C, Hennessy E, McKeague L. Adolescents' beliefs about the fairness of exclusion of peers with mental health problems. J Adolesc. 2015;42:59–67. https://doi.org/10.1016/j.adolescence.2015.03.008.

9. Balhara YPS, Yadav T. A comparative study of beliefs, attitudes and behaviour of psychiatric patients and their care givers with regards to magico-religious and supernatural influences. J Med Sci. 2012;12(1):10–7. https://doi.org/10.3923/jms.2012.I0.I7.

10. Charlson FJ, Diminic S, Lund C, Degenhardt L, Whiteford HA. Mental and substance use disorders in sub-Saharan Africa : predictions of epidemiological changes and mental health workforce requirements for the next 40 years. Open Access. 2014;9(10):1–11.

11. Falkenstrom F, Gee MD, Kuria MW, Othieno CJ, Kumar M. Improving the effectiveness of psychotherapy in two public hospitals in Nairobi. BJPsych Int. 2017;14(3):64–6.

12. Affairs S. The situation faced by young people in Kenya. Un-Published, 12–37. 2005. Retrieved from http://siteresources.worldbank.org. Accessed 26 Feb 2018.

13. Khasakhala L, Ndetei DM, Mathai M, Harder V. Major depressive disorder in a Kenyan youth sample: relationship with parenting behavior and parental psychiatric disorders. Ann Gen Psychiatry. 2013;12(1):15. https://doi.org/10.1186/1744-859X-12-15.

14. Muthee MW. Hitting the target, missing the point: youth policies and programmes in Kenya. Washington DC. 2010. Retrieved from https://www.wilsoncenter.org. Accessed 26 Feb 2018.

15. Philips B, Wennberg P, Werbart A. Ideas of cure as a predictor of premature termination, early alliance and outcome in psychoanalytic psychotherapy. Psychol Psychother. 2007;80(2):229–45. https://doi.org/10.1348/147608306X128266.

16. Weiner B. A cognitive (attribution)-emotion-action model of motivated behavior: an analysis of judgments of help-giving. J Pers Soc Psychol. 1980;39(2):186–200. https://doi.org/10.1037/0022-3514.39.2.186.

17. Werbart A. How do you understand and explain to yourself your problems and difficulties? British psychological society conference proceedings, 2006. p. 1–5.

18. Weiner B. An attributional theory of achievement motivation and emotion. Psychol Rev. 1985;92(4):548–73. https://doi.org/10.1037/0033-295X.92.4.548.

19. Galvin KM, Coope PJ. Making connections: reading in rational communication. 4th ed. Los Angeles: Roxbury Publishing Company; 2006.

20. Fritz Heider, Folkes V, Koletsky S, Graham J, Sherman SJ, Presson CC, Oliver R. The psychology of interpersonal relations. J Market. 1958;56:322. https://doi.org/10.1037/0022-3514.46.1.57.

21. Jones EE, Davis KE. From acts to dispositions: the attributional process in person perception. Adv Exp Soc Psychol. 1965. https://doi.org/10.1017/CBO9781107415324.004.

22. Kelley H. Attribution theory in social psychology. Nebraska Symp Motiv. 1976;15:192–238.

23. Weiner B, Perry RP, Magnusson J. An attributional analysis of reactions to stigmas. J Pers Soc Psychol. 1988;55:738–48. https://doi.org/10.1177/0146167295215004.

24. Försterling F. Attribution: an introduction to theories, research, and applications. Hove: Psychology Press; 2001.

25. Millman ZB, Weintraub MJ, Bentley E, DeVylder JE, Mittal VA, Pitts SC, Schiffman J. Differential relations of locus of control to perceived social stress among help-seeking adolescents at low vs. high clinical risk of psychosis. Schizophr Res. 2017. https://doi.org/10.1016/j.schres.2016.12.006.

26. Donaldson P, Best T, Langham ME, Browne M, Oorloff MA. Developing and validating a scale to measure the enacted and felt stigma of gambling. 2015. Retrieved from https://www.responsiblegambling.vic.gov.au. Accessed 26 Feb 2018.

27. Major B, O'Brien LT. The social psychology of stigma. Ann Rev Psychol 2005;56:393–421. https://doi.org/10.2307/3089335

28. Rüsch N, Angermeyer MC, Corrigan PW. Mental illness stigma: concepts, consequences, and initiatives to reduce stigma. Eur Psychiatry. 2005. https://doi.org/10.1016/j.eurpsy.2005.04.004.

29. Makanjuola V, Esan Y, Oladeji B, Kola L, Appiah-Poku J, Harris B, Gureje O. Explanatory model of psychosis: impact on perception of self-stigma by patients in three Sub-Saharan African cities. Soc Psychiatry Psychiatr Epidemiol. 2016;51(12):1645–54. https://doi.org/10.1007/s00127-016-1274-8.

30. Ssebunnya J, Kigozi F, Lund C, Kizza D, Okello E. Stakeholder perceptions of mental health stigma and poverty in Uganda. BMC Int Health Hum Rights. 2009;9:5. https://doi.org/10.1186/1472-698X-9-5.

31. Corrigan PW, Druss BG, Perlick DA. The impact of mental illness stigma on seeking and participating in mental health care. Psychol Sci Public Interest. 2014;15(2):37–70. https://doi.org/10.1177/1529100614531398.

32. Corrigan PW, Larson JE, Rüsch N. Self-stigma and the "why try" effect: impact on life goals and evidence-based practices. World Psychiatry. 2009;8(2):75–81. https://doi.org/10.1002/j.2051-5545.2009.tb00218.x.

33. Lingman M, Lydén J. Private theories about pathogenesis and cure among young psychiatric patients in Kenya—a thematic analysis. Linköpings universitet: Linköping; 2015.

34. Smith JA, Eatough V. Interpretative phenomenological analysis. Thousand Oaks: Sage Publications; 2007. p. 179–94. https://doi.org/10.4135/97818 48607927.n11.

35. Smith JA, Osborn M. Interpretative phenomenological analysis. In: Smith JA, editor. Qualitative psychology: a practical guide to research methods. 2nd ed. London: SAGE; 2008. P. 53–80.

36. Aslan Ş. The effect of self-emotion appraisal and external locus of control on problem-focused coping with stress. Munich: The Clute Institute; 2014. p. 599–606.

37. Mihaela PL, Magdalenaa SM, Loredanaa TS. A study on the relation between locus of control and creative attitudes in the structure of didactic competence. Procedia Soc Behav Sci. 2013;84:1381–5.

38. Bavojdan Rabani M, Towhidi A, Rahmati A. The relationship between mental health and general self-efficacy beliefs, coping strategies and locus of control in male drug abusers. Addict Health. 2011;3(3–4):111–8.

39. Gale CR, Batty GD, Deary IJ. Locus of control at age 10 years and health outcomes and behaviors at age 30 years: the 1970 British cohort study. Psychosom Med. 2008;70(4):397–403. https://doi.org/10.1097/PSY.0b013 e31816a719e.

40. Rudnick A, Montgomery P, Coatsworth-puspoky R, Cohen B, Forchuk C, Lahey P, Schofield R. Exploring positive pathways to care for members of the UK armed forces receiving treatment for PTSD: a qualitative study. Eur J Psychotraumatol. 2014;22(2):147–57. https://doi.org/10.3402/ejpt.v5.21759.

41. Rotter JB. Generalize d expectancies for internal versus external control of reinforcement. Psychol Monogr. 1966;80(1):1–28.

42. Wallston KA, Wallston BS, DeVellis R. Development of the multidimensional health locus of control (MHLC) scales. Health Educ Monogr. 19/8;6:160–70. https://doi.org/10.11//10901981/800600107.

43. Corrigan PW, Watson AC. The paradox of self-stigma and mental illness. Clin Psychol Sci Pract. 2002;9(1):35–53. https://doi.org/10.1093/clips y/9.1.35.

44. Corrigan PW. Empowerment and serious mental illness: treatment partnerships and community opportunities. Psychiatr Q. 2002;73(3):217–28. https://doi.org/10.1023/A:1016040805432.

45. Bede CA, Francis U. Demographic determinants of public perceptions of mental illness in heterogeneous communities of Lagos State Nigeria. Adv Soc Sci Res J. 2015;2(1):1–10. https://doi.org/10.14738/assrj.21.575.

46. Crocker J, Major B. Social stigma and self-esteem: the self-protective properties of stigma. Psychol Rev. 1989;96(4):608–30. https://doi.org/10.1037/0033-295X.96.4.608.

47. Ngui E, Khasakhala L, Ndetei D, Weiss Roberts L. Mental disorders, health inequalities and ethics: a global perspective. Int Rev Psychiatry. 2010;22:235–44. https://doi.org/10.3109/09540261.2010.485273.

48. Pescosolido BA. The stigma complex. Ann Rev Sociol. 2015;41:87–116. https://doi.org/10.1146/annurev-soc-071312-145702.The.

49. Furnham A, Chan E. Lay theories of schizophrenia—a cross-cultural comparison of British and Hong Kong Chinese attitudes, attributions and beliefs. Soc Psychiatry Psychiatr Epidemiol. 2004;39(7):543–52. https://doi.org/10.1007/s00127-004-0787-8.

50. Magliano L, Fiorillo A, De Rosa C, Malangone C, Maj M. Beliefs about schizophrenia in Italy: a comparative nationwide survey of the general public, mental health professionals, and patients' relatives. Can J Psychiatry (Revue Canadienne de Psychiatrie). 2004;49(5):322–30.

51. Angermeyer MC, Matschinger H. Causal beliefs and attitudes to people with schizophrenia: rend analysis based on data from two population surveys in Germany. Br J Psychiatry. 2005;186:331–4.

52. Nakane Y, Jorm AF, Yoshioka K, Christensen H, Nakane H, Griffiths KM. Public beliefs about causes and risk factors for mental disorders: a comparison of Japan and Australia. BMC Psychiatry. 2005;5(1):33. https://doi.org/10.1186/1471-244X-5-33.

53. Ikwuka U, Galbraith N, Nyatanga L. Causal attribution of mental illness in South-Eastern Nigeria. Int J Soc Psychiatry. 2013;60(3):274–9. https://doi.org/10.1177/0020764013485331.

54. Samouilhan T, Seabi J. University students' beliefs about the causes and treatments of mental illness. S Afr J Psychol. 2010;40(1):74–89. https://doi.org/10.1177/008124631004000108.

55. Thwaites R, Dagnan D, Huey D, Addis ME. The reasons for depression questionnaire (RFD): UK standardization for clinical and non-clinical populations. Psychol Psychother. 2004;77(Pt 3):363–74. https://doi.org/10.1348/1476083041839367.

56. Adewuya AO, Makanjuola ROA. Lay beliefs regarding causes of mental illness in Nigeria: pattern and correlates. Soc Psychiatry Psychiatr Epidemiol. 2008;43:336–41. https://doi.org/10.1007/s00127-007-0305-x.

57. Kyei JJ, Dueck A, Indart MJ, Nyarko NY. Supernatural belief systems, mental health and perceptions of mental disorders in Ghana. Int J Cult Ment Health. 2014;7(2):137–51. https://doi.org/10.1080/17542863.2012.734838.

58. Gureje O, Lasebikan VO, Ephraim-Oluwanuga O, Olley BO, Kola L. Community study of knowledge of and attitude to mental illness in Nigeria. Br J Psychiatry. 2005;186:436–41. https://doi.org/10.1192/bjp.186.5.436.

59. Astalin PK. Qualitative research designs: a conceptual framework. Int J Soc Sci Interdiscip Res. 2013;2(1):118–24.

60. Mulatu MS. Perceptions of mental and physical illnesses in North-western Ethiopia: causes, treatments, and attitudes. Journal of Health Psychology. 1999;4(4):531–49. https://doi.org/10.1177/135910539900400407.

61. Teferra S, Shibre T. Perceived causes of severe mental disturbance and preferred interventions by the Borana semi-nomadic population in southern Ethiopia: a qualitative study. BMC Psychiatry. 2012;12(1):79. https://doi.org/10.1186/1471-244X-12-79.

62. Mamah D, Striley CW, Ndetei DM, Mbwayo AW, Mutiso VN, Khasakhala LI, Cottler LB. Knowledge of psychiatric terms and concepts among Kenyan youth: analysis of focus group discussions. Transcult Psychiatry. 2013;50(4):515–31. https://doi.org/10.1177/1363461513499809.

63. Meyer B, Garcia-Roberts L. Congruence between reasons for depression and motivations for specific interventions. Psychol Psychother. 2007;80(Pt 4):525–42. https://doi.org/10.1348/147608306X169982.

64. Zafar SN, Syed R, Tehseen S, Gowani SA, Waqar S, Zubair A, Naqvi H. Perceptions about the cause of schizophrenia and the subsequent help seeking behavior in a Pakistani population—results of a cross-sectional survey. BMC Psychiatry. 2008;8:56. https://doi.org/10.1186/1471-244X-8-56.

65. Saravanan B, Jacob KS, Deepak MG, Prince M, David AS, Bhugra D. Perceptions about psychosis and psychiatric services: a qualitative study from Vellore, India. Soc Psychiatry Psychiat Epidemiol. 2008;43(3):231–8. https://doi.org/10.1007/s00127-007-0292-y.

66. Sunday E, Ibadan I. Mental health and psychotherapy. Through the eyes of culture: lessons for African psychotherapy. Trans Nr. 2016;15:1–11.

13

A program of family-centered care for adolescents in short-term stay groups of juvenile justice institutions

Inge Simons[1]*[iD], Eva Mulder[1,2], René Breuk[2], Kees Mos[3], Henk Rigter[1], Lieke van Domburgh[2,4] and Robert Vermeiren[1,4]

Abstract

Background: To provide successful treatment to detained adolescents, staff in juvenile justice institutions need to work in family-centered ways. As juvenile justice institutions struggled to involve parents in their child's treatment, we developed a program for family-centered care.

Methods: The program was developed in close collaboration with staff from the two juvenile justice institutions participating in the Dutch Academic Workplace Forensic Care for Youth. To achieve an attainable program, we chose a bottom-up approach in which ideas for family-centered care were detailed and discussed by workgroups consisting of group leaders, family therapists, psychologists, other staff, researchers, and a parent.

Results: The family-centered care program distinguishes four categories of parental participation: (a) informing parents, (b) parents meeting their child, (c) parents meeting staff, and (d) parents taking part in the treatment program. Additionally, the family-centered care program includes the option to start family therapy during detention of the youths, to be continued after discharge from the juvenile justice institutions. Training and coaching of staff are core components of the family-centered care program.

Conclusions: The combination of training and the identification of attainable ways for staff to promote parental involvement makes the family-centered care program valuable for practice. Because the program builds on suggestions from previous research and on the theoretical background of evidence-based family therapies, it has potential to improve care for detained adolescents and their parents. Further research is required to confirm if this assumption is correct.

Keywords: Family-centered care, Delinquent adolescents, Youth detention centers, Parental participation

Background

Treating incarcerated adolescents effectively requires involving their parents [22]. When treating delinquent youth, both protective and risk factors within the family domain must be addressed. Protective family factors include parental support, positive family interactions, personal assets of family members, future orientation of family members, and the family's support network [6, 15]. Risk factors include lack of parental monitoring or inept discipline, poor family functioning, maltreatment, low family affection and warmth, and parental problems such as drug (ab)use, psychopathology, and criminal activity [6, 21, 33, 47]. If the family of the delinquent adolescent is not given appropriate attention, poor family functioning is likely to persist, influencing the prospect of the youth to get involved in the juvenile justice system [8, 9, 20, 34].

Involving parents in juvenile justice is considered important for promoting positive child and family outcomes [7, 53]. Family-centered approaches were shown to decrease youth recidivism [13, 24]. A recent

*Correspondence: I.Simons@curium.nl
[1] Department of Child and Adolescent Psychiatry, Curium-Leiden University Medical Center, Post Box 15, 2300 AA Leiden, The Netherlands
Full list of author information is available at the end of the article

meta-analysis has shown that adolescents with severe behavior problems benefit more from family therapy compared to their peers with less severe behavior problems [49]. Notwithstanding the evidence, there is a lack of active and positive parental involvement in the juvenile justice system [35]. Intervention programs offered to adolescents in youth detention institutions all too often do not adequately address the youth's family [47]. Treatment instructions for involving parents of youths involved in the juvenile justice system are missing [7, 14, 29]. Until recently in the Netherlands, parents were kept at a distance and were hardly involved in their child's treatment during detention in a Juvenile Justice Institution (JJI) [39, 50]. The resulting gap between home and the JJI is likely to impair rehabilitation after detention. When families are not engaged in treatment during detention, it is difficult to convince them to take part in family-based outpatient treatment interventions [32].

Realizing the importance of involving parents, Dutch JJIs incorporated a few family-oriented activities in their usual care program. These activities included staff calling parents once a week or inviting parents to key meetings where the intervention plan for their child is being discussed [46]. Although promising, JJIs were found to not properly adhere to these instructions for involving parents [18]. Ways to involve parents were not systematically implemented in practice and staff were not properly trained in working with parents. Therefore, in 2011, the Netherlands Government issued a national position paper encouraging JJIs to improve parental participation [39]. This paper however only sketched a broad perspective, which needed to be detailed for implementation in everyday practice. Therefore, we took up the challenge to improve care in JJIs by developing the program for family-centered care (FC). Most youths in JJIs are initially detained in a short-term stay group, for a maximum period of 90 days, awaiting the final ruling of the juvenile judge. The judge may decide that the adolescent is to be released, or to be detained longer. In the latter instance, the adolescent usually is transferred to a long-term stay group for detention lasting many months or years [40]. We developed two versions of FC, one for short-term stay groups and one for long-term stay groups. The present paper discusses the short-term stay version.

Methods
The development of the FC program was one of the projects of the Academic Workplace Forensic Care for Youth (in Dutch: AWFZJ). The AWFZJ aims to bridge the gap between practice, research, education, and policy in forensic youth care by carrying out practice-based research. Two JJIs, two universities, two centers for child and adolescent psychiatry, and two universities of applied

sciences in the Netherlands collaborate in this workplace to improve care for forensic youth and to reduce recidivism. The AWFZJ aims to translate research results into practice. In our study protocol paper, we describe the full background and methods of our study on FC [40].

We have developed the FC program in close collaboration with staff from the two JJIs participating in the AWFZJ. The family work in our program was based on the theory and practice of two evidence-based therapies, i.e., multidimensional family therapy, MDFT [26] and functional family therapy, FFT [2]. Main points of the underlying theory are [25, 37, 44]:

- The problem behavior of the adolescent, delinquency in this instance, is shaped by risk and protective factors from all major social domains of which he or she is part: the person himself, family, friends and peers, school and work, leisure time environments, and justice and probation authorities, including the JJI staff. These domains influence each other constantly and all these domains must be targeted to achieve lasting treatment success. Reinforcing protective factors will serve as a buffer against the influence of risk factors.

- Most adolescent problem behavior consists of a combination of troubles, e.g., delinquency, substance abuse, truancy, and comorbid mental health problems. Epidemiological models have shown that these problem behaviors tend to reinforce each other, which jeopardizes treatment attempts. Therefore, JJI staff and therapists need to address the full array of problems, at the individual level of the adolescent, and any other level, including the family.

- Family therapy has a relational focus. Besides focusing on the family and family relationships, the therapist also works with the other social domains. According to theoretical notions, lack of knowledge about problem behavior among youths, parents, and staff, family malfunctioning, and poor communication between family members all have been found to contribute to the incidence and persistence of adolescent problem behavior. This calls for (psycho-)education, training family members to properly communicate with each other, and training the parents in parental skills, such as setting and enforcing home rules.

- Key to effective interventions is motivating the adolescent and the parents to take part in FC and eventually in family therapy. Treatment motivation cannot be taken for granted. Motivating the adolescent and parents to join FC activities and family interventions takes time and requires a thorough understanding of the pathways leading to problematic behavior. The theory underlying family therapy further encour-

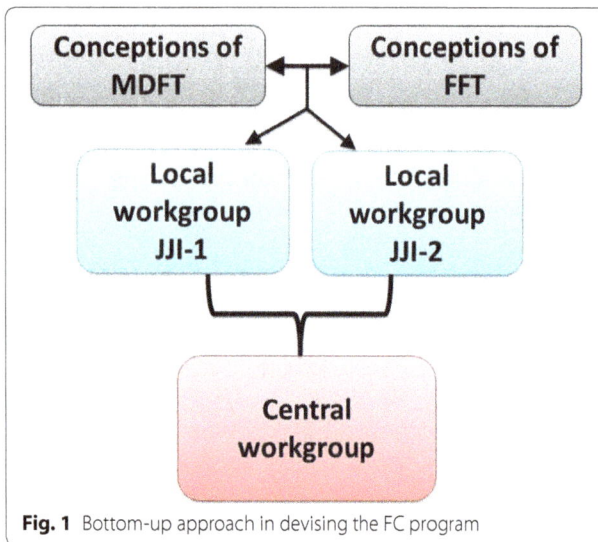

Fig. 1 Bottom-up approach in devising the FC program

ages the therapist to bond with both the adolescent and his parents in a committed, but neutral way. In other words, therapists—but also any other JJI staff—need to establish non-conflicting therapeutic alliances with both the youth and the parents.

We discussed the family therapy insights in workgroups of JJI group leaders, family therapists, psychologists, other JJI staff, and researchers. Based on these insights, ideas for FC were detailed and discussed. As applicability in practice was an important goal for the AWFZJ, we chose a bottom-up approach for developing the FC program. Each of the participating JJIs had a local workgroup, of which representatives took part in a central workgroup (see Fig. 1). One parent attended the meetings of the central workgroup as an advisory member on behalf of the Dutch parents association for children with developmental disorders and educational or behavioral problems. In the workgroups, we strived to translate the theoretical background of family therapy [37, 44] and the broad perspective from the national position paper [39] into practice by providing guidelines and directions for family-centered care. The FC program is compatible with the usual care programs in JJIs in which only a few family-oriented activities were already incorporated [46]. The workgroups also developed training workshops for JJI staff.

Results

The bottom-up workgroup sessions resulted in a manual describing how to deliver family-centered care in short-term stay groups in JJIs [31]. The manual starts by explaining the meaning of family-centered care: i.e., JJI staff actively involve parents in the guidance and treatment of their detained child. FC expects the entire institution to propagate family-centered care and all employees to embrace a systemic vision. In FC, staff work in a family-centered way. This starts as soon as the youth enters the JJI and continues throughout the stay. FC is integrated in all methods and procedures in the JJI and is therefore not considered to be a new form of therapy. Rather, FC changes practices for JJI staff regarding all youths and their parents. Therefore, FC is considered to be part of the basic program for delivering care in JJIs. Interventions within FC are selected according to the needs of adolescents and their parents. In FC, staff help families towards a better functioning. FC emphasizes that treatment gains during detention need to be maintained when the child returns home and recognizes that relapses are opportunities for change and growth. Therefore, staff help the adolescent to rehabilitate after discharge. Overall in FC, the trajectory during the youth's detention is transparent to the adolescents and his parents, and staff understand the complexity of family-centered care in a closed facility. Because of the high variation in duration of adolescents' stays, FC does not follow fixed time schedules; the activities are scheduled according to the needs of the adolescent and his parents during detention. FC offers much room for tailoring by group workers.

FC aims to improve parental participation rates, first by training staff in family-centered work according to the theoretical principles outlined above. The purpose of the training is for staff to increase systemic competencies and to develop a systemic perspective, i.e., being constantly aware of the importance and relevance of social domains, most notably the family, to prevent the youth from relapsing into problem behavior. In the systemic perspective, adolescents are seen as part of a family and this family is part of the solution for the current crisis.

Implementing FC introduces a different approach of treating detained adolescents. Involving parents in their child's everyday life and throughout their child's detention becomes routine in JJI procedures. This involvement is operationalized by the following activities: (a) informing parents; (b) parents meeting their child; (c) parents meeting staff; (d) parents taking part in the treatment program. Each activity will be explained in detail below. Through involving parents in every aspect of their child's detention, FC aims to increase youths' and parents' motivation for treatment interventions. Theories underlying family therapy see reconnection of the parents and child as a strong boost for treatment motivation. The four sets of activities in FC serve to reconnect the family members, and are therefore considered crucial for achieving positive treatment outcomes. If involving parents is routine and if staff establish working alliances with youths and parents, youth may be more willing to accept their parents' participation, both may feel more appreciated, and parents may be more motivated for participation.

Family-centered care: informing parents

In FC, parents are provided with adequate and timely information on procedures, developments, and events. Parents are contacted by telephone on the first day their child enters the JJI. The person best suited for making this call is the mentor; the group worker who has been assigned to the adolescent concerned. In this first contact, the mentor stresses that the best way to effectively treat the adolescent, is with the help of the parents. The mentor explains the importance of parents' involvement during their child's stay in the JJI. From there on, the mentor has at least weekly telephone contact with the parents to ensure that they monitor their child's behavior in the JJI and the progress made in achieving the treatment goals.

In addition to the calls by the mentor, the child's psychologist, or pedagogue (hereafter jointly referred to as psychologist), informs the parents about the nature of their child's problems, and about psycho-education and treatment opportunities.

Family-centered care: parents meeting their children

One goal of FC is to increase parents' motivation to visit their child frequently. By Dutch law, parents have a privileged status in visiting their children in a JJI. In FC, the opportunities for parents to visit their child are no longer restricted to the regular visiting hours, as parents are actively invited to engage in their child's everyday life in detention. Parental participation moves beyond seeing the youth in the visiting room. Parents are offered a tour through the JJI and are invited to attend activities of the so-called "living group" in which their child has been placed. Some of these activities that are open to parents are organized on a regular basis, such as family evenings. Other group-based activities are more spontaneous and less structured, tailored towards the needs of the youth and his parents. Examples of the latter are cooking and/or dining, game nights, or celebrations of birthdays or of diplomas obtained. Parents are encouraged to play a part in their child's everyday life in the JJI in the hope that the family bond will strengthen and communication will improve, through which trust can rebuild. This provides families with the opportunity to share positive experiences.

Family-centered care: parents meeting the staff

In the first week of detention, the mentor calls the parents and schedules a so-called family meeting for the third week, to be attended by the parents, the youth, the mentor, and the psychologist. If, based on the available information about the family, the meeting is expected to be complicated, the psychologist may consult a family therapist in advance. If needed, the latter is available to assist during the family meeting.

At the beginning of the family meeting, the psychologist first sits down with the parents alone to welcome them and to make them feel at ease. The psychologist stresses how important parents are for their child, and for the JJI to provide the best care and treatment. Spending time with the parents enables the psychologist to learn about the family history, and about family-based protective and risk factors, and other important domains shaping the adolescent's behavior. After half an hour, the mentor and the adolescent join the meeting. The second part of the family meeting allows the parent and child to interact with each other in a positive way (to be encouraged by the psychologist and the mentor). At the same time, it allows the psychologist to observe the family dynamics. This information will later be used in the treatment. A third part of the meeting serves to discuss the adolescent's problem behavior and the content of the treatment plan to be drafted. Shared-decision making is encouraged; input in this plan from the parents and the adolescent is required and essential for increasing treatment motivation. For as long as the adolescent stays in the JJI, the parents are invited to follow-up meetings with the psychologist, the mentor, and the adolescent to evaluate the progress according to this treatment plan.

Family-centered care: parents taking part in the treatment program

In FC, parents are always informed about their child's treatment program. Along the course of the adolescents' treatment, parents are invited to participate in their son's therapy sessions. Intervention programs such as aggression regulation training, social skills training, and offense analysis, often have their own terminology. To ensure that parents are able to communicate with their child about the therapy, parents join special sessions to learn the so-called "intervention language". Additionally, during the child's stay, staff pay attention to family relationships, communication, and dynamics, coaching both the adolescent and his parents towards more positive interactions.

In the first family meeting, JJI staff pay attention to the risk and protective factors influencing the problem behavior of the youth. Based on their findings, three trajectories are possible, see Fig. 2.

1. FC without family therapy.
2. In FC, family therapy starts during detention and continues after discharge.

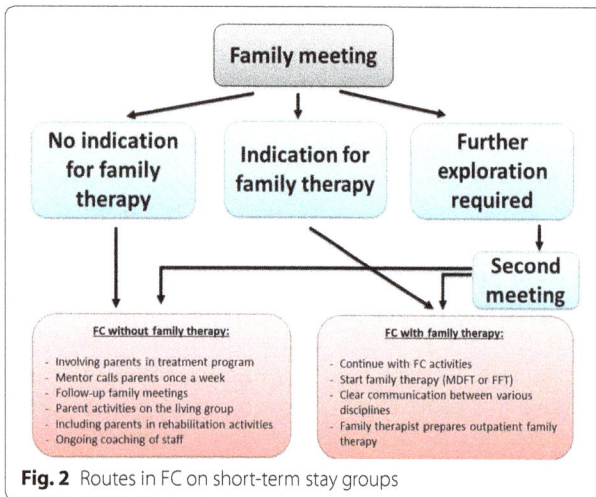

Fig. 2 Routes in FC on short-term stay groups

3. Further exploration is required to decide upon the appropriate trajectory.

If family therapy is not indicated (first route), staff involve parents according to the above-described principles of FC and invite parents for family activities as described in the program manual.

In the second route, family therapy (FFT or MDFT) starts as soon as possible and continues as outpatient therapy when the adolescent is discharged from the JJI. The type of family therapy to be chosen does not depend on theoretical considerations, but on the availability of either therapy within the JJI concerned. We assured that our FC program fits to both forms of family therapy. For the first residential phase, family therapy is adapted for use in closed settings such as JJIs [32]. The family therapist schedules frequent family sessions and individual sessions with the youth or the parents. Within FC, family therapists adhere to the MDFT or FFT manual, while there is some degree of flexibility regarding the frequency of sessions depending on the needs of adolescents and their parents. During detention, family therapy aims to improve the relationship and communication between the family members. When the youth returns home, real-life practice for improving family functioning begins.

In case further exploration of the family process is required as in the third route, a second meeting is scheduled on short notice to thoroughly assess the topics at hand. This route is applicable in three circumstances. In first instance, important family themes need to be discussed before juvenile discharge, e.g., crises within the family or questions about living arrangements other than with parents. In the second case, the psychologist has doubts about whether family therapy is indicated and needs another meeting to make an informed decision.

In last instance, family therapy is indicated but extra sessions are required to boost the family members' motivation to engage in family therapy. In all circumstances, the psychologist consults with the family therapist who is available to assist during or preparing for the second meeting.

Training staff in FC
The one-day training aims to familiarize staff with the principles of FC, to increase systemic competencies, and to ameliorate the implementation of family-centered work according to the FC manual. The training empowers staff to motivate parents for involvement. Once parents are engaged, bridges are built between family members and staff; between home and the JJI. During the training, special attention is paid to equip mentors of adolescents to motivate parents to visit their child in the JJI, as a mentor is the primary contact person for parents. Mentors are trained to contact, inform, and involve the parents. The training helps staff to adopt a systemic perspective and basic conceptions of family systems theory are explained. In the training, staff learn to see parents as supportive persons who do their best to deal with a difficult situation, and who are essential for establishing positive treatment outcomes. Staff learn about the two-way interaction patterns between parents and their children and how to build multiple therapeutic alliances, i.e., having a good bond with the youth and the parents alike, without taking sides.

Through role-playing exercises, group workers and psychologists train their skills in communicating with families, in person and through telephone contact. Additionally, family meetings are practiced through which staff experience how to establish multiple therapeutic alliances. The training provides staff with tools in reframing, improving the interrelationships between family members, increasing hope and motivation for change, and reducing negativity and blaming while improving positive communication between family members. Psychologists receive a specialized one-day workshop to enhance their skills required for the family-focused assessment during the family meeting.

The training program for staff includes bi-annual booster sessions to ensure that skills are practiced, improved, and fine-tuned. These booster sessions take up halve a day in which trainers repeat information from the original training and evaluate the current state of affairs regarding family-centered work in the teams. Teams of staff members reflect on which aspects of FC go well, and on which aspects need improvement. The trainers use this information to shape the training into a customized program tailored to the needs of a specific team.

Besides the training and booster sessions, FC prescribes team coaching supervised by a family therapist. This coaching takes place during the team meetings, which are scheduled every other week in the JJI. The first team meeting reserves one hour for so-called "intervision". During this intervision, group workers each present a problem or question regarding contact with parents on which he or she would like to receive feedback. One of the cases is selected for an in-depth discussion with colleagues, promoting systemic competencies and family-proof solutions for the problem. The other team meeting reserves one hour for discussing the case from a systemic perspective; attentive to the family the youth originated from and, in most instances, will return to.

Discussion

We succeeded in developing a program of family-centered care (FC) for adolescents in short-term stay groups of JJIs [31]. Our FC program changes the way in which parents are involved during their child's detention. The program moves beyond basic visitations for parents in the impersonal visiting room, towards parents being part of their child's everyday life in the JJI. In FC, parents are actively invited to play a prominent role during their child's detention and in their treatment. This involves being informed of every intervention, being part of decisions to be made, visiting the adolescent in his living group, taking part in living group activities, and joining meetings for parents. In addition, the FC program offers the opportunity to start family therapy during detention and to continue it on an outpatient basis after detention. Overall, training in FC changes the way in which JJI staff think about parents, which will be reflected in their work. The FC program is not only of interest for JJIs, but is easily translated to other residential settings as well. For example, the program has recently been adjusted for residential care institutions [41].

We expect FC to be successful because of its evidence-based background in which the program meets suggestions from previous studies. First and foremost, the FC program stimulates parental involvement, as is advocated by several previous researchers [1, 5, 13, 16, 52]. Other researchers stated that children should be seen as belonging to the families and that contact between children and family members should be considered as a right, not as a privilege [12, 36]. Residential care should persevere and, if possible, strengthen the connections between children and their family members [43]. Our FC program incorporated these views. Enabling parents to spend time with their child in the JJI provides families with the opportunity for positive experiences and to engage in positive communication, which in turn strengthens the family bond. This helps rebuilding trust and hope for the future

[27]. Second, the FC program emphasizes the importance of telephone contact with parents initiated by JJI staff on the first day of the child's detention. This first contact is the beginning of building a relationship between staff and parents and sets the stage for successful parental involvement [19]. Third, the family meeting enables staff to learn about parenting practices, family process, peer influence, and adolescent-specific characteristics [42]. As parents usually are the most reliable source of information about their children [13, 38], this meeting results in a better insight in the adolescent's problems. The family meeting might have an immediate therapeutic effect as well. If adolescents see how their offending behavior hurts family members, it is likely to increase their motivation for behavioral change and to promote a positive focus on the future [30]. Fourth, the FC program encourages shared decision-making, which has previously been identified as part of the central focus of family-centered care [43]. Fifth, the FC program emphasizes the importance of tailoring interventions to the risk and protective factors within the family and to the needs of the adolescent and his family, as suggested by previous research [23]. Sixth, the FC program offers the opportunity to start family therapy during detention which can continue on an outpatient basis, as is also previously advocated by other researchers [1, 48]. Finally, the program is part of a package deal including training of staff. One of the building blocks of implementing FC in practice is increasing systemic competencies among staff [4]. In FC training, staff learn about the mutual influence between youth problem behavior and family functioning, learn to see the family as part of the solution for the current crisis, and to build therapeutic alliances with parents. These themes and tools in the training are in line with recommendations for family-centered work [3, 10, 12, 14, 17, 28, 32, 50, 51], which might result in staff who are more sensitive in working with parents [45]. The training includes role-play exercises, enabling staff to train their skills in working with families, both in person and through telephone contact [19].

Before the start of our project, JJIs in the Netherlands reached unsatisfactory levels of parental participation [18, 39, 40, 50]. Bearing this in mind, we realized that our FC program did not only need to be strongly evidence-based, but also had to be attentive to the attainability of our program in practice. Our bottom-up approach contributed to achieving our aim, although this is not enough to reach successful implementation in practice. In order to truly work in a family-centered way, JJIs need to fully embrace a family-centered approach. Successful implementation is only possible if all layers and disciplines of the institution adopt a systemic view and develop skills in working with families [32]. Previous research has emphasized that the implementation of new interventions is challenging, especially in the case of family-focused interventions for youth with behavioral problems [5, 45]. Therefore, JJIs are encouraged to follow our bottom-up strategies to motivate staff for FC and to take the time to train staff in FC. The entire organization needs to be prepared for the implementation of a new program [11]. Overall, if implemented carefully, the FC program has great potential for improving care for detained adolescents and their families. Improved care through FC might contribute to positive treatment outcomes and FC ensures a better connection with outpatient care after detention. Careful and successful implementation is a requirement for FC to live up to its potential. Whether FC is able to improve care for detained adolescents and their families, will be examined in a practice-based mixed methods study [40]. In this study, we will address the following hypotheses comparing FC with usual care during detention: (1) FC increases parents' involvement with their detained child; (2) FC increases the motivation of the adolescent and his parents for accepting treatment and guidance by JJI staff and for taking part in family meetings; (3) FC adolescents show less problem behavior; (4) FC improves family interactions; (5) FC parents experience less parenting stress; (6) FC youths more often return to their family's home upon discharge; (7) FC enhances adolescents' and parents' satisfaction with the JJI; and (8) in FC groups, JJI staff members are more satisfied, feel more confident in their contact with parents, and more often incorporate the family perspective in their thinking [40].

Abbreviations
AWFZJ: Academic Workplace Forensic Care for Youth; FC: family-centered care; FFT: functional family therapy; JJI: Juvenile Justice Institution; MDFT: multidimensional family therapy.

Authors' contributions
KM and RB were project leaders in the workgroups for designing the program of family-centered care. The Dutch FC program is written by KM, RB, IS, and HR. IS drafted the current manuscript, which was critically reviewed by each of the authors. All authors read and approved the final manuscript.

Author details
[1] Department of Child and Adolescent Psychiatry, Curium-Leiden University Medical Center, Post Box 15, 2300 AA Leiden, The Netherlands. [2] Intermetzo-Pluryn, Post Box 53, 6500 AB Nijmegen, The Netherlands. [3] Youth Interventions Foundation, Post Box 37, 2300 AA Leiden, The Netherlands. [4] Department of Child and Adolescent Psychiatry, De Bascule-VUmc, Post Box 303, 1115 ZG Duivendrecht, The Netherlands.

Acknowledgements
The managements of the two participating JJIs within the AWFZJ supported the development of the program of family-centered care, for which we are grateful. We gratefully acknowledge the staff members in the workgroups for their suggestions regarding the program. Finally, thanks are gratefully extended to Winneke Ekkel for her help in improving the program by sharing her knowledge and experience.

Competing interests
The authors declare that they have no competing interests.

Funding
Our project was funded in 2010 by ZonMW, the Netherlands Organization for Scientific Research (NWO). Its ZonMW Project Number is 159010002.

References
1. Affronti ML, Levison-Johnson J. The future of family engagement in residential care settings. Resid Treat Child Youth. 2009;25:257–304. https://doi.org/10.1080/08865710903382571.
2. Alexander JF, Parsons BV. Functional family therapy: principles and procedures. Carmel: Brooks/Cole; 1982.
3. Alwon FJ, Cunningham LA, Phills J, Reitz AL, Small RW, Waldron VM. The Carolinas project: a comprehensive intervention to support family-centered group care practice. Resid Treat Child Youth. 2000;17(3):47–62. https://doi.org/10.1300/J007v17n03_08.
4. Barth RP. Residential care: from here to eternity. Int J Soc Welf. 2005;14:158–62. https://doi.org/10.1111/j.1468-2397.2005.00355.x.
5. Bekkema N, Wiefferink C, Mikolajczak J. Implementing the parent management training oregon model in The Netherlands. Emot Behav Difficulties. 2008;13(4):249–58. https://doi.org/10.1080/13632750802442136.
6. Boendermaker L, Ince D. Effectieve interventies tegen jeugddelinquentie. JeugdenCo Kennis. 2008;04:26–38.
7. Burke JD, Mulvey EP, Schubert CA, Garbin SR. The challenge and opportunity of parental involvement in juvenile justice services. Child Youth Serv Rev. 2014;39:39–47.
8. Coll KM, Juhnke GA, Thobro P, Haas R, Robinson MS. Family disengagement of youth offenders: implications for counselors. Fam J. 2008;16:359–63.
9. Delhaye M, Kempenaers C, Burton J, Linkowski P, Stroobants R, Goossens L. Attachment, parenting, and separation–individuation in adolescence: a comparison of hospitalized adolescents, institutionalized delinquents, and controls. J Genet Psychol. 2012;173:119–41.
10. Feinstein S, Baartman J, Buboltz M, Sonnichsen K, Solomon R. Resiliency in adolescent males in a correctional facility. J Correct Educ. 2008;59(2):94–105. https://doi.org/10.2307/23282791.
11. Fixsen DL, Naoom SF, Blase KA, Friedman RM, Wallace F. Implementation research: a synthesis of the literature. Tampa: University of South Florida (USF); 2005.
12. Garfat T. Fresh thinking about families: a view from residential care. Reclaiming Child Youth. 2011;20(3):5–7.
13. Garfinkel L. Improving family involvement for juvenile offenders with emotional/behavioral disorders and related disabilities. Behav Disord. 2010;36(1):52–60.
14. Gately G. Juvenile facilities strive to foster 'family engagement'. Juvenile Justice Information Exchange. 2014. https://jjie.org/2014/11/10/juvenile-facilities-strive-to-foster-family-engagement/107896/. Accessed 3 May 2017.
15. Gavazzi SM, Wasserman D, Partridge C, Sheridan S. The growing up FAST diversion program: an example of juvenile justice program development for outcome evaluation. Aggress Violent Behav. 2000;5(2):159–75.
16. Geurts EMW, Boddy J, Noom MJ, Knorth EJ. Family-centred residential care: the new reality? Child Fam Soc Work. 2012;17(2):170–9. https://doi.org/10.1111/j.1365-2206.2012.00838.x.
17. Goyette A, Marr K, Lewicki J-A. The family and community in milieu treatment: challenging the parameters of residential treatment. J Child Youth Care. 1994;9(4):39–50.
18. Hendriksen-Favier A, Place C, Van Wezep M. Procesevaluatie van YOU-TURN: introomprogramma en stabilisatie- en motivatieperiode. Fasen 1 en 2 van de basismethodiek in justitiële jeugdinrichtingen. Utrecht: Trimbos-instituut; 2010.
19. Herman KC, Borden LA, Hsu C, Schultz TR, Strawsine Carney M, Brooks CM, Reineke WM. Enhancing family engagement in interventions for mental health problems in youth. Resid Treat Child Youth. 2011;28(2):102–19. https://doi.org/10.1080/0886571X.2011.569434.
20. Hoeve M, Dubas JS, Eichelsheim VI, van der Laan PH, Smeenk W, Gerris JRM. The relationship between parenting and delinquency: a meta-analysis. J Abnorm Child Psychol. 2009;37(6):749–75.

21. Hoeve M, Smeenk W, Loeber R, Stouthamer-Loeber M, Van der Laan PH, Gerris JRM, Dubas JS. Long-term effects of parenting and family characteristics on delinquency of male young adults. Eur J Criminol. 2007;4(2):161–94.

22. Keiley MK. Multiple-family group intervention for incarcerated adolescents and their families: a pilot project. J Marital Fam Ther. 2007;33(1):106–24. https://doi.org/10.1111/j.1752-0606.2007.00009.x.

23. Kumpfer KL, Alvarado R. Effective family strengthening interventions. Juvenile Justice Bulletin. Family Strengthening Series. 1998.

24. Latimer J. A meta-analytic examination of youth delinquency, family treatment, and recidivism. Can J Criminol. 2001;43:237–53.

25. Liddle HA. Multidimensional family therapy: evidence base for transdiagnostic treatment outcomes, change mechanisms, and implementation in community settings. Fam Process. 2016;55(3):558–76.

26. Liddle HA, Dakof GA, Diamond G. Adolescent substance abuse: multidimensional family therapy in action. In: Kaufman E, Kaufman P, editors. Family therapy of drug and alcohol abuse. 2nd ed. Needham Heights: Allyn & Bacon; 1992.

27. Lyman RD, Campbell NR. Developmental clinical psychology and psychiatry. In: Treating children and adolescents in residential and inpatient settings, vol. 36. Thousand Oaks, CA: Sage Publications; 1996.

28. McDaniel R, McKinney B. Family-centered practices. Resid Group Care Q. 2005;6(1):7–8.

29. McLendon T, McLendon D, Hatch L. Engaging families in the residential treatment process utilizing family-directed structural therapy. Resid Treat Child Youth. 2012;29(1):66–77. https://doi.org/10.1080/08865 71X.2012.643679.

30. Mincey B, Maldonado N, Lacey CH, Thompson SD. Perceptions of successful graduates of juvenile residential programs: reflections and suggestions for success. In: Annual meeting of the American Educational Research Association, p. 1–31. https://doi.org/10.2307/23282643.

31. Mos K, Breuk R, Simons I, Rigter H. Gezinsgericht werken in Justitiële Jeugdinrichtingen op afdelingen voor kort verblijf. Zutphen: Academische Werkplaats Forensische Zorg voor Jeugd; 2014.

32. Mos K, Jong J, Eltink E, Rigter H. Wegwijzer voor toepassing van MDFT in justitiële jeugdinrichtingen en aansluitende ambulante zorg. Leiden: MDFT Academie; 2011.

33. Mulder E, Brand E, Bullens R, Van Marle H. Risk factors for overall recidivism and severity of recidivism in serious juvenile offenders. Int J Offender Ther Comp Criminol. 2011;55(1):118–35.

34. Nijhof KS, Van Dam C, Veerman JW, Engels RCME, Scholte RHJ. Nieuw Zorgaanbod: Gesloten jeugdzorg voor adolescenten met ernstige gedragsproblemen. Pedagogiek. 2010;30(3):177–91.

35. Peterson-Badali M, Broeking J. Parents' involvement in the youth justice system: rhetoric and reality 1. Can J Criminol Crim Justice. 2010;52(1):1–27.

36. Ridgely E, Carty W. Residential treatment: a resource for families. J Child Youth Care. 1998;11(4):77–81.

37. Rigter H, Liddle HA. Theoretische handleiding [MDFT—theory manual]. Leiden: MDFT Academy/Curium-LUMC/ErasmusMC; 2011.

38. Rosenbaum P, King S, Law M, King G, Evans J. Family-centred service: a conceptual framework and research review. Phys Occup Ther Pediatr. 1998;18:1–20. https://doi.org/10.1080/J006v18n01_01.

39. Sectordirectie Justitiële Jeugdinrichtingen. Visie op Ouderparticipatie in Justitiële Jeugdinrichtingen. Den Haag: Dienst Justitiële Inrichtingen, Ministerie van Veiligheid en Justitie; 2011.

40. Simons I, Mulder E, Rigter H, Breuk R, Van der Vaart W, Vermeiren R. Family-centered care in Juvenile Justice Institutions: a mixed methods study protocol. JMIR Res Protoc. 2016;5(3):e177. https://doi.org/10.2196/resprot.5938.

41. Simons I, van Domburgh L, Mos K, Breuk R, Rigter H, Mulder EA. Gezinsgericht werken in de residentiële jeugdzorg. Nijmegen: Academische Werkplaats Risicojeugd; 2017.

42. Slavet JD, Stein LAR, Klein JL, Colby SM, Barnett NP, Monti PM. Piloting the family check-up with incarcerated adolescents and their parents. Psychol Serv. 2005;2(2):123–32.

43. Small RW, Bellonci C, Ramsey S. Creating and maintaining family partnerships in residential treatment programs: shared decisions, full participation, mutual responsibility. In: Witthaker JW, Del Valle JF, Holmes L, editors. Therapeutic residential care with children and youth: developing evidence-based international practice. London: Jessica Kingsley Publishers; 2014. p. 156–71.

44. Spanjaard HJM, Breuk R. Theoretische Onderbouwing van Functional Family Therapy in Nederland. Amsterdam: FFT Nederland/De Bascule; 2013.

45. Stern SB, Smith CA. Reciprocal relationships between antisocial behavior and parenting: implications for delinquency intervention. Fam Soc. 1999;80(2):169–81. https://dx.doi.org/10.1606/1044-3894.659

46. Stuurgroep YOUTURN. YOUTURN Basishandleiding. Den Haag: Dienst Justitiële Inrichtingen; 2009.

47. Tarolla SM, Wagner EF, Rabinowitz J, Tubman JG. Understanding and treating juvenile offenders: a review of current knowledge and future directions. Aggress Violent Behav. 2002;7:125–43.

48. Trupin EJ, Kerns SEU, Cusworth Walker S, DeRobertis MT, Stewart DG. Family integrated transitions: a promising program for juvenile offenders with co-occurring disorders. J Child Adolesc Subst Abuse. 2011;20(5):421–36. https://doi.org/10.1080/1067828X.2011.614889.

49. Van der Pol T, Hoeve M, Noom M, Stams GJ, Doreleijers T, Van Domburgh L, Vermeiren R. The effectiveness of multidimensional family therapy (MDFT) in treating substance abusing adolescents with comorbid behavior problems: a meta-analysis. J Child Adolesc Psychiatry. 2017. https://doi.org/10.1111/jcpp.12685.

50. Vlaardingerbroek P. De justitiële jeugdinrichting en de ouders. In: van der Leun JP, editor. De vogel vrij. Den Haag: Boom Lemma uitgevers; 2011.

51. Walter UA, Petr CG. Family-centered residential treatment: knowledge, research, and values converge. Resid Treat Child Youth. 2008;25(1):2008. https://doi.org/10.1080/08865710802209594.

52. Whittaker JK, Holmes L, del Valle JF, Ainsworth F, Andreassen T, Anglin J, Zeira A. Therapeutic residential care for children and youth: a consensus statement of the international work group on therapeutic residential care. Resid Treat Child Youth. 2016;33(2):89–106. https://doi.org/10.1080/0886571X.2016.1215755.

53. Woolfenden SR, Williams K, Peat JK. Family and parenting interventions for conduct disorder and delinquency: a meta-analysis of randomised controlled trials. Arch Dis Child. 2002;86(4):251–6.

14

Suicidal deaths in elementary school students in Korea

Minha Hong[1], Han Nah Cho[2], Ah Reum Kim[2], Hyun Ju Hong[2,3] and Yong-Sil Kweon[2,4]*

Abstract

Background: The purpose of this study was to determine the characteristics of childhood suicidal deaths among elementary school students that occurred from 2011 to 2015 in Korea.

Methods: The report form of each suicide case by the teacher in charge to the Education Ministry was reviewed retrospectively.

Results: There were 19 suicidal deaths (12 boys, 7 girls) in elementary school students. The youngest case was a third grader (n = 1). Jumping from heights (n = 12) was the most frequently used method. Most suicides (n = 12) were committed in their homes.

Conclusion: These results highlight the alarming trend of early suicidal deaths and the importance of early suicide prevention strategies, especially in schools.

Keywords: Childhood, Suicide, Death, Characteristics

Background

Suicide rate in Korea is the highest among the organization for economic cooperation and development (OECD) countries; therefore, child and adolescent suicide is also a major concern in public health. Additionally, suicide ranks consistently among the leading causes of death in youth globally [1]. Although there is a growing research interest in suicide in the earlier period of life [2–4], we still have insufficient knowledge about childhood suicide. It has been assumed that children are prevented from engaging in deliberate acts to take their own life, due to their limited cognitive ability to understand death and/or plan a lethal attempt. [5, 6]. On the other hand, another view is that most children acquire the concept of death and suicide by the age of 8 and are capable of planning and executing suicide [7]. According to the National Statistical Office of Korea, the reported suicide cases among children aged 5–9 years varied from 0 to 7 per year since 1983, and the average suicide rate among those aged

10–14 years was 1.1–2.3 per 100,000. In the US, suicide is the second most common cause of death among those aged 10–14 years [8]. In Austria, the average suicide rate among children aged 10–14 years was 0.72 per 100,000 from 2001 to 2014 [9]. More research focused on specific age groups from a developmental perspective should be conducted to identify variables or correlates of child and adolescent suicides.

Previously published studies including elementary school aged children were very few [10–13], if any. Groholt et al. compared risk factors and characteristics for suicide between children (< 15 years) and adolescents (15–19 years), and reported that younger suicides were less likely to be preceded by mental disorder, suicidal ideation, or precipitating stress factors [13]. Loh et al. conducted a retrospective study on suicidal deaths in those aged 10–24 years between 2000 and 2004 in Singapore, and reported that 22 suicides were among those aged 10–14 years, while 65 were among those aged 15–19 [11]. Pomili et al. evaluated suicide among children and adolescents (aged 10–17 years), and reported that suicide rate was 0.91 per 100,000, with more suicides among boys (1.21 vs. 0.59) [14]. These studies were conducted

*Correspondence: yskwn@catholic.ac.kr
[4] Department of Psychiatry, Uijeongbu St. Mary's Hospital, College of Medicine, The Catholic University of Korea, 222 Banpo-daero, Seocho-gu, Seoul 16591, Republic of Korea
Full list of author information is available at the end of the article

mostly with the adolescent population, and not specifically with children.

As such, children and adolescents are mostly studied together, partly because of the rarity of absolute number of child and adolescent suicides. Most research on child and adolescent suicides is conducted on clinical samples, suicide survivors, and mainly on the adolescent population, and focused on mental illness and morbidity/mortality. To our knowledge, less information on suicides among elementary school aged children in Asia is available as yet. Besides, there have been no studies to our knowledge that focus on completed suicides of elementary school students, especially from teachers' perspectives. The studies of suicides in this age group could offer important information for prevention and interventions at schools. The purpose of this article is to present the descriptive data regarding suicidal deaths among elementary school children (aged 6/7–11/12 years) in Korea.

Methods

According to Korea education statistics service, the rates of elementary school enrollment during 2011–2015 are 99.1, 98.6, 97.2, 96.4, and 98.5%, respectively. That is, the rate of enrollment in elementary school is virtually one hundred percent. The ministry of education in Korea recognized the seriousness of suicides and reorganized the system. One of them is developing *Student Suicide Report* form (please see Additional file 1) to assess risk factors related to school life among suicide victims. Data were collected for each case by reviewing teachers' reports forms of suicides in elementary school. The report by the teacher in charge is mandatory for each suicide case in Korea.

This study is a retrospective review of the *Student Suicide Report* form (Additional file 1) about suicidal deaths of elementary school students in Korea between 2011 and 2015. As in other developed countries, elementary school education is compulsory for children aged 7(6)–12(11) years in Korea. The number of suicidal deaths in this study signifies the total number of suicides among the population of those aged 7–12 years in Korea. The records were examined with regard to gender, grade (at school), school life, and factors related to suicide, such as the method, site of suicide, previous experience of loss and attempts, and presence of a recognized stressful event. *Student Suicide Report* form (Additional file 1) consisted of two types of responses, one with a checklist and another one with a description. The researchers thoroughly checked both types of reports. Stressful events were extracted by the researchers from the description in the *Student Suicide Report* form. Descriptive statistical analysis was performed for all the data. This study was approved by the institutional review board of Hallym University Sacred Heart Hospital (2016-I044).

Results

A total of 19 suicide report forms of elementary school students' suicidal deaths during the 5 year period from 2011 to 2015 were reviewed. The majority of cases were among males (12, 63.2%). A boy in the third grade (n = 1) was the youngest case. Two cases were of fourth graders, followed by three cases of fifth graders, and 13 of sixth graders (Table 1).

Of 19 suicidal deaths, jumping from a height (n = 12, 63%) was the most frequently used method (Fig. 1). Hanging (n = 5, 27%) was the second most common method of suicide, followed by intoxication (n = 1, 5%) and unknown methods (n = 1, 5%) (Fig. 1). The majority of cases occurred at home (either inside or the terrace) (n = 12, 63%) (Fig. 2).

A suicide note was found in two cases (data not shown). Any contact (with family, friend, or teacher, etc.) before suicide was found in one case (data not shown). A history of self-mutilation was found in one case and suicide attempt was found in two cases (Table 2). The previous

Table 1 Characteristics of completed suicides among elementary school students between 2011 and 2015 [N (%)]

	Boys N = 12	Girls N = 7	Total N = 19
Grade			
3rd	1 (8.3)	0 (0.0)	1 (5.3)
4th	0 (0.0)	2 (28.6)	2 (10.5)
5th	1 (8.3)	2 (28.6)	3 (15.8)
6th	10 (83.3)	3 (42.8)	13 (68.4)
Residence			
Seoul	5 (41.7)	1 (14.3)	6 (31.6)
Busan	2 (16.7)	0 (0.0)	2 (10.5)
Daegu	3 (25.0)	0 (0.0)	3 (15.8)
Gyeonggi	0 (0.0)	2 (28.6)	2 (10.5)
Gangwon	0 (0.0)	1 (14.3)	1 (5.3)
Chungnam	0 (0.0)	1 (14.3)	1 (5.3)
Gyeongbuk	2 (16.7)	0 (0.0)	2 (10.5)
Jeonnam	0 (0.0)	2 (28.6)	2 (10.5)
Religion			
Christianity	3 (25.0)	1 (14.3)	4 (21.1)
Catholic	1 (8.3)	0 (0.0)	1 (5.3)
Buddhism	0 (0.0)	1 (14.3)	1 (5.3)
None	5 (41.7)	4 (57.1)	9 (47.4)
Unknown	3 (25.0)	1 (14.3)	4 (21.1)
Year of suicide			
2011	1 (8.3)	0 (0.0)	1 (5.3)
2012	2 (16.7)	1 (14.3)	3 (15.8)
2013	3 (25.0)	2 (28.6)	5 (26.3)
2014	5 (41.7)	2 (28.6)	7 (36.8)
2015	1 (8.3)	2 (28.6)	3 (15.8)
Living with both parents	9 (75.0)	5 (71.4)	14 (73.7)

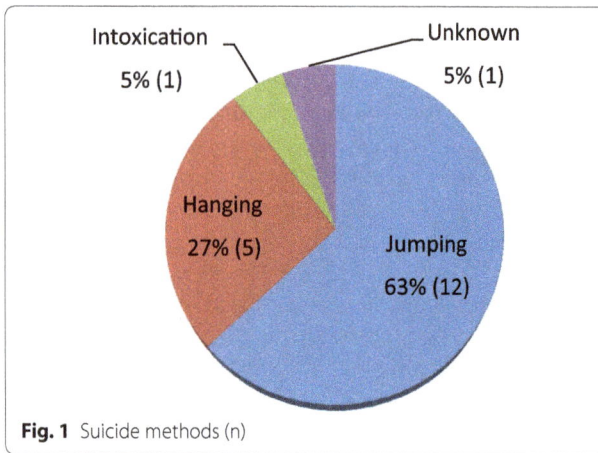

Fig. 1 Suicide methods (n)

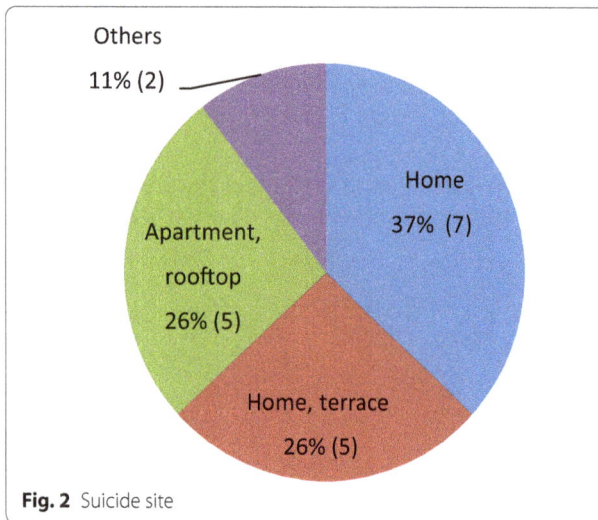

Fig. 2 Suicide site

Table 2 Previous experience of loss and attempts

	N	%
Prior history		
None	1	5.3
Self-mutilation	1	5.3
Suicide attempt	2	10.5
Unknown	15	78.9
Recent (within a year) experience of loss		
None	3	15.8
Yes	1	21.1
Unknown	15	78.9
Experience of suicide event		
None	2	10.5
Suicide of relatives	3	15.8
Unknown	14	73.7

apparent with increasing age [16], and that the youngest age of the case of suicidal death was about 9 years, who was a third grader [10, 12, 17]. Two recent systematic reviews of child suicides reported that youngest ages among cases of completed suicides was 8 years [10] and 9 years [3] respectively. Dervic et al. reported on seven suicides among children aged 5–9 years using data from Statistics Austria between 1970 and 2001 [6]. In our study, the youngest case was that of a boy in the third grade, whose exact age is not determined. We can assume that he might be 8–9 years old, because in Korea, children usually enter the elementary school at the age of 6–7 years. A recent research suggested that suicidal cognitions and behaviors in early childhood (ages 3–7 years) should be taken seriously as a marker of risk for ongoing suicidal ideation/behavior [18]. Considering that the children's understanding of suicide is related to cognitive maturity and experience [19, 20] and that the reported cases of suicidal deaths are shifting from adolescents to elementary school aged children, the populations with which suicide prevention strategies need to be conducted should be expanded.

In our study, the most common method of suicide was jumping from a height in both boys and girls. This is inconsistent with reports from other countries that hanging was the predominant method of suicide in children and young adolescents [3, 11, 21]. This is not surprising given that previous reports of greater prevalence of suicides by jumping from heights were in areas with more tall residential buildings [22], along with a high proportion of apartment residence and high population density in Korea. While the second most common method of suicide is using firearms in other countries [5, 21], it is not considered as a suicide method because they are forbidden by law in Korea. Another similar example is the

experience of loss within a year was found in one case and any experience of suicidal event in the past was found in three cases (Table 2).

In terms of stressful events around suicides, teachers were reported in the existence of stressful event in four cases, and there were ten cases of such stressful events identified by researcher (Table 3).

Discussion

This study provides representative data of suicidal deaths in elementary school students in Korea, given that the rate of enrollment in elementary school is virtually one hundred percent. The number of suicidal deaths was 19 in this study, signifying the total number of suicides among those aged 7–12 years in Korea.

The findings of this study are consistent with previous reports that the majority of those who died were male [10, 15], that the gender disparity becomes more

Table 3 Recognized stressful events

Reported recent stressful event	By teacher	By researcher
None	15 (79.0)	9 (47.4)
Yes	4 (21.0) Peer relational problem in group activity (1) Conflict within family (1) Parent counseling request (1) Rejection (1)	10 (52.6) Scolding from parents (3) Conflict within family (2) Divorce (1) Breaking window (1) Failing in basketball game's preliminary round (1) Rejection (1) Parent counseling request (1)

reduction in suicides using pesticides after 3-year phased bans of pesticides in Sri Lanka [23]. This finding implies that strict restrictions on access to lethal means in this population can be one strategy for suicide prevention [24].

Previous studies have noted that in terms of residence, Seoul, Busan, and Daegu city are metropolitan areas, whereas Gyeonggi, Gangwon, Chungnam, Gyeongbuk, and Jeonnam are non-metropolitan areas. The completed suicides accounted for more than half (57.9%) in metropolitan areas. Although Gyeonggi is a heterogeneous area where urban and regional characteristics coexist, it is considered to be metropolitan given that it is densely populated, close to Seoul, more industrialized, and has developed traffic systems and more tall buildings and apartments. Including Gyeonggi as metropolitan area, the completed suicide rate reaches almost 70%. Our findings are not consistent with previous studies suggesting that greater urban density was generally associated with lower suicide rates in adult and elderly population [25, 26]. One possible assumption is that the high relatively more children than elderly population are living in big cities and using jumping from a height as common method of suicide might make the difference. Disparity toward metropolitan areas in children can also be interpreted in the similar context as the suicide method.

In this study, the most frequent suicide site was the home, which is compatible with the previous results [27–29]. Other findings such as previous experience of loss and attempts and recognized stressful events, however, were not consistent with those of prior studies [2, 24]. This is partly due to the data source which reflects the perspective of the teacher in charge. Especially, stressful events related to the victim recognized by teachers and by researchers differ vastly. Presence of stressful events was recognized more by researchers (52.6%) than by teachers (26.3%). As shown in Table 3, both the teacher and researcher were aware of stressful events in four cases, such as conflicts within the family (1), parent counseling request from the school (1), rejection from friend (1), and being scolded by parent (1), which were recognized as peer relational problems in group activity

by the teacher. The researchers identified that there were precipitating factors such as arguments between family members or scolding from parents, divorce of parents, and failing in basketball game in six cases that were not recognized by teachers. This discrepancy of reporting between researcher and school teachers might result from a lack of understanding about child and adolescent mental health.

This study has several limitations. First, the sample size was small due to the number of completed suicide cases being 19, a common problem of single country suicide studies. Second, the study period was relatively short. Due to these limitations, we could provide only descriptive data, and not an inferential analysis. Finally, data source was mainly teachers' report forms. Thus, variables may reflect mainly teachers' perspectives. It is possible that school adjustment problems of students were overlooked by teachers.

Conclusion

The findings of this study provide valuable information about elementary school aged children, especially from the teachers' perspectives, and can be utilized in planning suicide prevention strategies at school. Further research is needed to investigate clinically significant variables and psychosocial factors using psychological autopsy.

Authors' contributions
MH and YK designed the study and made major contributions in writing the manuscript. HC and AK performed acquisition and analysis of data. HH performed interpretation and supervision. All authors read and approved the final manuscript.

Author details
[1] Department of Psychiatry, Myongji Hospital, Seonam University, College of Medicine, Goyang, Republic of Korea. [2] Hallym University Suicide and School Mental Health Institute, Hallym University, Anyang, Republic of Korea. [3] Department of Psychiatry, Hallym University Sacred Heart Hospital, College of Medicine, Hallym University of Korea, Anyang, Republic

of Korea. [4] Department of Psychiatry, Uijeongbu St. Mary's Hospital, College of Medicine, The Catholic University of Korea, 222 Banpo-daero, Seocho-gu, Seoul 16591, Republic of Korea.

Acknowledgements
None.

Competing interests
The authors declare that they have no Competing interests.

Funding
This study was supported by a Grant from the Jeollanamdo Office of Education from the Ministry of Education.

References

1. Organization WH. Preventing suicide: a global imperative. Geneva: World Health Organization; 2014.
2. Freuchen A, Groholt B. Characteristics of suicide notes of children and young adolescents: an examination of the notes from suicide victims 15 years and younger. Clin Child Psychol Psychiatry. 2015;20(2):194–206.
3. Dervic K, Brent DA, Oquendo MA. Completed suicide in childhood. Psychiatric Clin N Am. 2008;31(2):271–91.
4. Pfeffer CR, Conte HR, Plutchik R, Jerrett I. Suicidal behavior in latency-age children: an empirical study. J Am Acad Child Psychiatry. 1979;18(4):679–92.
5. Brent DA, Baugher M, Bridge J, Chen T, Chiappetta L. Age- and sex-related risk factors for adolescent suicide. J Am Acad Child Adolesc Psychiatry. 1999;38(12):1497–505.
6. Pfeffer CR. Childhood suicidal behavior. A developmental perspective. Psychiatric Clin N Am. 1997;20(3):551–62.
7. Tishler CL, Reiss NS, Rhodes AR. Suicidal behavior in children younger than twelve: a diagnostic challenge for emergency department personnel. Acad Emerg Med Off J Soc Acad Emerg Med. 2007;14(9):810–8.
8. Leading causes of death charts. 2014. https://www.cdc.gov/injury/wisqars/leadingcauses.html. Accessed 11 July 2017.
9. Laido Z, Voracek M, Till B, Pietschnig J, Eisenwort B, Dervic K, Sonneck G, Niederkrotenthaler T. Epidemiology of suicide among children and adolescents in Austria, 2001–2014. Wien Klin Wochenschr. 2017;129(3–4):121–8.
10. Beautrais AL. Child and young adolescent suicide in New Zealand. Aust NZ J psychiatry. 2001;35(5):647–53.
11. Loh C, Tai BC, Ng WY, Chia A, Chia BH. Suicide in young Singaporeans aged 10–24 years between 2000 to 2004. Arch Suicide Res Off J Int Acad Suicide Res. 2012;16(2):174–82.
12. Soole R, Kolves K, De Leo D. Suicide in children: a systematic review. Arch Suicide Res Off J Int Acad Suicide Res. 2015;19(3):285–304.
13. Groholt B, Ekeberg O, Wichstrom L, Haldorsen T. Suicide among children and younger and older adolescents in Norway: a comparative study. J Am Acad Child Adolesc Psychiatry. 1998;37(5):473–81.
14. Pompili M, Vichi M, De Leo D, Pfeffer C, Girardi P. A longitudinal epidemiological comparison of suicide and other causes of death in Italian children and adolescents. Eur Child Adolesc Psychiatry. 2012;21(2):111–21.
15. Freuchen A, Kjelsberg E, Lundervold AJ, Groholt B. Differences between children and adolescents who commit suicide and their peers: a psychological autopsy of suicide victims compared to accident victims and a community sample. Child Adolesc Psychiatry Mental Health. 2012;6:1.
16. Shaffer D, Gould MS, Fisher P, Trautman P, Moreau D, Kleinman M, Flory M. Psychiatric diagnosis in child and adolescent suicide. Arch Gen Psychiatry. 1996;53(4):339–48.
17. Groholt B, Ekeberg O. Suicide in young people under 15 years: problems of classification. Nord J Psychiatry. 2003;57(6):411–7.
18. Whalen DJ, Dixon-Gordon K, Belden AC, Barch D, Luby JL. Correlates and consequences of suicidal cognitions and behaviors in children ages 3 to 7 years. J Am Acad Child Adolesc Psychiatry. 2015;54(11):926–37.
19. Mishara BL. Conceptions of death and suicide in children ages 6-12 and their implications for suicide prevention. Suicide Lifethreat Behav. 1999;29(2):105–18.
20. Normand CL, Mishara BL. The development of the concept of suicide in children. OMEGA J Death Dying. 1992;25(3):183–203.
21. Dervic K, Friedrich E, Oquendo MA, Voracek M, Friedrich MH, Sonneck G. Suicide in Austrian children and young adolescents aged 14 and younger. Eur Child Adolesc Psychiatry. 2006;15(7):427–34.
22. Fischer EP, Comstock GW, Monk MA, Sencer DJ. Characteristics of completed suicides: implications of differences among methods. Suicide Lifethreat Behav. 1993;23(2):91–100.
23. Knipe DW, Chang SS, Dawson A, Eddleston M, Konradsen F, Metcalfe C, Gunnell D. Suicide prevention through means restriction: impact of the 2008-2011 pesticide restrictions on suicide in Sri Lanka. PLoS ONE. 2017;12(3):e0172893.
24. Gould MS, Kramer RA. Youth suicide prevention. Suicide Lifethreat Behav. 2001;31(Suppl):6–31.
25. Kim MH, Jung-Choi K, Jun HJ, Kawachi I. Socioeconomic inequalities in suicidal ideation, parasuicides, and completed suicides in South Korea. Soc Sci Med. 2010;70(8):1254–61.
26. Hong J, Knapp M. Geographical inequalities in suicide rates and area deprivation in South Korea. J Mental Health Policy Econ. 2013;16(3):109–19.
27. Lee CJ, Collins KA, Burgess SE. Suicide under the age of eighteen: a 10-year retrospective study. Am J Forensic Med Pathol. 1999;20(1):27–30.
28. Uzun I, Karayel FA, Akyildiz EU, Turan AA, Toprak S, Arpak BB. Suicide among children and adolescents in a province of Turkey. J Forensic Sci. 2009;54(5):1097–100.
29. Agritmis H, Yayci N, Colak B, Aksoy E. Suicidal deaths in childhood and adolescence. Forensic Sci Int. 2004;142(1):25–31.

15

Difficulties faced by university students with self-reported symptoms of attention-deficit hyperactivity disorder

Soo Jin Kwon[1], Yoonjung Kim[2*] (iD) and Yeunhee Kwak[2]

Abstract

Background: Attention-deficit hyperactivity disorder (ADHD) persists into adolescence and adulthood; however, few studies have analyzed the experiences of university students with ADHD. This study explored the difficulties experienced by university students with ADHD symptoms.

Methods: Between December 2015 and February 2016, face-to-face interviews were conducted with 12 university students with self-reported ADHD symptoms. Data were analyzed using thematic analysis.

Results: Difficulties in university life were classified into four main themes (lack of daily routine, unsatisfactory academic performance and achievement, reduced interpersonal skills, and continuing worries) and analyzed. University students with ADHD symptoms had difficulties coping with repeated cycles of negative thoughts and worries, irregular lifestyles due to poor time management, dissatisfaction with academic performance and interpersonal relationships, self-dissatisfaction, and decreased self-esteem.

Conclusion: To improve their university experience, students with ADHD should receive education about ways to stop worrying, to express emotions healthily, and to manage time efficiently.

Keywords: Attention-deficit hyperactivity disorder, Experience, Qualitative study, University students

Background

Attention-deficit hyperactivity disorder (ADHD) has as its major symptoms inattention, impulsivity, and hyperactivity [1]. The prevalence rates of ADHD have been increasing over the past decades [2]. The revised Diagnostic and Statistical Manual of Mental Disorders (DSM-5) includes diagnostic criteria for adult ADHD, which differ from those for childhood ADHD [1]. The DSM-5 includes more developmentally expansive criteria and is expected to have a marked impact on the diagnosis and treatment of adult ADHD. A cross-national study of 11,422 adults in the United States and Europe reported that the prevalence of adult ADHD was approximately 3.4% and was significantly higher in higher-income than in lower-income countries (4.2% vs. 1.9%, respectively)

[3]. Approximately 2–8% of university students have clinically significant ADHD symptoms [4]. Furthermore, studies in South Korea found that approximately 1.1% of adults had significant ADHD symptoms [5], and 7.6% of university students had ADHD [6].

Adults with ADHD have a lower quality of life than those without ADHD [7]. Similarly, college students with ADHD have a lower quality of life than do students without ADHD [8]; they have been shown to be more depressed and anxious, to be more easily angered or to suppress emotion, to have achieve less academically, and to be poorly supported in their relationships with their friends [9, 10]. ADHD symptoms have a negative impact on many aspects of life, including self-esteem, academic functioning, social functioning, and parent–child relationships [8, 11, 12]. Adults with ADHD are vulnerable to addiction; ADHD is often accompanied by addictive disorders [13] that are closely associated with sleep problems, leading to impairment in daily life [14].

*Correspondence: yoonjung@cau.ac.kr
[2] Faculty of Red Cross College of Nursing, Chung-Ang University, 84 Heukseok-Ro, Dongjack-Gu, Seoul 156-756, Republic of Korea
Full list of author information is available at the end of the article

In addition, adults with ADHD may experience frustration, depression, anxiety, difficulty in controlling emotions, interpersonal problems, and, in severe cases, personality disorders. They may often receive negative feedback from those around them and may exhibit suicidal behavior in response to repeated failures [4, 9, 10, 15–18]. Attending university is a particularly important period that affects future careers and overall social life; it is particularly challenging because of the adjustment to the new, unstructured environment that university students must make [19]. University students with ADHD experience a variety of academic, psychological, social, and mental problems [20]. Since university students with ADHD tend to have reduced life satisfaction and greater subjective pain than those without ADHD [21], there is a great need for ADHD treatment and interventions that support this vulnerable student cohort.

Although studies have been conducted to identify the support needs of university students with ADHD [18, 20], most of this research has focused on the experiences of students living in the United States, with little attention paid to diverse ethnic groups. To date, only a few studies have been conducted in Asia, making it difficult to generalize the findings to cross-national populations. The particular cultural demands faced by Korean university students, including the pressure to find a job and high parental expectations, may lead to difficulties such as mental health-related and self-centered behavioral problems [22, 23]. Given the low number of adults diagnosed with ADHD in Korea, the scarcity of related studies, and limited information about adult ADHD among the Korean population [10, 24], multifaceted studies and clinical approaches are needed to help Korean university students who have ADHD symptoms.

To adequately address and evaluate the difficulties that such students experience, the condition must be explored from their perspective. Therefore, the present study aimed to investigate the difficulties experienced by Korean university students with ADHD symptoms so as to provide the basic data needed to develop appropriate interventions.

Methods
Study design
Data were collected by conducting in-depth, individual interviews with university students with ADHD symptoms, and were analyzed using thematic analysis.

Participants
University students were recruited via an announcement posted on university bulletin boards. After signing the participation consent form, all volunteers were screened using the Korean version of the World Health Organization Adult ADHD Self-Report Scale (ASRS-v1.1) Symptom Checklist [25, 26]. Interviews were conducted with participants whose reported symptoms met more than four of the ASRS-v1.1 evaluation criteria [27]. A total of 12 participants (five men and seven women) were recruited, with a mean age of 22.2 years (range 20–29 years). Of these, two participants had been diagnosed with ADHD but were not receiving treatment at the time of the study; one participant had taken ADHD medication for approximately 2 years but had stopped taking it 3 years prior to enrolling in the study; the other participant was diagnosed with ADHD 8 years prior to enrolling in the study, had undergone counseling on four occasions, but had not received further treatment thereafter (Table 1).

Table 1 Participant demographic data (N = 12)

Number	Sex	Current age (years)	Current university year	Physician-diagnosed ADHD	Past medication
1	M	22	3	No	No
2	M	20	2	No	No
3	M	21	2	No	No
4	M	22	3	No	No
5	F	24	3	Yes	Yes
6	F	21	2	No	No
7	F	24	3	No	No
8	F	21	2	No	No
9	F	20	1	No	No
10	F	20	1	No	No
11	F	22	4	No	No
12	M	29	1	Yes	No

ADHD attention-deficit hyperactivity disorder

Data collection

Data were collected between December 2015 and February 2016. Interviews with individual participants were held at a venue of the participant's choice (the researcher's office or an empty classroom). The ASRS-v1.1 took approximately 5–10 min to complete and each interview lasted 60–100 min. The interview questions were semi-structured. The key question was "What difficulties do you experience with your ADHD symptoms?" Additional questions included the following: (a) How are you doing currently? (b) How do you deal with the difficulties associated with ADHD symptoms? (c) How do you think ADHD symptoms are going to affect your future? (d) Which aspects of your ADHD symptoms do you wish to improve? and (e) Do you have additional thoughts or information you would like to share with us? The participants were encouraged to describe their experiences fully and the interviews were recorded. Participants' nonverbal reactions and matters of importance, as determined by the interviewer, were written as comments in the filed notes. The recorded interviews were transcribed and analyzed.

Data analysis

The collected data were analyzed using thematic analysis, as described by Braun and Clark [28]. This six-phase method focuses on identifying and analyzing the meanings of common themes. In the present study, phase 1 involved familiarization with the data. Meaningful information on participant experiences and difficulties in relation to their ADHD symptoms were identified by repeated reading of the transcribed data. In phase 2, initial codes were generated from the data. A total of 155 meaningful descriptions were extracted and coded. In phase 3, we searched for themes within the data. The codes were compared with candidate themes, and all data regarding candidate themes were collected. Overall, 27 candidate themes were extracted. In Phase 4, the themes were reviewed, and the researcher verified whether the extracted themes fitted in with the overall data. In total, four themes and nine subthemes were extracted. In phase 5, these themes and subthemes were defined and named, and, in Phase 6, the content was checked and the results described in a report.

To ensure the trustworthiness of this qualitative research, the present study considered the paradigms of research credibility, transferability, dependability, and confirmability set forth by Lincoln and Guba [29]. The study was conducted in accordance with qualitative research procedures and attempted to exclude biases and maintain neutrality throughout the study period. Extracted themes and subthemes were confirmed with two participants. Data analysis and result extractions were performed in collaboration with a professor of nursing science who has experience in qualitative research.

Results

Theme 1. Lack of a daily routine

Each of the participants in this study lacked a daily routine, which manifested as having an irregular lifestyle and consistently breaking promises to themselves and others. Furthermore, it was noted that the difference between the strict high school environment of the Korean education system and the more lenient university setting disconcerted participants.

Having an irregular lifestyle

The participants reported that during high school, their daily lives were regulated by their parents and teachers; however, at university, there was an increase in individual freedom and their daily lives became less structured. For example, they had irregular sleeping and eating patterns, with periods of binge eating and excessive drinking. As a result of their unsettled lives, the participants felt that they were wasting their time and were failing to achieve their desired goals and stability. The participants also reported that during the first and second years of university, they did whatever they wanted to do and did not experience any instability-related problems. The participants did not begin to experience difficulties in daily life until later in their university career, at which point they tried to change their lifestyles, but failed. The following is an excerpt from one of the participants:

> *I used to be good at cleaning the house and did all my own cooking, but it did not last long. Now, I wake up in the afternoon and fall asleep when the sun rises. My life is very erratic (Participant 4).*

Plans not followed through

During their university careers, the participants made numerous attempts to learn new things or make plans to ensure regularity within their everyday lives, but they often gave up or failed to follow through on their intentions. Most of the participants received allowances from their families, but spent all their money on gifts for themselves or their friends. The participants would be embarrassed and reprimanded by their parents for failing to adhere to credit card limits. They recognized the need to change and enrolled in related support programs; however, they were repeatedly unable to alter their behavior and felt dejected. The following quotes are from two participants: "The funny thing is that I plan well but don't put in the work. Even when I do start, I don't finish as I intended to" (Participant 2) and "Since starting university, it seems that I am getting more and more haphazard.

I think that the increasing amount of study I need to do is more than I can cope with and so it's becoming pointless to plan" (Participant 11).

Theme 2. Unsatisfactory academic performance and achievement

The participants expressed dissatisfaction with their academic performance and achievement. Despite acknowledging their student duty to complete assignments and to study, they lacked motivation. Many of the participants procrastinated, resulting in unsatisfactory outcomes. In addition, there was great variability in participant concentration levels for activities such as classes, which require maintained interest.

Procrastination

The participants were aware that they had to prepare for assignments or examinations in advance, yet they often procrastinated. Even if they started an assignment well in advance of a deadline, they could not concentrate properly on the task. The participants often stayed up all night before an examination or assignment deadline, or resorted to only studying on the day of the examination. By procrastinating, the participants failed to leave enough time for assignment revisions but, reportedly, could concentrate more easily under time pressure. The following is an excerpt from one of the interviews:

I vaguely think that I should start to work hard for this assignment after a certain time point because the assignment is due. When the time comes, I slowly start to work, but even if I sit down in the morning, I only get started in the evening (Participant 4).

Difficulty prioritizing and completing tasks

When presented with multiple tasks to complete, the participants stated that they did not know which task to complete first and experienced difficulty in completing tasks efficiently. Participants found it difficult to complete tasks because they were trying to focus on multiple subjects and several individual and group assignments. Further, when working in a group setting, the participants often put in extra effort to avoid upsetting their peers, but their peers often had to revise their work because of its poor quality. Overall, since the participants did not start assignments on time and had to finish them hastily, completion rates, results, and grades were poor. The following excerpts are from two of the participants:

I've been involved in a lot of activities. Because of this, there have been a lot of things that I haven't been able to handle. I did try to study, but it didn't work out well. So, I've just done extracurricular

activities. I have a lot of regrets right now … The credits were very important for getting a job. It seems that I have never done my best in any assignment (Participant 5).

and "I feel like the pressure is getting so strong that I want to get it done anyhow, and fast. So, I don't think I can do anything properly now. I often think, 'Oh, why am I doing this?'" (Participant 6).

Interest-based participation

The students stated that they could only participate in campus activities, including classes, if activities were of interest to them. They stated that if they were taking an uninteresting class, they would be unable to focus and would instead waste time using their cell phones, scribbling, taking bathroom breaks, drinking beverages, or eating meals. The following excerpts are from two students: "I cannot keep still in a boring class. I intentionally don't participate in it. It's a waste of time. There are some professors who have interesting classes. I can take those classes" (Participant 11) and "If I listen [in a class] for about 10 min, I get more and more absent-minded. I stare at my watch, go to the bathroom although I do not want to go there, and play with my cell phone" (Participant 2).

Theme 3. Unskilled interpersonal relationships

The participants stated that they had experienced difficulties building and maintaining interpersonal relationships since childhood. Throughout their lives, they stated that they had suppressed their negative emotions, practiced avoidance, and displayed extreme reactions (such as sudden emotional outbursts) within their relationships. The participants reported that their daily university lives were not disrupted by their interpersonal relationships; however, they were aware that this could be problematic when they started working after graduation.

Extreme reactions

The participants expressed extremely negative emotions when they experienced difficult situations within interpersonal relationships. Some participants reacted by avoiding a certain situation or person, and by hiding negative emotions during conflicts. In general, participants avoided expressing negative emotions to others and were angry with their families for making them fearful of expressing their negative emotions. Participants reported that their relationships often deteriorated if they expressed negative emotions; therefore, they avoided people they did not like and kept silent when in their company. Yet, some participants reacted by having a sudden emotional outburst, including episodes of excitement, screaming, and anger. The following two excerpts are from study participants: "I don't want to see anyone I do not like, and because I don't want to face these situations, I just don't." (Participant 7) and.

I don't seem to be able to control my facial expression, although I can be patient in front of people. Sometimes I get angry at my friends or family, and I apologize to them afterwards when I feel relaxed or calm (Participant 3).

Difficulty building and maintaining relationships
Participants tried to overcome difficulties within interpersonal relationships by convincing themselves that they were fine with others or that their relationships were improving. However, failure to resolve conflicts within these relationships caused the participants to have difficulties developing deeper relationships with other people. Specifically, participants often encountered conflicts in relation to being late or absent for appointments. Further, the participants stated that their friends understood that they could occasionally not keep appointment times. Unlike high school, university affords students the opportunity to choose their own classes and make their own schedules; therefore, they have more freedom to live their lives without maintaining close relationships with other people. As a result, students often remain isolated and only interact with a small group of peers when necessary. The participants expressed difficulty in adjusting to certain subjects that required interactions with other people, with some participants even wanting to switch to subjects requiring fewer interpersonal relationships. The following quote is from one of the participants: "Interpersonal relationships were the most challenging for me. My biggest worry is always interpersonal relationships. I have always found maintaining deeper and longer relationships with others difficult" (Participant 6).

Theme 4. Continuous worry
Although the participants occasionally acted impulsively, they were generally introspective in their daily lives, and these thoughts caused worry. The participants tended to brood over past events and worried about things that had not happened yet. Furthermore, because of bad past experiences, the participants did not trust themselves in the future, thereby increasing their anxiety.

Obsession with past events
The participants tended to repeatedly think about and regret past events. Participants stated that if past events were associated with negative thoughts, then they often engaged in a perpetual cycle of worry. However, they did recognize that it was unnecessary to keep thinking

about the past and that it was not important to their current situation. The participants were mostly preoccupied with thoughts revolving around everyday matters, such as whether they satisfactorily submitted an examination paper, submitted their assignments without errors, closed the door properly, or whether or not there were problems in their relationships with other people. The following are excerpts from two participants: "I'm worried even though I think 'Oh, stop worrying. It's already over.'" (Participant 5) and "I am afraid I have a lot of worries about relationships with other people. When someone else does something wrong to me, I quickly forget it. However, when I do something wrong, I keep on remembering it" (Participant 9).

Self-distrust
The participants underestimated themselves because of negative past experiences. When they obsessed about past events, they often experienced anxiety and worry about the future. Specifically, the participants were concerned about finding professional fields or jobs that would be suitable for their perceived weaknesses. Participants expressed a desire to obtain an interesting job that would allow them to work independently, rather than collectively. However, the content of their future job was not concrete or realistic. Below are two interview excerpts: "I am afraid that overall, I fall short. If the average score of ordinary people is 50, I feel like I will score 40. Overall, I think I am a bit lacking in ability compared to other people" (Participant 3) and "I worry a lot about making mistakes. For example, I keep worrying that my answer sheet will not be properly submitted when I take an exam" (Participant 7).

Discussion
The present study aimed to analyze the difficulties experienced by university students with ADHD symptoms. A total of 12 eligible students were interviewed and four themes emerged during the analysis. The first theme was lack of a daily routine. University students with ADHD symptoms did not implement their plans well because of their inattention, impulsivity, and the lack of regularity within their daily lives. Hyperactivity, which is common in pediatric patients with ADHD, decreases markedly with age, such that superficial activity is maintained at a relatively reasonable level in adult patients with ADHD [30]. However, the present study shows that certain ADHD-related difficulties persist into adulthood, including impulsivity, inattention, difficulty in controlling emotions, and inability to systematize [15, 18]. In addition, previous studies have indicated that university students with ADHD symptoms have irregular sleeping hours and lower sleep quality [18, 31], and eat irregular meals

or occasionally partake in binge eating [31, 32]. These observations are consistent with the results of the present study. Many studies have shown that university students with an ADHD tendency or diagnosis have more difficulties with alcohol, smoking, and internet and smartphone addiction than do other students [6, 22, 26, 33, 34]. These outcomes further support the theory that university students with ADHD symptoms lack structure in their daily lives. Therefore, attention, support, and other appropriate interventions would help these students manage their daily life schedule, including their sleeping and eating behaviors, while coaching programs or organizational skills intervention programs may help them manage their time more efficiently [35, 36].

The second theme was unsatisfactory academic performance and achievement. Even if the students made plans to study in advance, they failed to prioritize and complete tasks. This resulted in unsatisfactory academic performance and achievement. The students made efforts to overcome these problems, but their concentration waned with lack of interest, and they struggled with repeated failures. Previous studies have reported that such students have difficulty planning and completing tasks as a result of procrastination or indecision, and thus do not manage their time well [37, 38]. Other studies have reported that university students with ADHD symptoms have low academic performance as a result of difficulties with concentrating on their studies and completing assignments, worries about studying and having high test anxiety, and not applying appropriate learning strategies, which all lead to problems with adjusting to university life [4, 9, 16–18, 21, 39]. Such difficulties in adjusting to university life can extend to difficulties in social functioning in adulthood. For example, these students may fail to secure employment or may find only low income employment [3, 40]. Therefore, programs promoting academic strategies and time management skills should be implemented to help these students improve their academic performance and educational achievements. As in previous studies, working memory training or self-monitoring can be applied to support their learning [41, 42]. In addition, our results indicate that these students should be encouraged to concentrate on their areas of interest, as this strategy might help them to better select and adapt to their future jobs.

The third theme was unskilled interpersonal relationships. The participants reported having extreme reactions in interpersonal relationships and experienced difficulties in forming and maintaining relationships as a result of this impulsivity. Previous studies have shown that university students with ADHD have higher levels of anger and greater difficulty in controlling emotions than their peers; therefore, these students often express anger in socially unacceptable ways [10, 33]. Furthermore, studies have reported that university students with ADHD tend to be more aggressive or confrontational in stressful situations than their peers; therefore, they often experience difficulties in forming relationships with other people [4, 10]. Since ADHD is associated with certain characteristics, such as inattentiveness and impulsivity, individuals diagnosed with ADHD tend not to pay enough attention to the feelings and desires of others, often interfering in a criticizing and controlling way, and causing conflict, disappointment, and distrust [10]. Research indicates that anger and aggressiveness negatively impact interpersonal relationships [43]. The establishment of self-identity and formation of personal relationships are important developmental tasks for university students. The lack of social skills in patients with ADHD is already known, but until now, the mechanisms leading to such difficulties have remained obscure; this study provides an understanding of why social skills are lacking. Impaired interpersonal competence can cause serious psychological maladjustment and low self-esteem, which have serious effects on life satisfaction [21]. It is, thus, important for college students with ADHD to be educated about how to express their negative feelings more healthily (rather than expressing extreme anger or displaying avoidance), to learn interpersonal skills, and to consider the effects that their ADHD symptoms can have on their relationships with others.

The final theme was continuous worry. This study found that although university students with ADHD symptoms tried to overcome these tendencies, they had high levels of self-distrust as a result of perpetually repeating cycles involving obsessing over past events and worrying about future failures. This can reduce their expectations for the future, gradually exacerbating their negative functioning. Previous studies have reported that university students with ADHD tendencies demonstrate a poorer adjustment to university life, exhibiting higher rates of depression and anxiety and lower than usual self-esteem and self-efficacy [6, 10, 21, 30, 44]. Patients with ADHD are known to have very poor tolerance for stress and dysfunctional coping styles [45]. As they are often inefficient and have difficulty adjusting to major life obligations, such as academic studies or occupations, these individuals are more likely than the general population to experience stress-causing negative life events [46, 47]. They may be very worried about repeated failures, the negative feedback they receive as a result of low academic performance, and interpersonal difficulties. These students are also more easily distracted. Time management is very important for enhancing self-efficacy and academic performance among university students [19]. Therefore, students should be taught effective time management skills to help them perform tasks efficiently and achieve a good work-life balance.

The final theme, the extent to which these students constantly worry about past mistakes and potential future ones, is important in this study. As a result of their history of repeated negative experiences and failed efforts, they come to distrust themselves and their ability to achieve their goals, which leads to further demoralization, loss of motivation, and progressive worsening of their functioning over time. Therefore, when providing interventions, it is necessary to repeatedly reduce negative feedback and to reinforce positive motivation for the future; this is an important implication arising from this study.

In summary, university students with ADHD symptoms have difficulties coping with repeated cycles of negative thoughts and worries, irregular lifestyles as a result of poor time management, dissatisfaction with academic performance and interpersonal relationships, and self-dissatisfaction. Although individual or group cognitive-behavioral therapy, mindfulness training, and coaching [20], may be helpful, it is necessary to consider the social and cultural environment of the subject based on the results of this study when applying and developing programs appropriate for them. To help these students live a healthy lifestyle at university, they should be properly diagnosed and educated about ADHD, how to prevent worrying, how to express emotions healthily, and how to effectively manage time. Social awareness of adult ADHD should also be enhanced.

This study has several limitations. First, the subjects were Korean university students; therefore, caution must be applied when generalizing these results to adults from other countries, cultures, and age groups. Further studies of university students or adults from different populations are needed. Second, participants were selected on the basis of self-reported ADHD symptoms; the experiences of and findings related to those formally diagnosed with ADHD or receiving ADHD treatment may differ. The findings of this study need to be captured and quantified using standardized rating instruments, and replicated in larger samples with fully diagnosed students. Despite these limitations, we believe that this study is important because it is the first to analyze difficulties from the perspective of Korean university students with ADHD symptoms. In addition, this study highlights the importance of developing intervention programs for such university students.

Conclusions

When the difficulties experienced by Korean university students with ADHD symptoms were analyzed, four main themes were identified, including lack of a regular daily routine, unsatisfactory academic performance and achievement, unskilled interpersonal relationships, and an ongoing tendency to worry. Students were aware of these difficulties and tried to overcome them by self-discipline. However, their self-esteem was lowered as a result of repeated cycles of inattentiveness and impulsivity. Therefore, to improve their experiences, university students with ADHD symptoms must develop insight into their diagnosis and be educated about ways to stop worrying and to effectively manage time. It is also important for universities to provide students with access to resources for life management.

Abbreviations

ADHD: attention-deficit hyperactivity disorder; DSM: diagnostic and statistical manual of mental disorders; ASRS: Adult ADHD Self-Report Scale.

Authors' contributions

SJK, YJK and YHK were responsible for study concept and design. SJK contributed to the collection of data. SJK and YJK were involved in the data analysis. SJK was responsible for drafting the manuscript, and all authors were involved in critical revisions of the manuscript. All authors read and approved the final manuscript.

Author details

¹ Nursing Science Research Institute, Chung-Ang University, Seoul, Republic of Korea. ² Faculty of Red Cross College of Nursing, Chung-Ang University, 84 Heukseok-Ro, Dongjack-Gu, Seoul 156-756, Republic of Korea.

Competing interests

The authors declare that they have no competing interests.

Funding

This study was supported by the National Research Foundation of Korea and funded by the Ministry of Science, ICT, and Future Planning of Korea (NRF-2015R1C1A1A02036634).

References

1. American Psychiatric Association. Diagnostic and statistical manual of mental disorders. 5th ed. Arlington: American Psychiatric Publishing; 2013.
2. Polanczyk GV, Willcutt EG, Salum GA, Kieling C, Rohde LA. ADHD prevalence estimates across three decades: an updated systematic review and meta-regression analysis. Int J Epidemiol. 2014;43:434–42.
3. Fayyad J, De Graaf R, Kessler R, Alonso J, Angermeyer M, Demyttenaere K, et al. Cross-national prevalence and correlates of adult attention-deficit hyperactivity disorder. Br J Psychiatry. 2007;190:402–9.

4. DuPaul GJ, Weyandt LL, O'Dell SM, Varejao M. College students
    with ADHD: current status and future directions. J Atten Disord.
    2009;13:234–50.
5. Park S, Cho MJ, Chang SM, Jeon HJ, Cho SJ, Kim BS, et al. Prevalence
    correlates and comorbidities of adult ADHD symptoms in Korea: results
    of the Korean epidemiologic catchment area study. Psychiatry Res.
    2011;186:378–83.
6. Kwak YS, Jung YE, Kim MD. Prevalence and correlates of attention-deficit
    hyperactivity disorder symptoms in Korean college students. Neuropsy-
    chiatr Dis Treat. 2015;11:797–802.
7. Agarwal R, Goldenberg M, Perry R, IsHak WW. The quality of life of adults
    with attention deficit hyperactivity disorder: a systematic review. Innov
    Clin Neurosci. 2012;9(5–6):10–21.
8. Pinho TD, Manz PH, DuPaul GJ, Anastopoulos AD, Weyandt LL. Predictors
    and moderators of quality of life among college students with ADHD. J
    Atten Disord. 2017. https://doi.org/10.1177/1087054717734645.
9. Advokat C, Lane SM, Luo C. College students with and without ADHD:
    comparison of self-report of medication usage study habits and aca-
    demic achievement. J Atten Disord. 2011;15:656–66.
10. Kim Y, Choi J, Yoo Y. College adjustment among first year students with
    ADHD symptoms. Cognit Behav Ther Korea. 2016;16:161–85.
11. Danckaerts M, Sonuga-Barke EJ, Banaschewski T, Buitelaar J, Döpfner
    M, Hollis C, et al. The quality of life of children with attention deficit/
    hyperactivity disorder: a systematic review. Eur Child Adolesc Psychiatry.
    2010;19:83–105.
12. Uneri OS, Senses-Dinc G, Goker Z. The quality of life (QoL) in attention
    deficit hyperactivity disorder (ADHD). In: Norvilitis JM, editor. ADHD-new
    directions in diagnosis and treatment. Shanghai: InTech; 2015.
13. Piñeiro-Dieguez B, Balanzá-Martínez V, García-García P, Soler-López B, CAT
    Study Group. Psychiatric comorbidity at the time of diagnosis in adults
    with ADHD: the CAT study. J Atten Disord. 2016;20:1066–75.
14. Stevens LJ, Kuczek T, Burgess JR, Hurt E, Arnold LE. Dietary sensitivi-
    ties and ADHD symptoms: thirty-five years of research. Clin Pediatr.
    2011;50:279–93.
15. Barkley RA, Murphy KR, Fischer M. ADHD in adults: what the science says.
    New York: Guilford Press; 2008.
16. Kim Y. The mediational effect of learning strategies on the relationship
    between ADHD symptoms and academic achievement. Cognit Behav
    Ther Korea. 2015;15:247–67.
17. Lefler EK, Sacchetti GM, Del Carlo DI. ADHD in college: a qualitative analy-
    sis. Atten Deficit Hyperact Disord. 2016;8:79–93.
18. Meaux JB, Green A, Broussard L. ADHD in the college student: a block in
    the road. J Psychiatr Ment Health Nurs. 2009;16:248–56.
19. Kim OS. The effects of time management on self-efficacy and academic
    achievement in college students. J Korean Fam Resour Manag Assoc.
    2013;17:1–17.
20. Fleming AP, McMahon RJ. Developmental context and treatment
    principles for ADHD among college students. Clin Child Fam Psychol Rev.
    2012;15:303–29.
21. Lee SJ. Relationship between symptoms of attention-deficit hyperactivity
    disorder and psychological maladjustment self-esteem life-satisfaction
    and academic achievement among college students. Korean J Educ Ther.
    2015;7:193–208.
22. Kim MK. Influence on university students' suicide ideation of job prepar-
    ing stress and problem drinking: moderating effect of resilience. J Korea
    Inst Youth Facil Environ. 2013;11:29–36 **(In Korean)**.
23. Park MJ, Kim JH, Jung MS. A qualitative study on the stress of university
    students preparing for employment. Korea J Couns. 2009;10:417–35.
24. Jeong HW, Chang MS, Kwak HW. Relationships among self-esteem
    depression and interpersonal problems in adult ADHD sub-clusters: path
    analysis and structural equation modeling. Korean J Cognit Biol Psychol.
    2011;23:153–69.
25. Kessler RC, Adler L, Ames M, Demler O, Faraone S, Hiripi E, et al. The World
    Health Organization Adult ADHD Self-Report Scale (ASRS): a short screen-
    ing scale for use in the general population. Psychol Med. 2005;35:245–56.
26. Kim JH, Lee EH, Joung YS. The WHO adult ADHD self-report scale: reliabil-
    ity and validity of the Korean version. Psychiatry Investig. 2013;10:41–6.
27. Kim DH, Lee KE, Lee YJ, et al. The association between smart phone addic-
    tion and attention-deficit hyperactivity disorder among some college
    students. J Korean Soc Matern Child Health. 2013;17:105–12.
28. Braun V, Clarke V. Using thematic analysis in psychology. Qual Res Psychol.
    2006;3:77–101.
29. Lincoln YS, Guba EG. Naturalistic inquiry. Newbury Park: Sage; 1985.
30. Kim JY, Kwak HW, Chang MS. Relationships among depression anxiety
    and quality of sleep in adults with ADHD tendency. Korea J Couns.
    2010;11:75–89.
31. Pagoto SL, Curtin C, Lemon SC, Bandini LG, Schneider KL, Bodenlos JS, Ma
    Y. Association between adult attention deficit/hyperactivity disorder and
    obesity in the US population. Obesity. 2009;17:539–44.
32. Merkt J, Gawrilow C. Health dietary habits and achievement motivation
    in college students with self-reported ADHD diagnosis. J Atten Disord.
    2016;20:727–40.
33. Blase SL, Gilbert AN, Anastopoulos AD, Costello EJ, Hoyle RH, Swart-
    zwelder HS, et al. Self-reported ADHD and adjustment in college: cross-
    sectional and longitudinal findings. J Atten Disord. 2009;13:297–309.
34. Kim TM, Suk KH. Relationships between adult ADHD and internet addic-
    tion: focus on the mediating effects of interpersonal problems. Korean J
    Health Psychol. 2014;19:813–28 **(In Korean)**.
35. LaCount PA, Hartung CM, Shelton CR, Stevens AE. Efficacy of an
    organizational skills intervention for college students with ADHD symp-
    tomatology and academic difficulties. J Atten Disord. 2015. https://doi.
    org/10.1177/1087054715594423.
36. Prevatt F. Coaching for college students with ADHD. Curr Psychiatry Rep.
    2016;18:110.
37. Asherson P, Chen W, Craddock B, Taylor E. Adult attention-deficit hyperac-
    tivity disorder: recognition and treatment in general adult psychiatry. Br J
    Psychiatry. 2007;190:4–5.
38. Biederman J, Faraone SV, Spencer TJ, Mick E, Monuteaux MC, Aleardi M.
    Functional impairments in adults with self-reports of diagnosed ADHD:
    a controlled study of 1001 adults in the community. J Clin Psychiatry.
    2006;67:524–40.
39. Cheung KK, Wong IC, Ip P, Chan PK, Lin CH, Wong LY, et al. Experiences
    of adolescents and young adults with ADHD in Hong Kong: treatment
    services and clinical management. BMC Psychiatry. 2015;15:95.
40. Spencer TJ, Biederman J, Mick E. Attention-deficit/hyperactivity disorder:
    diagnosis lifespan comorbidities and neurobiology. J Pediatr Psychol.
    2007;32:631–42.
41. Gropper RJ, Gotlieb H, Kronitz R, Tannock R. Working memory training in
    college students with ADHD or LD. J Atten Disord. 2014;18:331–45.
42. Scheithauer MC, Kelley ML. Self-monitoring by college students
    with ADHD: the impact on academic performance. J Atten Disord.
    2017;21:1030–9.
43. Solanto MV. Cognitive-behavioral therapy for adult ADHD. Seoul: Sigma
    Press; 2013 **(In Korean)**.
44. Roh HL, Shin EJ. Relationship between prevalence of attention deficit
    hyperactivity disorder symptoms and depression of college students. J
    Korea Acad Indus Coop Soc. 2015;16:1937–45.
45. Barkley RA. Attention-deficit hyperactivity disorder: a handbook for
    diagnosis and treatment. 4th ed. New York: Guilford Press; 2014.
46. Lee DY, Lee CS, Park JW, et al. Study of relation among stress adult
    attention-deficit hyperactivity disorder symptoms and suicide idea in
    conscripts. J Korean Soc Biol Ther Psychiatry. 2011;17:250–6 **(In Korean)**.
47. Barkley RA. Attention-deficit hyperactivity disorder: a handbook for
    diagnosis and treatment. 3rd ed. New York, NY: Guilford Press; 2006

16

Elucidating adolescent aspirational models for the design of public mental health interventions: a mixed-method study

Sauharda Rai[1]*[iD], Safar Bikram Adhikari[1], Nanda Raj Acharya[1], Bonnie N. Kaiser[2] and Brandon A. Kohrt[1,2,3,4]

Abstract

Background: Adolescent aspirational models are sets of preferences for an idealized self. Aspirational models influence behavior and exposure to risk factors that shape adult mental and physical health. Cross-cultural understandings of adolescent aspirational models are crucial for successful global mental health programs. The study objective was elucidating adolescent aspirational models to inform interventions in Nepal.

Methods: Twenty qualitative life trajectory interviews were conducted among adolescents, teachers, and parents. Card sorting (rating and ranking activities) were administered to 72 adolescents aged 15–19 years, stratified by caste/ethnicity: upper caste *Brahman* and *Chhetri*, occupational caste *Dalit*, and ethnic minority *Janajati*.

Results: Themes included qualities of an ideal person; life goals, barriers, and resources; emotions and coping; and causes of interpersonal violence, harmful alcohol use, and suicide. Education was the highest valued attribute of ideal persons. Educational attainment received higher prioritization by marginalized social groups (*Dalit* and *Janajati*). Poverty was the greatest barrier to achieving life goals. The most common distressing emotion was 'tension', which girls endorsed more frequently than boys. Sharing emotions and self-consoling were common responses to distress. Tension was the most common reason for alcohol use, especially among girls. Domestic violence, romantic break-ups, and academic pressure were reasons for suicidality.

Conclusion: Inability to achieve aspirational models due to a range of barriers was associated with negative emotions—notably tension—and dysfunctional coping that exacerbates barriers, which ultimately results in the triad of interpersonal violence, substance abuse, and suicidality. Interventions should be framed as reducing the locally salient idiom of distress tension and target this triad of threats. Regarding intervention content, youth-endorsed coping mechanisms should be fortified to counter this distress pathway.

Keywords: Children, Adolescents, Interpersonal violence, Low-income countries, Stigma, Idioms of distress, Cultural models, Substance abuse, Suicide, Nepal

Background

Adolescent aspirational models influence behavior choices and exposure to risk and protective factors, which ultimately shape adult mental and physical health [1]. Aspirational models are sets of preferences for an idealized self, towards which an adolescent strives, and they are often the reference by which adolescents determine their self-esteem and self-worth [2]. Aspirational models are developed through the interaction of individual experience, local social networks, and exposure to media representations of success [3, 4]. Aspirational models can be applied to recent advances in conceptualizing adolescent interventions in the field of global mental health [5–7].

*Correspondence: sauharda.rai@gmail.com
[1] Transcultural Psychosocial Organization Nepal (TPO Nepal), Anek Marga, Baluwatar, Kathmandu, Nepal
Full list of author information is available at the end of the article

Effective youth interventions to promote self-esteem and wellbeing are considered best practices in the most recent World Bank guidelines for disease control and prevention (DCP-3). Interventions during adolescence are also associated with life-long positive physical and mental health outcomes [8, 9]. However, there is no one-size-fits-all life course model for youth around the globe, and therefore youth interventions need to be adapted based on local needs, desires, culture, and available resources [8, 10]. There is also a wide variation both between and within countries regarding adolescent mental health, and thus it is necessary to understand local risk and protective factors during adolescence [10, 11].

Research on health and wellbeing of adolescents has increased in recent years. The United Nations Sustainable Development Goals and Global Strategy for women's, children's, and adolescent health have pushed this agenda forward [12, 13]. More specifically, there is a need for research on adolescent mental health within low- and middle-income countries (LMICs) [14, 15].

In Nepal, prior studies have explored prevalence rates and risk factors for adolescent mental health problems [16–18]. However, studies have neither addressed how adolescents aspire toward idealized selves nor explored the perceived barriers and resources associated with achieving these goals. We aimed to elucidate adolescent aspirational models in a region of rural Nepal with high rates of adult mental illness [19, 20], with the aim to identify content for mental health interventions.

Setting

Nepal is ranked among the least developed countries, with a human development index of .54 and per-capita income of 2400 USD in 2014. Per 2011 national census data, children from 0 to 17 years constitute 44.4% of the population of 26.3 million [21]. Political instability, a recent history of violent conflict, structural violence including gender- and caste/ethnic-based discrimination, low quality of infrastructure, limited access to quality education and health services, and lack of employment opportunities are barriers to achieving physical and mental health throughout the country. Although a decade has passed since the People's War (1996–2006), the country has only recently established a new constitution, which remains highly contentious amid an environment of escalating ethnic disputes, including calls for ethnic federalist redistricting. The fact that almost 1260 people leave the country every day for foreign employment and 24.7% of the gross domestic product is contributed by remittance from these migrants demonstrates the limited in-country resources [22].

The study was set in Jumla, a mountainous district in northwestern Nepal with an area of 2531 km^2. The

district has a population of 108,921, with an average household size of 5.6 [21]. The literacy rate is 55% (male—68% and female—41%), and agriculture is the major occupation. The district is divided into 30 Village Development Committees (VDCs) and has one hospital, the Karnali Academy of Health Sciences Hospital (KAHS), 9 health posts, and 26 sub-health posts. Only 29% of households have access to electricity, and 98% of them use firewood for cooking. Seasonal migration to India is common. Until 2007, Jumla was only connected to the outside world through air travel or three-day walk to the nearest road. Karnali Highway opened in 2007, and though it is functional only during good weather, it has been instrumental in changing the life of people in the district by integrating local, regional, national, and international economies [23].

Jumla's population is predominantly Hindu (98%). The Hindu caste system, as practiced in Jumla, influences social interactions, life trajectories, and mental health [24]. The caste system in Nepal was formalized by the government through the legal code of 1854, known as the *Muluki* Ain, which divides social groups into high vs. low and pure vs. impure categories. On top of the caste hierarchy are Brahman, the priestly castes, followed by Chhetri/Thakuri castes. Unlike the rest of Nepal, the Chhetri castes in Jumla and surrounding areas are divided into alcohol-drinking *Matwali* and alcohol-abstaining *Tagdari Chhetri* groups. Dalit (previously known as "untouchable") castes are at the bottom of the Hindu hierarchy [25]. Finally, there are Janajati, ethnic minority groups, the majority of whom are not Hindu [26].

In Jumla, Dalits have been found to have a higher prevalence of depression and anxiety compared to other groups, explained by their low economic status and greater exposure to stressful life events. As in other parts of the world, female gender has been found to be a strong predictor of poor mental health in Jumla [20, 26].

In terms of defining emotions and idioms of distress, some work has already been done in Nepal [27–29]. Definitions are often multifaceted, with common categorizations involving local version of the concepts of heart-mind (Nepali: *man*), brain-mind (*dimaag*), spirit (*saato*), and social status (*ijjat*). Expressions of emotion, especially regarding the brain-mind, are also related to stigma [27]. Alongside these ethnopsychological terms is the use of English terms like "tension" to define emotions [28, 29].

Methods

The initial phase of the study involved development of interview guides based on previous ethnographic studies, formative interviews with similar populations, and literature reviews of adolescent life choices and burden of mental health problems [30–33]. The first phase of data collection involved a life trajectory interview (LTI) conducted with 20 adolescents, teachers, and parents. This was then followed by a ranking and rating activity conducted with 72 adolescents.

Data collection was completed in collaboration with Transcultural Psychosocial Organization (TPO) Nepal. The first author, a native Nepali with a background in field research and familiarity working in the study site, conducted the initial life trajectory interviews and card sorting activity and trained the other TPO researchers at Jumla. Both other TPO researchers (2nd and 3rd author) had more than 4 years of research experience and training in qualitative and quantitative methods, as well as ethics of research with vulnerable populations. These field researchers were also certified psychosocial counselors and provided first-hand psychosocial counseling to participants whom they screened as having some form of mental health and psychosocial problems. Data collection occurred from September 2014 through May 2015. In this study, adolescents were defined as people from 15 to 19 years of age. The age group was selected because this range captured the cultural notion of adolescent in Nepal [30].

A. Life trajectory interview (LTI)

The LTI was designed to understand the link between large-scale structural conditions and social processes with individual outcomes. It investigates how life-course models mediate the relationship between adolescent development and later psychiatric conditions [34, 35]. Six themes were included:

1. Understanding the ideal person [*raamro maanche*]
2. Life goals
3. Barriers and resources
4. Emotions and coping
5. Interpersonal conflict
6. Alcohol and suicide.

These six themes were chosen based on prior research in the study site. Because preventing adolescent suicide was a broader aim of our work in Nepal, we prioritized themes related to youth suicide and mental health. Suicide is the single leading cause of mortality among women of reproductive age [36], and in Jumla, the area where this study was conducted, 85% of suicides among women occur before the age of 25 years [37]. Work on suicide and mental health in this region of the country and elsewhere in Nepal has highlighted the importance of alcohol use, interpersonal conflict, thwarted life goals,

emotional dysregulation, and lack of coping skills as risk factors [38–40]. The six themes were piloted in four initial interviews conducted jointly by the first and last authors and through ethnographic observation in Jumla.

The *"ideal person"* theme explored the respondent's understanding of an ideal person. It described the general qualities of an ideal person through an individual, social, and cultural perspective. *"Life purpose and goals"* explored the life purpose of the respondent and the general adolescent population in Jumla. It also explored the similarities and differences in life goals with their parents and ways to balance them. *"Barriers and resources"* looked at the possible internal and external barriers that were likely to occur in their life and the resources to address it. *"Emotions"* looked at the different positive/negative emotions they experience and ways to cope with them. We especially looked at "tension," which is an English idiom for stress and psychological distress increasingly used in South Asia by both adult and adolescent populations [28, 29]. For *"Coping,"* we wanted to make the distinction between two different themes: sharing feelings (*man ko kura satne*: sharing things in the heart-mind), which is considered a positive behavior by adolescents, and venting/projecting negative emotions onto others (*aru lai rish pokhne*: throwing anger onto someone else) as a dysfunctional way of channeling feelings. *"Interpersonal conflicts"* explored difficult and abusive social relationships. *"Alcohol, substance use, and suicide"* addressed substance use attitudes and behaviors among adolescents in Jumla.

Each interview took 60–90 min, and a debriefing form was written after every interview. Most interviews were digitally recorded with participant's consent. Four participants did not provide consent for recording, so detailed notes were taken for those interviews. Of the four not consenting for audio recording, three were adolescents who did not feel comfortable being recorded. One teacher did not consent for recording because of fear that the recording could be obtained by persons other than the researchers. Although not explicitly stated, the history of political violence during the Maoist revolution in the area (1996–2006) may have influenced comfort with audio recordings. In particular, Maoists had targeted teachers leading to particular sensitivity of these participants. Interviews were transcribed directly into English. Coding was done using Nvivo Version 10 using thematic analysis [41]. The first author coded all the interviews with a codebook developed jointly by the first, second, and senior author based on close reading of transcripts.

Altogether, 10 themes and 74 sub-themes were identified, which became the basis for the card ranking and rating tasks. The themes were:

1. Qualities of an ideal person (*Raamro maanchhe*)—8 sub-themes
2. Life goals—8 sub-themes
3. Barriers for life goals—7 sub-themes
4. Resources for life goals—4 sub-themes
5. Positive emotions/thoughts—6 sub-themes
6. Negative emotions/thoughts—7 sub-themes
7. Coping mechanisms—9 sub-themes
8. Causes of violence—9 sub-themes
9. Causes of alcoholism—7 sub-themes
10. Causes of suicide—9 sub-themes.

In accordance with recommendations for transparency and availability of qualitative data while protecting anonymity of participants [42], examples of qualitative coding queries are presented in Additional file 1.

B. Card sorting (ranking and rating task)

Cultural consensus analysis is a set of techniques used to understand how people in a cultural group make sense of information within a domain [43, 44]. Common methods used in cultural consensus analysis include free listing, ranking, and pile sorts. We employed a modified ranking and rating card sort that allowed for a visual display of preferences, timeline, thoughts, and frequency related to the ten themes identified in the life trajectory interviews [45, 46].

The 10 themes were written on separate sheets of poster paper, and index cards were developed for the 74 sub-themes. For each theme, the participant was given the set of corresponding index cards and was asked to rank the items based on preference, timeline, thoughts and/or frequency. For example, in Fig. 1 the participant was given a set of seven cards, and the respondent first chose the cards that were relevant for their life; this respondent included all cards. Then the respondent ranked the index cards by assigning a number to each card. Finally, the respondent indicated how likely they were to experience those barriers in their life by placing them in the specified area of the chart. Here, keeping the index cards on the left means the items were less likely to happen, and on the right, it meant the items were more likely to happen in their life. They had the choice of discarding cards that were not relevant to them. The charts were then photographed, and scores were entered by overlaying a visual matrix onto the photographs.

Before using this with study participants, the procedure was pilot tested with research staff at TPO Nepal to evaluate its acceptability, feasibility, and comprehensibility.

Ethnicity and gender were the two main demographic factors examined to test associations with ranking and rating data. These two factors were evaluated for

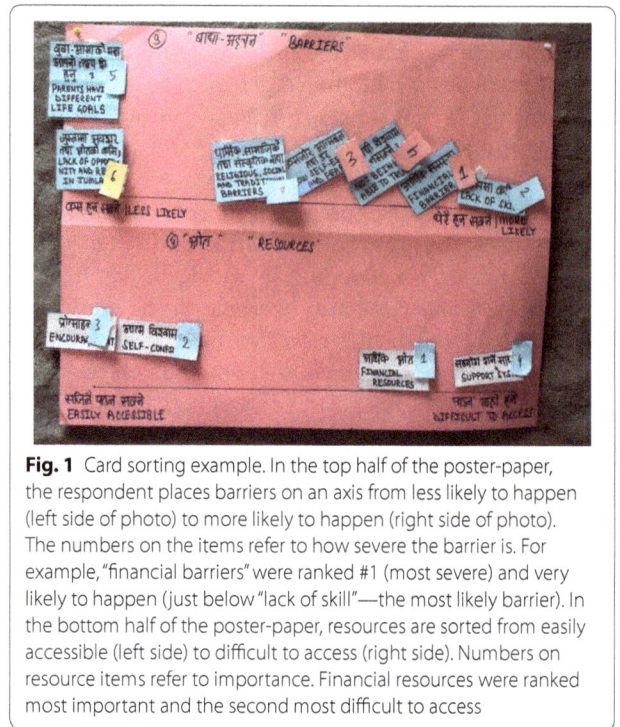

Fig. 1 Card sorting example. In the top half of the poster-paper, the respondent places barriers on an axis from less likely to happen (left side of photo) to more likely to happen (right side of photo). The numbers on the items refer to how severe the barrier is. For example, "financial barriers" were ranked #1 (most severe) and very likely to happen (just below "lack of skill"—the most likely barrier). In the bottom half of the poster-paper, resources are sorted from easily accessible (left side) to difficult to access (right side). Numbers on resource items refer to importance. Financial resources were ranked most important and the second most difficult to access

associations with the eight themes: quality of an ideal person, life goals, barriers, frequency of emotion, coping mechanisms, causes of violence, alcohol use, and suicide. Demographic factors were tested separately for their significance using one-way ANOVA tests. A statistical significance of $p < .05$ was used. SPSS [Statistical Package for the Social Sciences Version 24 (IBM/SPSS, 2016)] was used for statistical analysis. All quantitative data are available in Additional file 1.

Results

Twenty respondents participated in the life trajectory interviews (LTIs) (see Table 1). Sixty percent were female. The majority (75%) of respondents were adolescents, and the remaining 15% were teachers and 10% parents. The participants represented the four major castes/ethnicities in Jumla—Brahman (35%), Chhetri (20%), Dalit (30%) and Janajati (15%). Adolescents included both students (n = 10) and youth who had dropped out of school (n = 5).

Seventy-two adolescents participated in the card sorting exercise, with equal representation of boys and girls. As it was necessary for the participants to read the index card and charts, only school-going or literate adolescents were selected. One-third of the ranking sample was high-caste (Brahman or Chhetri), one third was low caste Dalit, and one third was Janajati (Table 1).

Table 1 Sample characteristics

	Life trajectory interviews (n = 20)	Card sorting (n = 72)
	n (%)	n (%)
Gender		
Male	8 (40%)	36 (50%)
Female	12 (60%)	36 (50%)
Caste		
Brahman	7 (35%)	13 (18.1%)
Chhetri	4 (20%)	12 (16.7%)
Dalit	6 (30%)	23 (31.9%)
Janajati	3 (15%)	24 (33.3%)
Group		
Adolescent	15 (75%)	72 (100%)
Teacher	3 (15%)	–
Parent	2 (10%)	–

Qualities of an ideal person

An ideal person (Nepali: *raamro maanche*) was someone whom respondents aspired to be. LTI responses included attributes for thoughts, behaviors, education, and physical features. More than half of respondents reported education to be the most important characteristic of an ideal person (Table 2). Among the four caste groups, Dalit adolescents saw "socially acceptable behavior" as the most important character of an ideal person, and Brahmans saw it as the least important (caste/ethnicity group difference ANOVA, $F = 4.25, p = .008$). In contrast, Brahman adolescents endorsed being physically healthy and good looking as the most important characteristic ($F = 3.99, p = .011$).

Life goals

Results from card sorting and LTIs revealed that the greatest importance was placed upon education and obtaining government jobs. All participants in card sorting chose education as one of their life goals, of which 75% selected it as the most important. Importance of education was highest among Dalit respondents and lowest among Brahman respondents ($F = 7.49, p = .001$). Government jobs, locally termed as "*lok Shewa*," refers to being a bureaucrat or becoming a police officer or army soldier. Chhetri respondents ranked the importance of government jobs higher than Dalit respondents ($F = 3.81, p = .013$). For example:

> "I want to study a lot first. I want to study up to a higher level, go to different places, understand and learn many things and ultimately become a nurse."—15-year-old Dalit Female

> "My child's first priority is to study, become a great person, stand on her own feet and get married only after she achieves this. I will support this." 45-year-old Brahman Parent, Female

Migration and marriage were among the least prioritized life goals. Migration was predominantly a goal for those who wanted to travel within the country to obtain higher education. Migration for work was not prioritized. LTIs revealed that marriage was seen as a goal only after education was completed. Among the five adolescents who had dropped out of school, two of them (1 male and 1 female) were married and had dropped out of school after marriage. Continuing traditional family occupations (e.g., farmer, Hindu Brahman priest, Dalit blacksmith, Dalit cobbler) was the second lowest ranked life goal but was found to be statistically significant, with more girls wanting to continue their family tradition than boys ($F = 4.14; p = .047$). For example:

> "I have given up trying to convince my parents [to change their traditional beliefs]. But when I am menstruating, I do not have to sleep in the cowshed. I can sleep at home but cannot go downstairs, and my parents take me to hospital if I have lot of pain. It is slowly changing."—17-year-old Janajati Female

Barriers to life fulfillment

The greatest barrier in fulfilling life goals came in the form of poor finances and low self-esteem. Financial resources were required for continuing education, learning new skills, and added labor. The participants also noted lack of skills, opportunities, and institutions to continue education as possible barriers:

> "I have written songs and want to record an album, but there is no such opportunity and resources here in Jumla. There is no place to even getting trained in singing, and I cannot go to Nepaljung [nearest city] to do all these."—18-year-old Dalit Male who was an aspiring singer

Religious and cultural barriers scored the lowest in terms of barriers to achieving life goals.

Emotional distress

The English-language term '*tension*' was the most frequently endorsed negative emotion among the adolescents. As discussed in "Methods" section, this English language term is increasingly used in South Asia to denote stress and psychological distress, whereas other emotional terms were in Nepali. Girls rated the frequency of tension higher than boys ($F = 5.27, p = .025$).

Table 2 Card sort results (n = 72)

	Rank[a]	Mean	SD	Gender		Ethnicity	
				F	p value	F	p value
Qualities of ideal person	(1–8)						
Educated	1	6.80	1.80	.61	.43	.64	.59
Socially acceptable behavior	2	5.46	1.50	.50	.48	4.25	.008**
Positive thinking	3	4.65	2.30	1.15	.29	.21	.89
Helping others	4	4.49	2.44	.84	.36	.84	.48
Keeping family happy	5	4.13	2.48	.11	.74	1.36	.26
Self-satisfaction	6	3.92	2.19	.01	1.00	.39	.76
Physically healthy/good looking	7	2.87	2.72	2.34	.13	3.99	.01*
Religious	8	2.73	2.45	.29	.59	.51	.68
Life goals	(1–8)						
Better education	1	7.42	1.13	.68	.41	7.49	.001**
Getting a job	2	6.17	1.24	3.10	.08	3.81	.01*
Following your dreams	3	5.65	1.76	2.83	.09	.55	.65
Earning money	4	5.07	1.57	.44	.50	1.30	.28
Business	5	3.77	2.09	.01	.92	1.75	.16
Migration	6	3.48	1.91	.06	.43	.72	.55
Continue family tradition	7	3.48	1.50	4.14	.05*	1.17	.33
Marriage	8	2.73	1.53	.41	.52	1.17	.33
Barriers	(1–7)						
Finance	1	5.46	1.88	2.50	.12	1.28	.29
Low self-esteem	2	4.59	1.91	.13	.72	.75	.52
Skills	3	4.57	1.94	.09	.75	1.46	.23
Lack of opportunity	4	4.18	1.48	1.85	.18	.53	.66
Trust	5	3.68	2.04	.31	.58	.81	.49
Different life goals with parents	6	3.51	1.92	.38	.54	.89	.45
Religious/cultural barriers	7	3.18	2.01	1.16	.29	2.40	.07
Frequency of emotions	(1–7)						
Tension	1	6.00	2.34	5.27	.03*	1.98	.12
Sadness	2	4.49	2.23	2.01	.10	.33	.80
Embarrassment	3	4.25	2.77	.16	.68	.75	.52
Anger	4	4.01	2.74	.01	.89	1.31	.28
Inferiority	5	3.71	2.31	1.62	.21	1.32	.27
Fear	6	3.70	2.72	.85	.36	.19	.89
Self-guilt	7	3.36	2.72	.02	.87	.19	.90
Coping mechanism	(1–9)						
Sharing	1	6.08	2.17	.10	.70	2.84	.04*
Self-consoling	2	6.08	2.01	.21	.06	.42	.74
Thinking continuously	3	4.37	2.38	.03	.60	.55	.65
Staying alone	4	4.31	2.36	1.96	.16	4.73	.005**
Crying	5	3.85	2.49	.003	.96	.91	.44
Venting	6	3.77	1.96	3.99	.05	.82	.49
Acceptance	7	3.65	2.45	4.56	.04*	1.17	.32
Alcohol	8	1.58	2.16	.03	.85	1.43	.26
Suicidal thoughts	9	1.09	1.84	.17	.68	1.93	.15

Table 2 continued

	Rank[a]	Mean	SD	Gender		Ethnicity	
				F	p value	F	p value
Causes of violence	(1–9)						
Bad habits	1	6.75	2.33	1.25	.27	.12	.94
Alcohol	2	6.26	2.65	1.26	.26	1.35	.26
Financial issues	3	6.10	2.29	.66	.42	1.76	.16
Less coping/tolerance	4	5.52	2.63	.56	.46	3.49	.02*
Inequality	5	4.89	2.22	1.14	.29	.86	.46
Misunderstanding	6	4.86	2.22	.39	.53	.46	.71
Culture/traditional reasons	7	4.73	2.19	.09	.76	.37	.77
Not obeying parents	8	4.47	2.15	1.40	.24	.62	.60
Unhealthy competition	9	3.70	2.64	1.88	.17	.54	.65
Reasons for alcohol use	(1–7)						
Tension	1	6.29	2.04	8.07	.006**	.29	.83
Friend circle	2	5.93	2.16	.07	.79	.98	.40
Family environment	3	4.34	2.78	.09	.77	.84	.47
To have fun	4	4.29	2.42	2.30	.13	.96	.42
To relax	5	3.74	2.17	.07	.79	.75	.52
Tradition	6	3.64	2.82	.84	.36	1.11	.35
Cultural traditions	7	3.08	2.52	.31	.58	.99	.40
Causes of suicide	(1–9)						
Domestic violence	1	5.65	2.33	.30	.58	.41	.74
Love tragedies (romantic break-up)	2	5.60	2.49	.18	.67	.50	.68
Exam pressure	3	4.94	2.37	2.26	.14	1.22	.31
Alcohol problems	4	4.62	2.62	.16	.69	.57	.64
Financial issues	5	4.57	2.61	.16	.69	1.42	.25
Relationship issues (other than romantic relationships)	6	4.47	2.07	.20	.65	.69	.56
Social status	7	3.18	2.33	.01	.96	.17	.92
Interpersonal conflict	8	2.71	2.13	.29	.59	.77	.51
Lack of social support	9	2.65	2.48	.98	.33	1.24	.30

[a] Lower numbers refer to higher ranking for importance or frequency (e.g., a '1' for qualities of ideal person refers to the highest ranked quality; a '1' for frequency of emotion refers to the most commonly experienced distressing emotion)

* p value: < .05, ** p < .001

Sadness and embarrassment were also noted as other frequent manifestations of emotional distress:

> "I get 'tension' when I am practicing my run—especially while running up and down the hill. I already have a hearing problem, and I get 'tension' that there will be no one to take care of me and nothing to do with my life if I fall and break my legs and hands."—18-year old Brahman Female

Coping

Sharing with friends/families and self-consoling were the most common forms of coping mechanism in Jumla. There were caste differences regarding how people coped through sharing. Brahman respondents described sharing the most (F = 2.84, p = .04) and staying alone

the least (F = 4.73, p = .005), with Chhetri respondents saying the opposite, staying alone the most and sharing the least. Gender differences were found in expressions of emotion. Boys endorsed more acceptance of their emotions than girls did (F = 4.56 p = .036). For example:

> "Whenever I face difficulties and get negative thought, I share it with my sisters. I also do pooja [prayers] and share my happiness and difficulties with God."—15-year-old Brahman Female

> "When I am worried, I call my brothers immediately because I suppose they will say something to me and ask why I am feeling like that. I will tell them openly because they have been supporting me for very long. Then my brother convinces me

and asks me not to think like that. So, I am always searching for my cellphone to call my brother during times like that."—17-year-old Janajati Female

Many adolescents utilized self-consoling to cope with their problems and emotions.

"When I have bad thoughts, I look at my friends and observe what they do to remove those thoughts. By looking at them I know what I should do to remove them and gets convinced that it is not just me but others too who are having those negative thoughts."—15-year-old Chhetri Female

Causes of violence

Bad habits including gambling and domestic feuds topped the list in major causes of violence in Jumla, followed by alcohol use. Caste differences were noted pertaining to thresholds for physical retaliation with violence. Janajati respondents were found to have the lowest threshold to respond with physical violence when engaged in altercations with others (F = 3.49, p = .021).

"When people drink alcohol, they use bad and foul language. Those people who are not drunk cannot tolerate someone speaking with a foul mouth to them and then the fighting starts. Drunk people start physically assaulting people they are quarreling with."—16-year-old Janajati Male

Reasons for alcohol use

Tension and a coercive peer and family environment were described as the major causes of alcohol use. Females were found to be more prone to drinking than men because of tension (F = 8.07, p = .006). Cultural drinking practices scored lower for harmful alcohol use:

"These days people from all caste/ethnicity have started to drink. They drink openly or secretly. There is a liquor store opposite to the place where I work, and I see lot of people coming there to buy alcohol."—18-year Dalit Male

Causes of suicide

Domestic violence, break-ups in romantic relationships, and academic exam pressure were the top three causes of suicide named. High rates of domestic violence resulting from alcohol use were reported in the LTIs, which in turn was described to be the leading cause of suicide. The participants also described their difficulty in coping with relationship problems and immense pressure they get to do well in their school leaving certificate (SLC) exams, which occur at the end of 10th grade and are the major determinant of admittance to further education.

"My father drinks alcohol and beats my mother. I get stressed about it and cannot concentrate in school too. So, I think that it is better to die then live like this."—16-year-old Dalit Female

"I think when I don't study well, how will I become a nurse, and when I don't become a nurse, how will I live my life? Also, I won't be capable to do other works, so I feel like it is better to die than to live."—16-year-old Dalit Female

Discussion

Utilizing a mixed-methods approach, we conducted qualitative life trajectory interviews and administered a card sorting task to elucidate aspirational models among adolescents in rural northwestern Nepal. We developed a framework to integrate the qualitative and quantitative findings to understand adolescent aspirational models (Fig. 2). We found that education was the most highly valued attribute of ideal persons. Educational attainment received higher prioritization by *Dalit* castes and *Janajati*, whereas *Brahman* caste youth gave education less priority. Poverty was identified as the greatest barrier to achieving life goals among all groups. The most common distressing emotion was *'tension'*. Girls reported *'tension'* more frequently than boys, and girls were most likely to drink alcohol because of *'tension'*. Sharing emotions and self-consoling were common behavioral response to emotional distress. *Brahman* youth were more likely to endorse coping with emotions by sharing their feelings with others, Boys reported drinking for social pleasure with peer groups. Domestic violence, 'love tragedies' and SLC exam pressure were the most common reasons for suicide.

An emphasis on education emerged as the central focus for aspirational models. This was closely connected with academic stress to do well on the SLC examination and then to use one's academic success to achieve the goal of securing a stable government job. Less priority was given to the constructs of cultural practices and traditional jobs such as farming, especially among boys. Lietchy highlighted the conflict between being modern or traditional among Kathmandu youth [4]. Young people in Jumla seemed to struggle with pursuing identity goals of being both "modern" and "traditional" simultaneously. For example, they discussed fighting against the negative aspects of traditional practices, though the study data show that these barriers did not hinder achieving their life goals. They also admitted that traditional beliefs are not absolute, and it was necessary to balance tradition and modernity, especially with their older family members. Poverty was commonly seen as a bigger barrier than traditional values and practices. Similarly, tension among girls and peer pressure among boys were more dominant

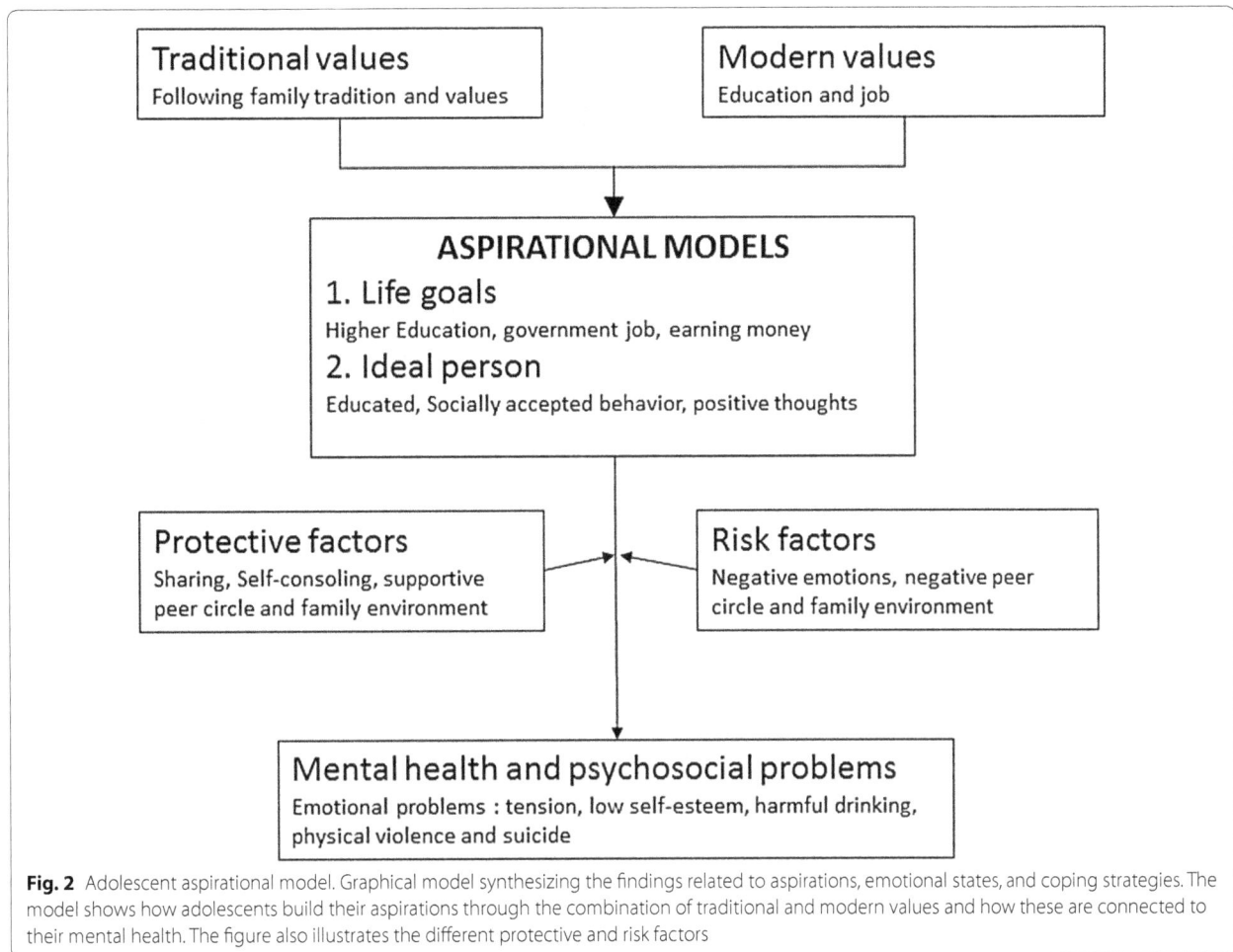

Fig. 2 Adolescent aspirational model. Graphical model synthesizing the findings related to aspirations, emotional states, and coping strategies. The model shows how adolescents build their aspirations through the combination of traditional and modern values and how these are connected to their mental health. The figure also illustrates the different protective and risk factors

causes of harmful alcohol use than traditional practices were.

This also challenges some of our pre-existing expectations about rural youth aspirational models. We had thought that Jumla, often stereotyped as a traditional society, would have respondents emphasizing traditional rituals and practices. However, our current data showed their emphasis on education and employment and less focus on migration and marriage.

The focus on education as the major quality of an ideal person and the most sought-after life goal reinforces previous findings in a similar population in Nepal, among whom the promise of education led them towards youth radicalization and becoming child soldiers. Adolescents (especially girls) were found to join armed groups (Maoists in Nepal) because they did not see any hope of education in their community and were seeking alternative ways to become empowered and educated [47, 48]. This highlights the need to design interventions to increase educational opportunities for these populations, with a special focus on girls.

"Tension" could also be a key target for intervention. The English term, translated into Nepali as "tannab," has already built up its own unique meaning in Nepali. In her study among mothers in Nepal, Clarke described tension as "having many thoughts in mind and being distracted, worried, despairing and unable to do work" [28]. This emotion stood out as the most complex and common difficulty for the adolescents in our study. It was also identified as the major reason for alcohol use especially among girls, who reported higher levels of tension than adolescent males. Interventions should focus on developing pathways for adolescents to cope with tension.

Sharing and self-consoling, considered as positive coping mechanisms, were the two most commonly used coping practices and reported to be the most effective. In post-conflict areas such as this, developing resiliency skills could be a key in developing positive mental health [49]. Studies among vulnerable groups in Nepal have shown that developing resiliency can have better outcomes and is feasible in the context of LMIC settings like Nepal [50]. Locally grounded community-based groups can be a potential intervention target for improving these practices. It could include groups like classrooms, child clubs and youth groups. Classroom-based interventions have already been started and practiced in Nepal, showing effectiveness among particular sub-groups. For example, one classroom-based intervention increased pro-social behavior among girls, which may be associated with enhanced use of sharing emotion distress and support with other girls [18].

Peer group interventions could be an excellent choice focusing on coping with emotions and behavioral changes. In rural Nepal, it has been found that children's behavior problems are caused by negative peer influence and poor family environment [16]. Developing a positive peer circle is also equally important, as deviant peer groups were found to be one of the major reasons for adolescents to start using alcohol. In parallel, multilevel support and engagement are equally important. In another study conducted among children in rural Nepal, Adhikari and colleagues suggested using a similar kind of intervention that includes multi-level groups such as peer groups [16]. A peer group model combined with parents and a school support system can also be an important way to address suicide [51]. In his study among adolescents living in extremely impoverished communities, Farrell found that increased peer support reduced risk of suicide attempts [52]. Studies in LMICs have concluded that there is moderate to strong evidence of success of school-based interventions in promoting mental health of young people—enhancing their emotional and behavioral wellbeing, including improved self-esteem and coping skills [6, 53]. Peer group interventions can be conducted in a school-based setting in places like Jumla, where community-based children organizations (e.g. child clubs, sports clubs) are not as common as in other places. A school-based approach is well supported, with other studies among adolescents acknowledging its feasibility, effectiveness, and acceptability [15, 54–56]. In Nepal, interventions targeting other public health domains have demonstrated the success of peer support models among different castes [57].

In the same community where this study was conducted, dialectical behavior therapy (DBT) has been adapted for adult women with prior suicidal and other self-injurious behavior [58]. The adolescent aspirational models identified here could be used to adapt adult DBT for adolescent populations, which is a key period to intervene to prevent future suicidal behavior [8].

In Jumla, mental health support for the whole population, not only adolescents, is nearly absent. This is a problem globally. Although neuropsychiatric illnesses represent a large percentage of disability adjusted life

years in LMICs, mental health services in national health systems in these countries are extremely weak [59]. People with mental health problems have the lowest rates of treatment for their health conditions, and integration into primary health care has been advocated as a potential solution [60]. Thus, it would be worthwhile to explore integration of adolescent mental health services into primary health care in Jumla. Such programs have already been implemented for adult mental health care in other rural areas of Nepal [61–63].

Studies have shown that in the context of LMICs, there is a need to identify and design interventions that are culturally relevant and sensitive to differences across caste and genders [64, 65]. Differences among the participant's caste, gender, age and educational status will help to guide the design of culturally salient interventions and inform future research across these domains of mental health. In our study, Dalits were found to be most interested in attaining higher education but were least interested in government jobs. This reflects the Dalits' perception that it would be difficult for them to access and fit in government jobs, which are mostly dominated by Brahman and Chhetri. Discrepancies were noted even within the higher caste group in terms of coping mechanisms. Chhetri chose to stay alone the most and not share their feelings and emotions with others. Interestingly, girls were found to be using more aggressive forms of coping than boys by venting their emotions on others. Girls were also more prone to tension and more likely to start drinking to cope with tension. These differences point to the need to avoid making assumptions about caste groups and gender when designing interventions. Salient caste/ethnic and gender features across different regions need to be assessed while designing these interventions.

Limitations

Due to the card sorting activity's requirement of literacy, the largest limitation of this study was the inability to include adolescents who were illiterate. Thus, to generalize the findings of this study, this limitation should be considered. Another limitation of this study is regarding the limited number of options during card sorting. Choices during card sorting were derived from the initial interviews, and the participants did not have the choice to add options that were unique. Variation in adolescent aspiration models and differences among caste and gender exists substantially between different regions and communities. Therefore, findings from this study should not be over generalized beyond Jumla without conducting ample ethnographic work in other communities to support these findings.

Conclusion

Based on the findings from the card sorting activity and interviews, we ascertain that there is a need for a model of cultural intervention for adolescents in Jumla that focuses on developing peer/parent/school groups, education and job opportunities, self-esteem, and access to resources, as well as reducing tension, stress, alcohol use, and relationship problems. Research in Jumla has shown that there is an association between childhood stressors and adult depression through a gene-by-environment pathway [19]. Thus, it is important to intervene among these groups to reduce the burden of adult mental health problems. While traditional and cultural aspects cannot be separated from intervention, it is important to incorporate their changing patterns among the young and educated adolescents of Jumla. Pathways of sharing and resiliency should be further developed and strengthened. Focus of intervention should be equally on group as well as individual.

Abbreviations

DCP: disease control and prevention; LMIC: lower and middle income countries; HDI: human development index; CBS: Central Bureau of Statistics; VDC: Village Development Committee; WHO: World Health Organization; TPO: Transcultural Psychosocial Organization; KAHS: Karnali Academy of Health Sciences; NHRC: Nepal Health Research Council; LTI: life trajectory interview; SPSS: Statistical Package for the Social Sciences; SLC: school leaving certificate.

Authors' contributions

SR drafted the manuscript. SR and BAK designed the study and research tools. SR, SBA, and NRA performed data collection. SR and BNK performed data analysis. BAK supervised the study and revised the manuscript. All authors reviewed the final manuscript. All authors read and approved the final manuscript.

Author details

[1] Transcultural Psychosocial Organization Nepal (TPO Nepal), Anek Marga, Baluwatar, Kathmandu, Nepal. [2] Duke Global Health Institute, Duke University, Durham, NC, USA. [3] Department of Psychiatry and Behavioral Sciences, George Washington University, Washington, DC, USA. [4] Department of Psychiatry, Duke University, Durham, NC, USA.

Acknowledgements

Transcultural Psychosocial Organization (TPO) Nepal assisted in research implementation and grant administration. Upasana Regmi and Megan Ramaiya provided their helpful suggestions and support during the piloting of the study. Anvita Bhardwaj and Dristy Gurung provided critical review of the manuscript. The authors thank Ganesh Rokaya and the residents of Jumla for their cooperation and support of the study.

Competing interests

The authors declare that they have no competing interests.

Funding

This study was funded by HopeLab, http://www.hopelab.org, Redwood, California. The funder had no role in conducting the study, analyzing the data, or preparing the manuscript.

References

1. Clarke P, Marshall V, House J, Lantz P. The social structuring of mental health over the adult life course: advancing theory in the sociology of aging. Soc Forces. 2011;89(4):1287–313.
2. Bandura A. Social foundations of thought and action: a social cognitive theory. Bergen: Prentice-Hall, Inc; 1986.
3. Dickerson DL, Brown RA, Johnson CL, Schweigman K, D'Amico EJ. Integrating motivational interviewing and traditional practices to address alcohol and drug use among urban American Indian/Alaska native youth. J Subst Abuse Treat. 2016;65:26–35.
4. Liechty M. Suitably modern: making middle-class culture in a new consumer society. Princeton: Princeton University Press; 2003.
5. Patel V, Flisher AJ, Nikapota A, Malhotra S. Promoting child and adolescent mental health in low and middle income countries. J Child Psychol Psychiatr. 2008;49:313–34.
6. Fazel M, Patel V, Thomas S, Tol W. Mental health interventions in schools in low-income and middle-income countries. Lancet Psychiatry. 2014;1(5):388–98.
7. Petersen I, Swartz L, Bhana A, Flisher AJ. Mental health promotion initiatives for children and youth in contexts of poverty: the case of South Africa. Health Promot Int. 2010;25:daq026.
8. Dunne T, Bishop L, Avery S, Darcy S. A Review of Effective Youth Engagement Strategies for Mental Health and Substance Use Interventions. J Adolesc Health. 2016;60:487–512.
9. Patel V, Chisholm D, Parikh R, Charlson FJ, Degenhardt L, Dua T, Ferrari AJ, Hyman S, Laxminarayan R, Levin C. Addressing the burden of mental, neurological, and substance use disorders: key messages from disease control priorities. Lancet. 2016;387(10028):1672–85.
10. Cheng Y, Li X, Lou C, Sonenstein FL, Kalamar A, Jejeebhoy S, Delany-Moretlwe S, Brahmbhatt H, Olumide AO, Ojengbede O. The association between social support and mental health among vulnerable adolescents in five cities: findings from the study of the well-being of adolescents in vulnerable environments. J Adolesc Health. 2014;55(6):S31–8.
11. Patton GC, Coffey C, Cappa C, Currie D, Riley L, Gore F, Degenhardt L, Richardson D, Astone N, Sangowawa AO. Health of the world's adolescents: a synthesis of internationally comparable data. Lancet. 2012;379(9826):1665–75.
12. Cordon O. Global strategy for women's, children and adolescents' health in the post-2015 sustainable development goals (SDGs). In: 2015 APHA Annual Meeting and Expo (Oct 31–Nov 4, 2015): 2015: APHA; 2015.
13. Griggs D, Stafford-Smith M, Gaffney O, Rockström J, Öhman MC, Shyamsundar P, Steffen W, Glaser G, Kanie N, Noble I. Policy: sustainable development goals for people and planet. Nature. 2013;495(7441):305–7.
14. Nagata JM, Ferguson BJ, Ross DA. Research priorities for eight areas of adolescent health in low-and middle-income countries. J Adolesc Health. 2016;59(1):50–60.
15. Balaji M, Andrews T, Andrew G, Patel V. The acceptability, feasibility, and effectiveness of a population-based intervention to promote youth health: an exploratory study in Goa, India. J Adolesc Health. 2011;48(5):453–60.
16. Adhikari RP, Upadhaya N, Gurung D, Luitel NP, Burkey MD, Kohrt BA, Jordans MJD. Perceived behavioral problems of school aged children in rural Nepal: a qualitative study. Child Adolesc Psychiatry Mental Health. 2015;9(1):1.
17. Burkey MD, Ghimire L, Adhikari RP, Wissow LS, Jordans MJD, Kohrt BA. The ecocultural context and child behavior problems: a qualitative analysis in rural Nepal. Soc Sci Med. 2016;159:73–82.
18. Jordans MJD, Komproe IH, Tol WA, Kohrt BA, Luitel NP, Macy RD, De Jong JT. Evaluation of a classroom-based psychosocial intervention in conflict-affected Nepal: a cluster randomized controlled trial. J Child Psychol Psychiatr. 2010;51:818–26.

19. Kohrt BA, Worthman CM, Ressler KJ, Mercer KB, Upadhaya N, Koirala S, Nepal MK, Sharma VD, Binder EB. Cross-cultural gene – environment interactions in depression, post-traumatic stress disorder, and the cortisol awakening response: FKBP5 polymorphisms and childhood trauma in South Asia: GxE interactions in South Asia. Int Rev Psychiatry. 2015;27(3):180–96.

20. Kohrt BA, Hruschka DJ, Worthman CM, Kunz RD, Baldwin JL, Upadhaya N, Acharya NR, Koirala S, Thapa SB, Tol WA. Political violence and mental health in Nepal: prospective study. Br J Psychiatry. 2012;201(4):268–75.

21. Central Bureau of Statistics Nepal. National Population and Housing census 2011. In: National Report; 2012.

22. Sharma S, Pandey S, Pathak D, Sijapati-Basnett B. State of migration in Nepal. Nepal: Centre for the Study of Labour and Mobility Kathmandu; 2014.

23. Gaire K, Beilin R, Miller F. Withdrawing, resisting, maintaining and adapting: food security and vulnerability in Jumla, Nepal. Reg Environ Change. 2015;15(8):1667–78.

24. Kohrt BA. Vulnerable social groups in postconflict settings: a mixed methods policy analysis and epidemiology study of caste and psychological morbidity in Nepal. Intervention. 2009;7(3):239–64.

25. Sharma PR. The State and Society in Nepal: Historical Foundations and contemporary trends. Kathmandu: HImal Books; 2004.

26. Kohrt BA, Speckman RA, Kunz RD, Baldwin JL, Upadhaya N, Acharya NR, Sharma VD, Nepal MK, Worthman CM. Culture in psychiatric epidemiology: using ethnography and multiple mediator models to assess the relationship of caste with depression and anxiety in Nepal. Ann Hum Biol. 2009;36(3):261–80.

27. Kohrt BA, Hruschka DJ. Nepali concepts of psychological trauma: the role of idioms of distress, ethnopsychology and ethnophysiology in alleviating suffering and preventing stigma. Cult Med Psychiatry. 2010;34(2):322–52.

28. Clarke K, Saville N, Bhandari B, Giri K, Ghising M, Jha M, Jha S, Magar J, Roy R, Shrestha B. Understanding psychological distress among mothers in rural Nepal: a qualitative grounded theory exploration. BMC psychiatry. 2014;14(1):1.

29. Chase LE, Welton-Mitchell C, Bhattarai S. "Solving Tension": coping among Bhutanese refugees in Nepal. Int J Migrat Health Soc Care. 2013;9(2):71–83.

30. Kohrt BA, Maharjan SM. When a child is no longer a child: Nepali ethnopsychology of child development and violence. Stud Nepali History Soc. 2009;14(1):107–42.

31. Karki R, Kohrt BA, Jordans MJD. Child led indicators: pilot testing a child participation tool for psychosocial support programmes for former child soldiers in Nepal. Intervention. 2009;7(2):92–109.

32. Liechty M. Media and markets: youth identities and the experience of modernity in Kathmandu, Nepal. In: Amit-Talai V, Wulff H, editors. Youth cultures: a cross-cultural perspective. New York: Routledge; 1995. pp. 166–201.

33. Thapa S, Mishra V. Mass media exposure among urban youth in Nepal. Asia Pac Popul J. 2003;18(1):5–28.

34. Brown RA, Hruschka DJ, Worthman CM. Cultural models and fertility timing among cherokee and white youth in appalachia: beyond the mode. Am Anthropol. 2009;111(4):420–31.

35. Brown RA, Worthman CM, Costello EJ, Erkanli A. The Life Trajectory Interview for Youth (LTI-Y): method development and psychometric properties of an instrument to assess life-course models and achievement. Int J Methods Psychiatric Res. 2006;15(4):206–15.

36. Suvedi BK, Pradhan A, Barnett S, Puri M, Chitrakar SR, Poudel P, Sharma S, Hulton L. Nepal Maternal Mortality and Morbidity Study 2008/2009: summary of preliminary findings. Kathmandu: Family Health division, Department of Health Services, Ministry of Health, Government of Nepal; 2009.

37. Hagaman AK, Khadka S, Lohani S, Kohrt B. Suicide in Nepal: a modified psychological autopsy investigation from randomly selected police cases between 2013 and 2015. Soc Psychiatry Psychiatr Epidemiol. 2017;52(12):1483–94.

38. Bhardwaj A, Bourey C, Rai S, Adhikari R, Worthman CM, Kohrt BA. Interpersonal violence and suicidality among former child soldiers and war-exposed civilian children in Nepal. Global Mental Health. 2017. https://doi.org/10.1017/gmh.2017.31.

39. Ramaiya MK, Fiorillo D, Regmi U, Robins CJ, Kohrt BA. A Cultural adaptation of dialectical behavior therapy in Nepal. Cogn Behav Prac. 2017;24(4):428–44.

40. Kohrt BA, Bourey C. Culture and comorbidity: intimate partner violence as a common risk factor for maternal mental illness and reproductive health problems among former child soldiers in Nepal. Med Anthropol Q. 2016;30(4):515–35.

41. Braun V, Clarke V. Using thematic analysis in psychology. Qual Res Psychol. 2006;3(2):77–101.

42. Tsai AC, Kohrt BA, Matthews LT, Betancourt TS, Lee JK, Papachristos AV, Weiser SD, Dworkin SL. Promises and pitfalls of data sharing in qualitative research. Soc Sci Med. 2016;169:191–8.

43. Borgatti SP. Elicitation techniques for cultural domain analysis. Enhanc Ethnogr Methods. 1999;3:115–51.

44. Weller SC. Cultural consensus theory: applications and frequently asked questions. Field Methods. 2007;19(4):339–68.

45. Bernard HR. Research methods in anthropology: Qualitative and quantitative approaches. Lanham: Rowman Altamira; 2011.

46. Mammen JR, Norton SA, Rhee H, Butz AM. New approaches to qualitative interviewing: development of a card sort technique to understand subjective patterns of symptoms and responses. Int J Nurs Stud. 2016;58:90–6.

47. Kohrt BA, Yang M, Rai S, Bhardwaj A, Tol WA, Jordans MJ. Recruitment of child soldiers in Nepal: mental health status and risk factors for voluntary participation of youth in armed groups. Peace Conflict J Peace Psychol. 2016;22(3):208.

48. Morley CA, Kohrt BA. Impact of peer support on PTSD, hope, and functional impairment: a mixed-methods study of child soldiers in Nepal. J Aggress Maltreatment Trauma. 2013;22(7):714–34.

49. Levey EJ, Oppenheim CE, Lange BC, Plasky NS, Harris BL, Lekpeh GG, Kekulah I, Henderson DC, Borba CP. A qualitative analysis of factors impacting resilience among youth in post-conflict Liberia. Child Adolesc Psychiatry Mental Health. 2016;10(1):26.

50. Kohrt BA, Worthman CM, Adhikari RP, Luitel NP, Arevalo JMG, Ma J, McCreath H, Seeman TE, Crimmins EM, Cole SW. Psychological resilience and the gene regulatory impact of posttraumatic stress in Nepali child soldiers. Proc Natl Acad Sci. 2016;113(29):8156–61.

51. Miller AB, Esposito-Smythers C, Leichtweis RN. Role of social support in adolescent suicidal ideation and suicide attempts. J Adolesc Health. 2015;56(3):286–92.

52. Farrell CT, Bolland JM, Cockerham WC. The role of social support and social context on the incidence of attempted suicide among adolescents living in extremely impoverished communities. J Adolesc Health. 2015;56(1):59–65.

53. Barry MM, Clarke AM, Jenkins R, Patel V. A systematic review of the effectiveness of mental health promotion interventions for young people in low and middle income countries. BMC Public Health. 2013;13(1):835.

54. Das JK, Salam RA, Lassi ZS, Khan MN, Mahmood W, Patel V, Bhutta ZA. Interventions for adolescent mental health: an overview of systematic reviews. J Adolesc Health. 2016;59(4):S49–60.

55. Oman RF, Vesely SK, Aspy CB, Tolma EL. Prospective associations among assets and successful transition to early adulthood. J Inf. 2015;105(1):e51–6.

56. DeSocio J, VanCura M, Nelson LA, Hewitt G, Kitzman H, Cole R. Engaging truant adolescents: results from a multifaceted intervention pilot. Prev School Failure Alter Educ Children Youth. 2007;51(3):3–9.

57. Posner J, Kayastha P, Davis D, Limoges J, O'Donnell C, Yue K. Development of leadership self-efficacy and collective efficacy: adolescent girls across castes as peer educators in Nepal. Global Public Health. 2009;4(3):284–302.

58. Ramaiya MK, Fiorillo D, Regmi U, Robins CJ, Kohrt BA. A cultural adaptation of dialectical behavior therapy in Nepal. Cogn Behav Prac. 2017;24:428–44.

59. Akol A, Engebretsen IMS, Skylstad V, Nalugya J, Ndeezi G, Tumwine J. Health managers' views on the status of national and decentralized health systems for child and adolescent mental health in Uganda: a qualitative study. Child Adolesc Psychiatry Mental Health. 2015;9(1):54.

60. Herrenkohl TI, Lee JO, Kosterman R, Hawkins JD. Family influences related to adult substance use and mental health problems: a developmental analysis of child and adolescent predictors. J Adolesc Health. 2012;51(2):129–35.

61. Jordans M, Luitel N, Pokhrel P, Patel V. Development and pilot testing of a mental healthcare plan in Nepal. Br J Psychiatry. 2016;208(s56):s21–8.

62. Kisa R, Baingana F, Kajungu R, Mangen PO, Angdembe M, Gwaikolo W, Cooper J. Pathways and access to mental health care services by persons living with severe mental disorders and epilepsy in Uganda, Liberia and Nepal: a qualitative study. BMC psychiatry. 2016;16(1):305.

63. Angdembe M, Kohrt BA, Jordans M, Rimal D, Luitel NP. Situational analysis to inform development of primary care and community-based mental health services for severe mental disorders in Nepal. Int J Mental Health Syst. 2017;11(1):69.

64. Harms S, Jack S, Ssebunnya J, Kizza R. The orphaning experience: descriptions from Ugandan youth who have lost parents to HIV/AIDS. Child Adolesc Psychiatry Mental Health. 2010;4(1):6.

65. Martínez-Hernáez A, Carceller-Maicas N, DiGiacomo SM, Ariste S. Social support and gender differences in coping with depression among emerging adults: a mixed-methods study. Child Adolesc Psychiatry Mental Health. 2016;10(1):2.

17

What do young adolescents think about taking part in longitudinal self-harm research? Findings from a school-based study

Joanna Lockwood[1,2]* ⓘ, Ellen Townsend[3], Leonie Royes[3], David Daley[1,2] and Kapil Sayal[1,2]

Abstract

Background: Research about self-harm in adolescence is important given the high incidence in youth, and strong links to suicide and other poor outcomes. Clarifying the impact of involvement in school-based self-harm studies on young adolescents is an ethical priority given heightened risk at this developmental stage.

Methods: Here, 594 school-based students aged mainly 13–14 years completed a survey on self-harm at baseline and again 12-weeks later. Change in mood following completion of each survey, ratings and thoughts about participation, and responses to a mood-mitigation activity were analysed using a multi-method approach.

Results: Baseline participation had no overall impact on mood. However, boys and girls reacted differently to the survey depending on self-harm status. Having a history of self-harm had a negative impact on mood for girls, but a positive impact on mood for boys. In addition, participants rated the survey in mainly positive/neutral terms, and cited benefits including personal insight and altruism. At follow-up, there was a negative impact on mood following participation, but no significant effect of gender or self-harm status. Ratings at follow-up were mainly positive/neutral. Those who had self-harmed reported more positive and fewer negative ratings than at baseline: the opposite pattern of response was found for those who had not self-harmed. Mood-mitigation activities were endorsed.

Conclusions: Self-harm research with youth is feasible in school-settings. Most young people are happy to take part and cite important benefits. However, the impact of participation in research appears to vary according to gender, self-harm risk and method/time of assessment. The impact of repeated assessment requires clarification. Simple mood-elevation techniques may usefully help to mitigate distress.

Keywords: Self-harm, Adolescence, Ethics, Longitudinal, Multi-methods, Mood-mitigation

Background

Self-harm, here defined as any act of self-poisoning or self-injury irrespective of motivation or suicidal intent [1], is a common and significant health concern in adolescence. Average lifetime prevalence of self-harm in community-based samples of adolescents in Europe and Australia has been estimated at 17.8% [2], with rates comparable internationally [3]. While self-harm for many is about preserving rather than ending life [4] it is nonetheless strongly linked to completed suicide, with 40–60% of those who die by suicide having a history of self-harm [5]. Youth who self-harm are also at increased risk of mental health difficulties and multiple life problems such as increased alcohol use and relationship difficulties [6, 7]. Adolescents who self-harm thus represent an extremely vulnerable group.

Adolescence—the developmental period spanning 12–25 years of age—is an important time to focus research on self-harm as these years are likely to include the onset (12–14 years), peak (15–24 years) and start of remittance of the behaviour [8–10]. Rates of self-harm behaviour are three times higher in adolescents than adult populations [11]. Much self-harm research to date

*Correspondence: llxjll@nottingham.ac.uk
[1] Division of Psychiatry & Applied Psychology, Institute of Mental Health, University of Nottingham, University of Nottingham Innovation Park, Triumph Road, Nottingham NG7 2TU, UK
Full list of author information is available at the end of the article

has focused on mid to late adolescence. This approach is important given high rates of self-harm in this age group [12], but this focus may also be a consequence of the additional ethical and procedural challenges involved in research with younger age groups, and a reluctance on the part of ethics committees and Institutional Review Boards (IRBs) to sanction self-harm research in those perceived to be at heightened vulnerability. Yet, research at earlier stages of adolescence is important to understand how and why self-harm first develops [13]. Moreover, recent reports suggest that increasing rates of self-harm across adolescence show the steepest rise in girls under 16 years of age [14], suggesting that early adolescence is a period of particular concern in adolescent self-harm. Most young people who self-harm do not seek clinical support [2], and this is particularly the case in young adolescents (aged 12–14 years) where community-based cases of self-harm outnumber hospital presentations by up to 20 times [15]. School-based studies thus provide a vital opportunity to engage with an early adolescent population at risk of self-harm who may otherwise remain hidden. Work which strengthens the evidence base for the ethical suitability of self-harm studies in younger age groups in school-based samples can help to reframe the calculation of risk for future research in this critical area.

Ethical challenges—overstated risks?

For researchers and regulatory bodies rightfully mindful of the need to balance the delivery of research objectives against ensuring participant wellbeing [16, 17], a key concern is that asking participants about self-harm/suicidality may introduce, reinforce or exacerbate such acts, or cause undue psychological distress [16]. In fact, reviews of the evidence, which have pooled findings across adult and adolescent populations, have suggested that asking about such issues is not associated with negative outcomes [18, 19] and may, in fact, confer benefits for those at most risk [20]. This is important for anonymous survey-based studies where a direct gauging of impact is impossible.

Response from school-based youth to self-harm studies

Relatively few studies have sought to understand the impact that being asked specifically about self-harm has on school-based respondents. Hasking and colleagues [21] examined whether completing a survey about non-suicidal self-injury (NSSI), suicidality, and wider psychological constructs was perceived as either enjoyable or upsetting/worrying, in school-based students aged 12–18 years. Overall, the majority of participants enjoyed participation at baseline and at 1-year follow-up with only a minority finding participation to be upsetting/

worrying, but those who had thought about or experienced self-harm were more likely to have had this response. Notably, Hasking and colleagues found that girls were more likely than boys to find the survey upsetting, but also more likely than boys to report enjoying participation. There may be a nuanced gendered distinction in reactions to sensitive research that warrants further analysis. It is important, given the greater prevalence of self-harm in girls relative to boys [14], to establish further if this gendered distinction is moderated by the likelihood that an individual has a history of self-harm i.e. whether vulnerability is conferred by self-harm status, by gender, or an interaction between the two. Other school-based studies have similarly found that while overall participation in a research survey is viewed positively there are nonetheless links between increased vulnerability and likelihood of reporting distress [22, 23]. Importantly, these studies point to factors such as being "interested" in the topic [22] or finding it "worthwhile" [23] which partially mitigate this distress, and similar findings have been found in a study with young adults [24]. Notably, one of these studies only included boys from a select-entry school [22] which limits how generalisable these findings are to a general school population; the other [21], gathered reactions to questions on suicide, drug use and sexual abuse, issues which could arguably have a different personal resonance than self-harm in a younger population. Nonetheless these studies suggest that there may be an important distinction when making a judgment of impact in self-harm research, between having an emotional response and a cognitive evaluation of that response, and highlight that more evidence, particularly examining gender differences is now needed.

Establishing short-term risk

Not all studies have found that those at highest risk are more likely to experience distress. In suicide research [20], high risk students with raised depressive symptomatology who answered survey questions about suicide were less likely to report distress or suicidality immediately afterwards and 2 days later than high risk participants in a control group who were not asked these questions. Hence, asking about suicidality apparently conferred short-term benefits to those at most risk. In support, Mathias and colleagues [25] in a sample of mainly 14 year olds with experience of in-patient psychiatric care reported a dose–response effect where adolescents with greater severity of suicidal ideation reported greatest reduction in ideation in repeated assessments over 6-month intervals [25]. These studies are important in establishing the impact of participation in research over time for young samples, albeit in research focused on suicide or with clinical groups. Notably, within self-harm research, the potential salutary effects of study participation over time for the most vulnerable was supported in a University-based sample over a 3 week period [24], but not in a school-based sample over a 1-year period [20]. Hasking and colleagues [20] demonstrated that a deterioration in psychological functioning over time (i.e. increased vulnerability) was associated with a change in evaluation of study participation from a positive to a negative valence at 1-year follow-up. Given that clinical decisions may often be based on short-term assessment of risk—hours, days, weeks, rather than years—short-term follow-up studies may improve the clinical relevance of study data [26, 27]. It is therefore important to test the impact of participation in a self-harm study with a school-based population using a short-term prospective design. Such prospective examination will also be important in establishing if school-based youth with and without self-harm experience differ in their response to repeated assessment. Of note, Muehlenkamp and colleagues [28] found that University participants without self-harm experience were less amenable to repeat participation.

Current study

The current study sought further understanding of how school-based adolescents with and without experience of self-harm felt about taking part in a longitudinal study about self-harm. Specifically, the impact of study participation on early adolescents (aged 15 years and under) was sought. Other self-harm/suicide studies that have included youth of this age have predominantly targeted participants across a broader span of adolescence [19–21, 25]. Given evidence that the pattern of risk for adolescent self-harm may differ in early, mid and late adolescence it is important to distinguish between these developmental stages [14, 15]. As male and female respondents have been shown to differ in response to research participation [21], and are known to differ in prevalence of self-harm [15] a nuanced examination of responses to participation based on gender and self-harm status was also sought. Given that prospective studies with short follow-up phases are recommended for clinically relevant research [26, 27], this study seeks to evaluate the impact of asking young people to take part in a longitudinal study over a short time period (10–12 weeks) and strike a balance between being sufficiently short-term to enable clinical relevance, but also sufficiently spaced in time to be accommodated within a dense school timetable. Recent research has recommended taking steps to reduce any potential negative impact of study involvement on youth [21]. Mood elevation techniques have been employed following lab-based self-harm research [28, 29] and studies using other methods [7, 30] and are also recommended in

online settings [24, 31]. An additional aim of the present study was to evaluate the use of a simple mood elevation tool that can easily be incorporated into a paper-based survey. A multi-method exploratory approach combined quantitative and qualitative analysis to augment understanding and maximise interpretation of findings [32]. Specifically the present research asked (1) Does participation in a longitudinal self-harm survey have an impact on participant mood? (2) How do young people rate and describe their experience of participation? (3) Do young people engage with a simple mood elevation device following participation in a self-harm survey? As our multi-method examination is largely exploratory no testable predictions were made. Responses across these outcomes (mood impact/survey rating/survey description/engagement with a mood elevation device) were compared for the sample overall and according to self-harm status and gender.

Methods

Participants

Participants were recruited from three secondary schools in the East Midlands of England to a broader study on impulsivity and self-harm. The study ran from October 2016 until February 2017. Parents of students in years 9 and 10 (aged 13–15 years) were sent an information sheet and opt-out consent form via electronic parent mail and asked to discuss the study with their child. School assemblies and tutor sessions, held before data collection, reinforced information and participant rights. Reminder messages were sent to parents 1 week before data collection.

A total of 710 students were invited to take part. Parental consent was withdrawn from $n = 18$ (2.5%). In addition, 46 students (6.5%) did not take part due to withdrawing assent ($n = 11$), other school commitments, or absence. The total number of participants completing the survey at baseline was thus 646. Recruitment was spread across schools (198:218:230). The mean age of participants was 13.5 years, (SD = .61) and 94% of the sample were aged 13–14 years. The sample was 51% male, 46% female, with 3% not stating a gender. The majority (81%) identified their ethnicity as white. Of the baseline participants, 594 completed the follow-up survey. Average follow-up time was *12.1 weeks, SD = 1.15*. The retention rate of 92% compares favourably with other school-based longitudinal studies [21]. Reasons for attrition ($n = 52$) at follow-up included spoiled or missing codes from completed papers $n = 27$ (52%); parent removed consent for follow-up $n = 3$ (5.7%); and unspecified absence $n = 22$ (42%). Distributions of gender (male 50%, female 47%, 3% unspecified) and ethnicity (white 84%) were similar at follow-up. Main analysis focuses on those who participated at both time points.

Materials and measures
Questions about self-harm behaviour
Participants were provided with a definition of self-harm based on NICE (National Institute for Health and Clinical Excellence) guidelines [33]: "Self-harm is hurting yourself on purpose such as cutting, hitting, biting, burning or self-poisoning (such as swallowing too many pills or other dangerous substances), *no matter what the reason.* Self-harm is not hurting yourself by accident." This definition reflects a lack of categorical distinction between self-harmful behaviour with or without suicidal intent [34]. Participants were asked two questions modified from the Lifestyle and Coping Questionnaire [LCQ: 2]: "Have you ever seriously *thought* about trying to harm yourself on purpose in some way but *not* actually done so?" and "Have you ever on purpose harmed yourself in some way?" A modified version of the LCQ has been used in other school-based studies [35]. Analyses for the present study are based on answers to the two self-harm questions indicated above. However, the full survey included a number of additional questions relating to self-harm which asked participants for information about how recently and frequently they self-harm; to provide a description and reason for their most recent episode; and to quantify the typical length of time between first having the urge to self-harm and completing the act. Participants were also asked two questions about help-seeking behaviour in school. All participants were asked to provide an answer to the self-harm questions, even if this was to write "not relevant". This ensured that all participants completed each section and sought to reduce the visible distinction between those with and without experience of self-harm during testing.

Current mood rating scale
Participants were asked to rate current mood state on a visual analogue scale (VAS) at the start and end of the survey. This approach has been used in qualitative self-harm research with adolescents [36]. The VAS had response options ranging from 0 (illustrated by a sad face and additional text "I feel really sad and down in the dumps") to 10 (illustrated by a happy face and "I feel really happy"). At the midpoint a neutral face and the words "I'm not feeling happy or sad" represented a score of 5. Participants were asked to mark their current mood on the scale. Comparison of pre- and post-survey VAS ratings provided an estimate of the immediate emotional impact of participation.

Survey rating
Participants were asked to rate their experience of taking part in the survey by selecting from provided response options, which were positively-valenced (interesting, enjoyable); negatively-valenced (upsetting, annoying); or neutral (fine), or by supplying their own term of reference in an open-response section. Multiple response choices were not prohibited.

Open questions about the survey
An open response question asked participants to "Describe your thoughts about taking part in the survey and any feelings the content may have raised".

Doodle activity page
The final survey page contained cute animal images, cartoons, exam howlers, jokes, a space to write a joke, and doodle/colour-in spaces. New doodles and imagery were included at follow-up to maintain interest and novelty. Participants were invited to engage with this page once they had completed the survey, or wished to withdraw, with the following invitation: "The survey has now finished. Thanks for taking part! Time to chill... Check out the following page." "Engagement" was defined as a demonstrable sign of actively engaging with the activities and spaces on the doodle page by drawing/doodling/colouring in/writing on the page etc. This page aimed to recalibrate mood, which may have been lowered through participation. Evidence suggests that looking at cute images of animals, cartoons and emotive texts are effective at eliciting positive mood [37, 38].

Procedure
Ethical approval was obtained from the Division of Psychiatry and Applied Psychology Research Ethics subcommittee at The University of Nottingham. All survey materials were trialled, piloted and modified with a youth advisory panel with lived experience of self-harm. On the day of the baseline study consented students were provided with an information sheet, assent form and envelope. Study procedures, rights of withdrawal and limits of confidentiality and anonymity were explained by the researcher (in person or by video) or by individual tutors according to a set script. Participants generated a unique identification (ID) code and wrote this on their survey. In order that surveys could be linked to a student if responses indicated concern for safety, students were asked to include their ID code on a signed assent form and envelope, and to seal the form inside the envelope. Sealed envelopes and surveys were collected and stored separately. Procedures were repeated at follow-up. Data collection took place during designated lesson time.

Students sat individually within class groups and were instructed not to discuss answers. All students received a resource sheet detailing sources of support in school and appropriate outside agencies. Survey responses were screened within 24 h of data collection for safeguarding reasons.

Analysis approach

Data were analysed using SPSS v24 for Windows. Paired sample T tests were used to examine differences in mood scores pre- to post-survey at baseline and at follow-up for the sample overall. Between-subjects ANOVAs were used to examine effects of self-harm status (yes—a reported history of self-harm vs. no—no reported history of self-harm) and gender (Boys vs. Girls), and the gender*self-harm status interaction, for influence on mood-change scores (post VAS score–pre VAS score) at baseline and follow-up. For statistically significant interactions, simple main effects and pairwise comparisons were examined using a corrected p value to control for multiple comparisons ($p=.025$). For non-significant interactions, main effects analyses were performed. Chi square analysis was used to compare distributions of categorical ratings of the survey (positive/negative/neutral)—these were compared for those with and without lived experience of self-harm at baseline and follow-up. Analysis of standardised residuals identified where observed ratings in each category differed from those expected by chance (positive or negative residuals >1.96). Qualitative responses were coded using thematic analysis [39]. Thematic analysis is a flexible form of pattern recognition which allows themes to be derived inductively (from the data) and deductively (from past literature and theory) in order to best capture and summarise a phenomenon of interest. A sample of transcribed responses were independently read and coded inductively by JL and LR. A coding frame that integrated inductively- and deductively-derived codes was then developed by JL, verified via discussion, and applied to the full data set. The coding frame contained labels, descriptions and examples of codes and themes [40]. Themes were identified and refined into main themes and sub-themes. A third researcher blind to study aims independently tested the applicability of data-to-theme allocation from randomly selected extracts with percentage consensus agreement of 83%. Consensus of 70% or above is deemed necessary for themes to be judged as coherent and valid [40].

Results

Initial analysis

Completers v non-completers

Initial analysis compared the 594 participants who completed both the baseline and follow-up surveys (completers) with the 52 who only provided baseline data (non-completers). Chi square tests revealed that groups did not differ by gender ($p=.287$) or ethnicity ($p=.497$). However, groups differed according to school ($p<.001$). Groups did not differ in terms of self-harm incidence ($p=.313$); or thoughts ($p=.121$). Nor were they more likely to have rated the survey at baseline as a negative rather than a positive experience ($p=.734$). Mann–Whitney U tests revealed no difference between groups in the distribution of mood-change scores pre- to post-survey ($p=.367$).

Incidence of self-harm thoughts and behaviour

At baseline, 30.4% of participants indicated having had thoughts of self-harm and 23.6% indicated lifetime self-harm. At follow-up, rates of self-harm thoughts were similar to baseline (30.6%), and reported incidence of lifetime self-harm was 27.6%. Of the additional 29 respondents indicating self-harm behaviour at follow-up, 25 reported first onset of behaviour between the baseline and follow-up assessment.

Did current emotional rating scores change following completion of the survey?

A 2×2 between subjects ANOVA revealed a statistically significant interaction between gender and self-harm status on mood-change score from pre to post survey completion at baseline $F(1,467)=4.673$, $p=.031$, partial $\eta^2=.010$. Simple main effects analysis revealed there was no significant overall effect for self-harm status ($p=.755$); however, there was an overall statistically significant difference in mean mood change scores by gender. Specifically, mood change scores differed between boys with a self-harm history and girls with a self-harm history, $F(1,467)=8.189$, $p=.004$, $\eta^2=.017$ (Bonferroni corrected). There was no significant difference between boys and girls who had not self-harmed ($p=.447$). Table 1 presents mean VAS scores at both baseline and follow-up for boys and girls with and without self-harm, and the complete sample. Findings suggest that completing the survey had a negative impact on mood for girls who had self-harmed (post-survey mood scores were lower than pre-survey scores), but conversely a positive impact on mood for boys who had self-harmed (post-survey scores were higher than pre-survey scores). A second ANOVA compared mood change scores pre-to-post survey for boys and girls across levels of self-harm status at follow-up. This time there was no statistically significant interaction between gender and self-harm status $F(1,427)=.379$, $p=.538$, partial $\eta^2=.001$. Main effects analysis revealed no statistically significant main effect of gender $F(1,427)=1.278$, $p=.259$, partial $\eta^2=.003$; or main effect of self-harm status $F(1,427)=.021$, $p=.884$,

Table 1 Mean pre-survey and post-survey mood scores at baseline and follow-up

Self-harm status	Gender	Baseline			Follow-up		
		N	VAS pre-	VAS post-	N	VAS pre-	VAS post-
SH no	Boys	199	7.09 (1.82)	7.21 (1.99)	176	7.03 (1.89)	6.72 (2.24)
	Girls	164	6.72 (1.86)	6.68 (2.15)	138	6.67 (1.76)	6.67 (2.01)
SH yes	Boys	43	5.93 (2.29)	6.35 (2.28)[a]	45	6.12 (2.22)	5.48 (2.44)
	Girls	65	4.97 (1.77)	4.79 (1.85)[a]	72	5.33 (2.13)	4.58 (2.24)
Overall		491	6.60 (1.97)	6.54 (2.18)	489	6.49 (1.9)	6.22 (2.3)[b]

The table presents means for the VAS (visual analogue scale) ratings provided at the start (VAS pre-) and at the end (VAS post-) of each survey assessment for the sample overall, and by self-harm Status and Gender. Standard deviations are shown in parentheses

"SH yes" denotes lifetime incidence of self-harm. "SH no" denotes no reported history of self-harm

[a] A significant interaction between mean mood-change score for boys and girls at the level of SH yes $F(1467) = 8.189$, $p = .004$, $\eta^2 = .017$ which survives Bonferroni correction at $p = .025$

[b] A statistically significant difference between VAS pre- and VAS post-survey scores, $t = 3.807$, $p < .0001$

$partial$ $\eta^2 = .000$. Hence, neither gender nor self-harm status influenced mood change scores at the follow-up timepoint (See Table 1).

How did participants rate the survey?

Table 2 presents proportions of participants rating each survey in positive ("interesting", or "enjoyable"), neutral ("fine"), and negative ("annoying" or "upsetting") terms. Most participants at baseline rated the survey in positive/neutral terms overall (79.7%) and across gender and self-harm status. However, comparing groups by self-harm status: Chi square analysis revealed that the ratings differed between those with and without self-harm χ^2 $(2) = 37.606$, $p < .001$. Inspection of standardised residuals revealed that those who did not endorse self-harm had lower levels of negative ratings than would be expected by chance; while those with self-harm experience had higher levels of negative ratings, and lower levels of positive ratings than would be expected by chance. The most common negative responses cited by those without lived experience of self-harm were "annoyance" (n = 17, 4.3%) and "boring/pointless" (n = 13, 3.3%). By contrast, the most common response for those endorsing self-harm was feeling "upset" (n = 23, 16%) with a few respondents reporting finding the survey annoying (n = 9, 6.3%) or "boring/pointless" (n = 4, 2.8%). However, it is important to note that most participants did not report negative responses. Comparing ratings by gender did not reveal a significant difference in response ($p = .184$).

At follow-up, the survey was again rated in positive/neutral terms by the majority overall (73.5%) and across self-harm status and gender. However, an increased percentage of respondents gave the survey a negative response at follow-up, compared to baseline, and this was driven in part by an increase in those finding the survey "boring" or "pointless" (8.7 v. 3.1%

at baseline). Chi square analysis revealed that the distribution of positive, negative and neutral ratings did not differ according to self-harm status ($p = .071$). The most common negative response cited by those without self-harm was "boring" (increased to 10.4% from 3.3%) with "annoying" selected by an increased 6.9% compared to 4.3% at baseline. Similarly, the most common response for those with self-harm was now "annoying" (14.2%) with feeling "upset" reduced from 16 to 10.3%. Notably, for those endorsing self-harm the percentage of negative evaluations was lower at follow-up than at baseline while positive evaluations were proportionally higher at follow-up; the opposite pattern of response was reported in those without self-harm experience for whom positive ratings decreased and negative ratings increased in comparison to baseline. Of the 25 participants who revealed a first incidence of self-harm between assessments, most rated the survey as a positive/neutral experience at baseline (83%) and follow-up (60%), although again the response pattern reflected an increase in negative ratings by follow-up, and the highest proportion of negative response for any category of respondent. Again, when comparing ratings by gender, no significant difference in response was observed at follow-up ($p = .545$).

What did participants think about taking part in the survey?

Responses to the item "Please share your thoughts about taking part in the survey, and any feelings the context may have raised" were refined into six themes (three positive, two negative and one neutral) using thematic analysis [39]. No main thematic differences emerged between time-points. Main themes, subthemes, and frequencies of endorsement are shown in Fig. 1.

Table 2 Proportions of participant ratings for positive, neutral and negative evaluation of the survey at baseline and follow-up

	Baseline					Follow-up				
	N	Positive (%)	Neutral (%)	Positive/neutral (%)	Negative (%)	N	Positive (%)	Neutral (%)	Positive/neutral (%)	Negative (%)
Overall	582	170 (28.6)	309 (52.0)	479 (79.7)	103 (17.3)	578	136 (23.5)	300 (51.9)	436 (73.5)	142 (23.9)
SH yes	119	25 (18.5) −	64 (47.4)	183 (60.6)	46 (34.8) +++	155	30 (19.4)	77 (46.5)	107 (69.0)	48 (31.0)
SH no	439	145 (32.6)	240 (55.3)	391 (86.1)	54 (12.1) − −	423	106 (25.1)	223 (51.3)	329 (77.7)	94 (22.2)
Girls	273	73 (26.7)	147 (49.0)	220 (76.2)	53 (19.4)	270	60 (22.2)	148 (54.8)	208 (77.0)	62 (23)
Boys	293	96 (32.8)	153 (52.2)	249 (84.3)	44 (15.0)	292	74 (25.3)	147 (50.3)	221 (76.0)	71 (24.3)

−/+ Standardised residual score of > 1.96; − −/+ + standardised residual score of > 2.58; − − −/+ + + standardised residual score of > 3.29 at p < .01 (.05/5)

"SH yes" denotes lifetime incidence of self-harm, "SH no" denotes no reported history of self-harm

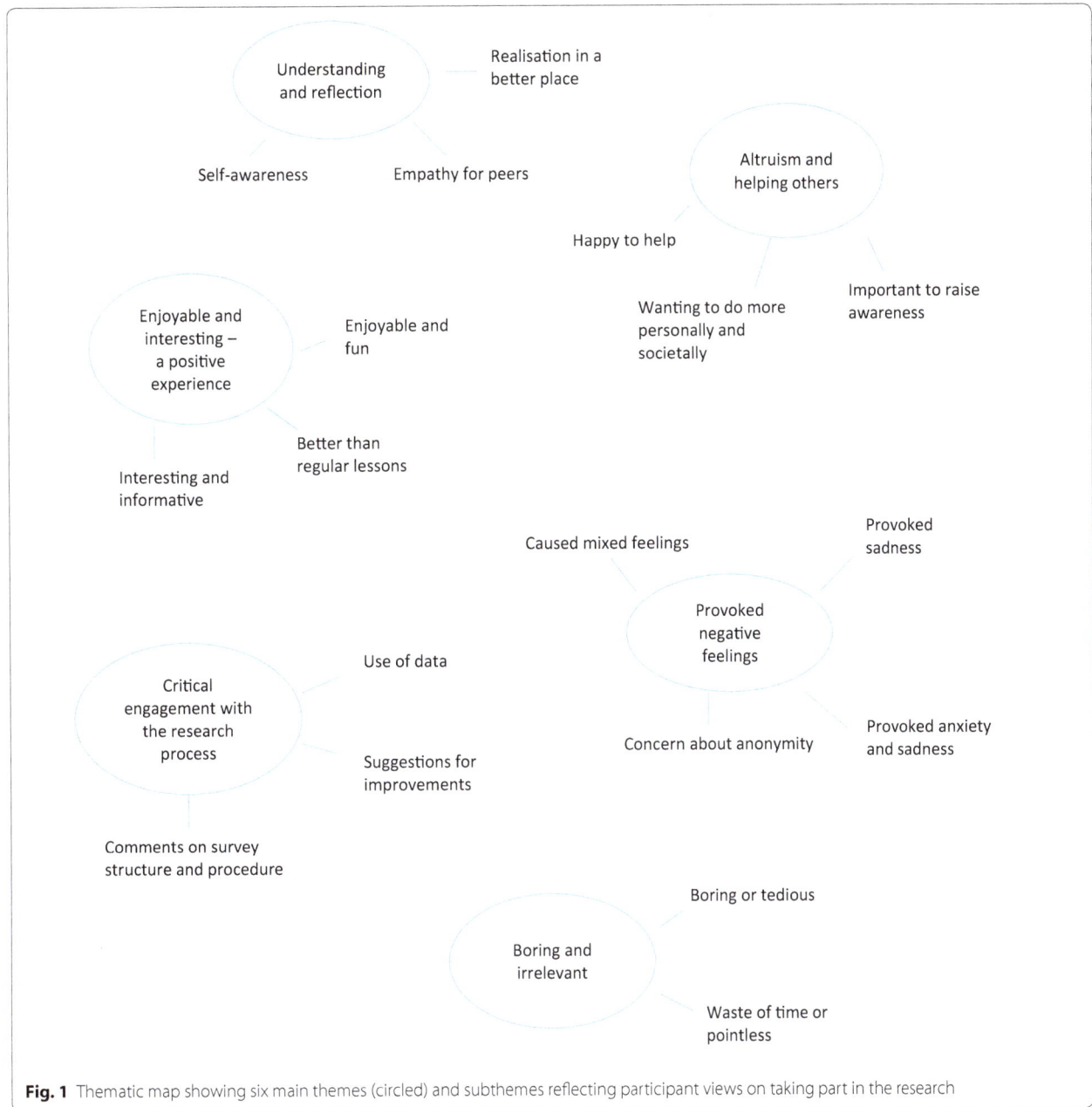

Fig. 1 Thematic map showing six main themes (circled) and subthemes reflecting participant views on taking part in the research

Theme: Understanding and reflection

Young people valued the greater self-awareness and understanding gained from participation: *"It's a really good and interesting way to gain information and think about your life."* (F, aged 14, SH). Participants felt that they "knew themselves better" from the experience and enjoyed the opportunity for self-reflection: *"I think it [taking part] brings you more in touch with your feelings and allows you to get presence and really think."* (M, aged 13, no SH). For some it was greater understanding of others that was important: *"It makes me more aware of the*

emotional health of my peers." (F, aged 13, no SH.) Taking part was a chance to offload and also provided relief: *"It's made me feel relieved that I have let out how I feel"* (F, aged 13, SH). Some found value in realising they were in a good place: *"I realise now that I enjoy lots of things and I am a better and happier person that I used to be."* (F, aged 13, SH); *"It's just reminded me how much happier I am now than when I was so sad, so that's good."* (F, aged 15, SH). This theme was the most consistently endorsed overall with endorsement from 50 participants at baseline (28% of responses) and 30 participants at follow-up

(18% of responses). Overall, a slightly higher numbers of girls (n = 44) than boys (n = 36) endorsed this theme.

Theme: Altruism and helping others

Being able to help others was a source of value: *"I hope my input will help people for the better."* (F, aged 13, no SH); *"It's ok, and didn't upset me and I'm happy to help."* (M, aged 13, SH). The benefits were often linked to contributing to research: *"I feel happy I have taken part in some useful research."* (F, aged 13, no SH). Students felt it was important to raise awareness of mental health: *"I think that it is good that people are recognising that mental health in young teenagers, especially students, is a big deal."* (F, aged 14, SH). Some wanted further opportunities and support to discuss such issues: *"I think we should get lessons in PSHE [Personal, Social and Health Education] about self-harm and depression and suicide as it is a bit of a stigma topic and it shouldn't be."* (F, aged 14, no SH). A number of students felt that schools could do more to facilitate peer support: *"I don't know how to help people who self-harm and feel that this is something that schools should teach."* (F, aged 13, no SH). This was the second most consistently endorsed theme overall, endorsed by 33 participants at baseline (18.5% of responses) and 28 participants at follow-up (17% of responses). Endorsement was similar overall between boys (n = 31) and girls (n = 30).

Theme: Enjoyable and interesting—a positive experience

For some participants the process of taking part in the research was enjoyable in itself: *"I thought it was quite fun, like Christmas!"* (F, aged 13, no SH). *"It was good, I would do it anytime"* (M, aged 13, SH). For others there were additional perceived benefits, like missing class: *"Don't mind, gets us out of lessons."* (M, aged 13, no SH). Students felt happy to have been asked their opinions: *"I think it is good that people are researching our age group and giving us a say."* (F, aged 14, SH). Some were pleased to be involved with a University study: *"I think it is cool that the University is asking us."* (F, aged 13, no SH). Participants reported enjoying the survey in similar numbers at baseline (n = 26, 15%) and follow-up (n = 27, 16%). More girls than boys endorsed this theme at baseline (n = 17 vs. n = 9), a pattern reversed at follow-up (n = 12 girls vs. n = 15 boys).

Theme: Provoked negative emotions

Some students indicated that thinking about self-harm in others made them feel sad: *"I find it quite upsetting to know that people can feel some of the options."* (F, aged 15, no SH). For some, the survey was a difficult reminder of past actions: *"It made me feel upset, because I remembered that time."* (F, aged 13, SH). However, this was often a mixed emotional response: *"I felt upset because it reminded me of what I used to do, but happy because I have passed that stage in my life."* (F, aged 13, SH). Some voiced feelings of anxiety, particularly about anonymity and confidentiality: *"I feel really anxious and in a panic because anyone could read this."* (F, aged 13, SH). This theme was endorsed by similar numbers at baseline (n = 24, 13% of responses) and follow-up (n = 23, 14% of responses). Notably, at both time points, more girls than boys endorsed this theme—(n = 22 vs. n = 2) at baseline and (n = 17 vs. n = 6) at follow-up.

Theme: Boring or irrelevant

Some participants simply found the survey to be "pointless" or a "waste of their time". Feelings that the survey was "boring", or "repetitive" were increasingly cited at the follow-up assessment: *"Boring because we have already done it."* (M, aged 13, no SH). For some, the lack of personal relevance was a source of annoyance: *"It's annoying as it is not relevant and depressing."* (F, aged 14, no SH). A small number of participants endorsed this theme, with 6 participants at baseline (3% of responses) and 12 participants at follow-up (7% of responses). This response was predominantly a male phenomenon with all but two references to boredom or irrelevance coming from boys.

Theme: Critical engagement with the research process

Participants offered thoughts on how the research could be improved. Some suggested that the survey did not go far enough: *"The questions were very clear, but needed more depth."* (M, aged 14, no SH), or had, *"surprisingly little content about self-harm"* (M, aged 13, no SH). Others felt the survey should have included broader questions on "drugs and alcohol" or "sexuality". Some queried what would happen with their data: *"It would be interesting to see what research you would do with the results, or what solutions you would have to problems."* (M, aged 13, no SH). Some questioned the validity of a survey: *"I think that people who have self-harmed wouldn't say it on a survey because if you self-harm you don't tell anyone."* (F, aged 13, no SH). Others wondered whether participants would be able to adequately assess their responses: *"People may not be able to evaluate what they think."* (F, aged 13, SH). This final theme was the most commonly identified response at follow-up, with endorsement rising from 17 participants (10% of responses) at baseline to 34 participants (21% of responses) at follow-up. More boys endorsed this theme than girls overall, although proportions were similar at each time point (n = 10 boys and n = 7 girls at baseline; n = 19 boys and n = 15 girls at follow-up).

Did participants engage with the final doodle page?

Just over half of the participants (55% baseline and 60% follow-up) chose to tangibly engage with the doodle page (e.g. doodled, filled in speech bubbles, offered a joke). At baseline a higher proportion of participants with self-harm engaged (76%) than those without (55%), but this was not a significant difference $\chi^2 (2)=2.303, p=.129$. At follow-up by contrast, a significantly higher proportion of those without self-harm (63 v 50%) tangibly engaged with this page, $\chi^2 (1)=8.045, p=.005$. There were no differences in proportions of interactions with the doodle page between boys and girls. The distribution of mood-change scores (pre- to post-survey) differed between those who did and did not complete the final activity page at baseline (Mann–Whitney $U=26,139.5, z-2.570 \ p=.010$). Those engaging with the page reported a small decrease in emotional rating (mean change in score $-.19$), while those not engaging reported a small increase in emotional rating (mean change in score $+.05$). However, distributions did not differ at follow-up ($p=.294$). Students commented on the final doodle page in the open response section: *"I'm rating the survey a 10 because of the cats"* (Did not say, aged 13, no SH). *"I love doing these surveys. I feel relieved to write down how I feel and I love the doodle page at the end!"* (F, aged 13, SH thoughts). A number of young people suggested that the final page had made them feel better: *"I feel strange, nervous, also confused and hurt, but relieved. Thanks for the doodles – it helped calm me down"* (F, aged 13, SH).

Discussion

Overall, the present findings suggest, that for the majority, participation in research on self-harm was not perceived as a negative experience by young adolescents and did not impact negatively on mood. Participants described important benefits such as increased self-awareness, a chance to off-load, and helping others. However, subtle differences were observed according to gender, self-harm status and across time-points. Firstly, emotional rating (VAS) scores indicated that, following participation, respondents largely rated their mood at the positive (happy) end of the scale. But there were notable differences between the most vulnerable boys and the most vulnerable girls in their immediate emotional reaction to participation, as indicated by the VAS. For boys with self-harm, participation led to an improvement in mood; whereas for girls with self-harm, participation led to a deterioration in mood. The finding that high-risk boys found a mood-based benefit from involvement resonates with some previous studies [19, 24, 25] which indicate that participation can confer benefit for those at greatest risk. Although notably, this pattern of findings was not supported at follow-up. These findings suggest

however, that in terms of immediate emotional reaction, conferred benefits are less likely to be found for girls who self-harm. As such, studies may need to be particularly alert to the immediate emotional impact of research participation on vulnerable girls.

The survey rating data revealed that the majority of participants judged taking part as a positive/neutral experience at both baseline and follow-up. Positive/neutral evaluations far outweighed negative evaluations for boys and girls and those with and without self-harm at both time points. Closer analysis at baseline revealed significant differences in the pattern of emotional responses felt between those with and without self-harm experience: a higher proportion of those endorsing self-harm found participation to be a negative experience and a smaller proportion rated the survey positively compared with those who did not self-harm. This suggests an increased vulnerability in response for those with lived experience of self-harm. However, differences in response distributions between these groups were not observed at follow-up. In most cases, at the second assessment, participants reported fewer positive/neutral evaluations and more negative reactions to the survey (which may be in line with the overall VAS follow-up findings) but there was one notable exception. For those endorsing self-harm, a larger proportion found the survey to be a positive or neutral experience at the second compared to first time of assessment, and negative reactions to the survey for this subset actually decreased over time. This resulted in a smaller percentage point difference in positive/neutral ratings and negative ratings between those who had and had not self-harmed. The finding of an increased positive outcome over time for those at higher risk of self-harm again chimes with previous research [25, 28] suggesting that those at greatest vulnerability may gain greatest long-term benefit from on-going participation.

The contrasting responses found from those with and without self-harm experience across VAS and survey ratings may relate to the perceived relevance of the survey for individual respondents. At follow-up, an increased number of negative reactions to participation for those not endorsing self-harm related to boredom, a lack of personal bearing and annoyance at being asked to complete a survey twice—findings which were supported in the qualitative analysis. These reactions featured far less for those with lived experience of self-harm. Relevance may drive the benefit gained from longitudinal engagement with this topic, although this does not rule out finding the survey emotionally impactful (as demonstrated by lower VAS scores). Qualitative findings suggest the increase in positive ratings at follow-up in part may relate to a possible therapeutic benefit derived from an on-going opportunity to "offload" and self-reflect. This may be particularly important for groups typically unlikely to have disclosed their behaviour [2] or lacking opportunity to discuss and describe it. It could also be argued that exposure to the topic at baseline may have desensitised participants for the follow-up assessment. The effects of this could be greatest for those with lived experience who may have felt a greater emotional response to the topic at the outset. The sharp increase in negative evaluations of the survey for those without lived experience at follow-up suggests it will be important for future research to explore the impact of research participation for those who are psychologically healthy, as well as those at greater risk, over repeated assessment, particularly where follow-up is relatively short. In particular, increased rates of annoyance mainly for those not endorsing self-harm behaviour (see also [28], but also across the sample overall, should be recognised and mitigated where possible.

The findings also highlight the varied nature of individual response to participation. Engaging with a sensitive topic may cause understandable distress for some (such as the lowering of mood found for girls with self-harm), but it does not necessarily follow that this is evaluated as a "negative" outcome. Markedly, many participants coupled positive and negative ratings, separating emotional responses from a cognitive evaluation (e.g. *nervous* yet *interesting; uncomfortable,* but *fine; difficult* yet *worthwhile).* Given the complexity of the behaviour, it is not surprising that respondents selected multiple categories to describe their response. This suggests that it is important for ethical guidelines around self-harm research to recognise that potential benefits and potential risks from involvement are not necessarily mutually exclusive.

Although there was no statistical distinction between boys and girls when comparing survey ratings, analyses indicated differences in emotional response to survey participation according to both VAS scores and thematic analysis, where a qualitatively different reaction to survey participation from girls, who did describe feeling upset, was found to boys, who broadly did not. Further qualitative research may help to clarify these gender differences in response to participation. The qualitative findings largely support those found by Hasking and colleagues [20] in their school-based sample. A novel thematic finding in this study was the large endorsement for a critical engagement in the research process indicating that many young people are not only supportive of research endeavour but are keen to reflect on, question and challenge the process.

This study also provides insight into the use of a simple mood recalibration doodle page. A small majority of participants chose to engage with this page, though rates of engagement varied across groups. At baseline, those whose mood decreased the most (participants endorsing self-harm) had a higher rate of engagement with the page. At follow-up, those who reported an increase in negative survey ratings (participants not endorsing selfharm) were more likely to demonstrably engage. It could be argued that those feeling the greatest negative impact from participation may more readily seek out recalibration, but more work should seek to evaluate the impact of such mitigation tools in community samples using longitudinal designs. The present study did not provide an experimental test of mitigation or specifically elicit participants' reactions to the doodle page. We can not know to what extent the page was helpful for those who nonetheless left no physical indication of engagement. However, large numbers of participants did demonstrably engage and many chose to reference this in open responses. Undoubtedly for some, the page helped to calm emotions. Moreover, the study's advisory youth panel strongly endorsed the doodle page. Importantly, the page brought an additional and unexpected ethical advantage. The self-penned jokes, doodles, or direct comments written directly on the survey script by participants who also used the page to offer reassurance to the research team that they were feeling all right, had a positive impact on researcher wellbeing. Collecting data on self-harm has an inevitable impact on researchers but the evaluation of this impact is under-researched. The need to better document and discuss harm minimisation for researchers has been discussed elsewhere [31, 41] and sharing potential practical solutions is advocated.

Key strengths of this study include the focus on a community-based sample of early adolescents (aged 13–14) for whom self-harm risk is heightened [15] and the additional insight offered on how both male and female participants, with and without self-harm experience, respond differentially to study involvement. Given recommendations for short-term prospective examinations of self-harm risk in youth [26, 27] this study provides important ethical encouragement, via multiple and converging methods, that short-term assessment (at least in terms of weeks) does not confer added risk to the majority of participants. In addition, novel insight is provided into the role of a simple mood enhancement tool. The low attrition (8%) compares favourably with previous school-based research [21]. High willingness to complete a follow-up survey may be seen as an additional marker of a study's acceptability. Nonetheless, the influence of the school-based setting must be recognised. Schools, as an "adult-owned territory" [42] hold an inherent power asymmetry within which children generally participate in compulsory activities [43]. Thus, despite clear efforts to emphasise participant rights to withdraw, a learned compliance can compromise the voluntary principles of participation [44]. There are limitations to the conclusions that can be reached from this study. We did not explicitly ask participants at follow-up how they felt after completing the baseline assessment and we can not examine if reported reactions were transitory. Neither did we explicitly ask participants if they found the research to be worthwhile. A small number of students (4%) indicated initiating self-harm behaviour between assessment points. This compares with rates reported in other prospective school-based studies of 2.6 and 6.0% [13, 45]. While the development of self-harm observed here may follow the natural trajectory of self-harm, the design of the study does not allow us to rule out any causal iatrogenic link. These questions would be usefully addressed in future studies. The present study largely assesses self-harm in terms of a lifetime presence of behaviour. While this broad indicator of self-harm status was adequate in distinguishing differences in response, meaningful information about the impact of study involvement is likely to be gained from a finer grained analysis of self-harm status in which the recency or frequency of behaviour is accounted for. Notably, those indicating the most recent onset of self-harm (i.e. first time behaviour occurring between assessment points) recorded a high proportion of negative responses at the follow-up assessment (40%). Those with current versus historical self-harm may differ in both emotional response and cognitive appraisal of that response. Further research should explore these ideas.

Conclusions

This study contributes important information on the impact of research participation on young adolescents using quantitative and qualitative data to augment understanding. Participation was, for the most part, reported to have been a positive and beneficial experience, and many valued the chance to critically engage with the research process. Those with self-harm experience, and in particular girls who self-harm, displayed an increased vulnerability compared to those who did not self-harm (lower mood ratings following participation, a larger proportion of negative ratings) but, nonetheless, most evaluated their participation in positive or at least neutral terms. However, further work is needed to understand the impact of repeated assessment on those with and without lived experience for whom research reactions qualitatively differ. Many young people felt that having an opportunity to discuss mental health in school was important and may confer unique benefits for those who self-harm. School settings are potentially well placed to accommodate appropriate response to risk and provide support. Ensuring that any school-based support is appropriate and effective is critical

however. Evidence-based school programmes such as the Signs of Self-Injury Programme [46], for example, which are designed to educate about self-harm and offer skills to staff and students to respond to self-harm may offer a promising and systematic way forward [47]. Prospective research on adolescent self-harm is ethically viable in schools, but the inclusion of a simple mood-elevating tool may be an additional and easily incorporated means of mood elevation, and beneficial to participants and researchers.

Abbreviations

NICE: National Institute for Health and Clinical Excellence; LCQ: Lifestyle and Coping Questionnaire; VAS: visual analogue scale; F: female; M: male; SH: self-harm; PSHE: Personal, Social and Health Education; IRB: Institutional Review Board.

Authors' contributions

JL conceptualised the study, performed the analysis, and drafted the initial manuscript. LR provided additional qualitative analysis. ET, KS, and DD were involved in designing the study and editing the manuscript. All authors read and approved the final manuscript.

Author details

[1] Division of Psychiatry & Applied Psychology, Institute of Mental Health, University of Nottingham, University of Nottingham Innovation Park, Triumph Road, Nottingham NG7 2TU, UK. [2] Centre for ADHD and Neurodevelopmental Disorders Across the Lifespan, Institute of Mental Health, University of Nottingham, Nottingham, UK. [3] Self-Harm Research Group, School of Psychology, University of Nottingham, Nottingham, UK.

Acknowledgements

Thanks to Stephanie Sampson for support in qualitative reliability testing. The authors gratefully acknowledge the schools and participants involved in this study, and the advisory youth panel.

Competing interests

The authors declare that they have no competing interests.

Funding

This work is supported by the Economic and Social Research Council [Grant ES/J500100/1]. The funding body was not involved in the design of the study, the collection, analysis or interpretation of data, or the writing or approval of the manuscript.

References

1. Kapur N, et al. Non-suicidal self-injury v. attempted suicide: new diagnosis or false dichotomy? Br J Psychiatry. 2013;202(5):326–8.
2. Madge N, et al. Deliberate self-harm within an international community sample of young people: comparative findings from the Child & Adolescent Self-harm in Europe (CASE) Study. J Child Psychol Psychiatry. 2008;49(6):667–77.
3. Muehlenkamp J, et al. International prevalence of adolescent non-suicidal self-injury and deliberate self-harm. Child Adolesc Psychiatry Ment Health. 2012;6:10.
4. NICE, N.I.f.H.a.C.E. Self-harm: the short-term physical and psychological management and secondary prevention of self-harm in primary and secondary care. Clinical guidelines, No. 16. Leicester: British Psychological Society; 2004.
5. Owens D, Horrocks J, House A. Fatal and non-fatal repetition of self-harm: systematic review. Br J Psychiatry. 2002;181:193–9.
6. Mars B, et al. Clinical and social outcomes of adolescent self harm: population based birth cohort study. BMJ. 2014;349:g5954.
7. Townsend E, et al. Self-harm and life problems: findings from the Multicentre Study of Self-harm in England. Soc Psychiatry Psychiatr Epidemiol. 2016;51(2):183–92.
8. Whitlock J. Self-injurious behavior in adolescents. PLoS Med. 2010;7(5):e1000240.
9. Morey Y, Mellon D, Dailami N, Verne J, Tapp A. Adolescent self-harm in the community: an update on prevalence using a self-report survey of adolescents aged 13–18 in England. J Public Health. 2016;39(1):58–64.
10. Moran P, et al. The natural history of self-harm from adolescence to young adulthood: a population-based cohort study. Lancet. 2012;379(9812):236–43.
11. Ogle RL, Clements CM. Deliberate self-harm and alcohol involvement in college-aged females: a controlled comparison in a nonclinical sample. Am J Orthopsychiatry. 2008;78(4):442–8.
12. Whitlock J, Eckenrode J, Silverman D. Self-injurious behaviors in a college population. Pediatrics. 2006;117(6):1939–48.
13. Stallard P, et al. Self-harm in young adolescents (12–16 years): onset and short-term continuation in a community sample. BMC Psychiatry. 2013;13:328.
14. Morgan C, et al. Incidence, clinical management, and mortality risk following self harm among children and adolescents: cohort study in primary care. BMJ. 2017;359:j4351.
15. Geulayov G, et al. Incidence of suicide, hospital-presenting non-fatal self-harm, and community-occurring non-fatal self-harm in adolescents in England (the iceberg model of self-harm): a retrospective study. Lancet Psychiatry. 2017;5(2):167–74.
16. Lakeman R, Fitzgerald M. The ethics of suicide research. Crisis. 2009;30(1):13–9.
17. Lakeman R, Fitzgerald M. Ethical suicide research: a survey of researchers. Int J Ment Health Nurs. 2009;18(1):10–7.
18. Dazzi T, et al. Does asking about suicide and related behaviours induce suicidal ideation? What is the evidence? Psychol Med. 2014;44(16):3361–3.
19. DeCou CR, Schumann ME. On the iatrogenic risk of assessing suicidality: a meta-analysis. Suicide Life Threat Behav. 2017. https://doi.org/10.1111/sltb.12368.
20. Gould MS, et al. Evaluating iatrogenic risk of youth suicide screening programs: a randomized controlled trial. JAMA. 2005;293(13):1635–43.
21. Hasking P, Tatnell RC, Martin G. Adolescents' reactions to participating in ethically sensitive research: a prospective self-report study. Child Adolesc Psychiatry Ment Health. 2015;9:39.
22. Langhinrichsen-Rohling J, et al. Sensitive research with adolescents: just how upsetting are self-report surveys anyway? Violence Vict. 2006;21(4):425–44.
23. Robinson J, et al. Does screening high school students for psychological distress, deliberate self-harm, or suicidal ideation cause distress—and is it acceptable? Crisis. 2011;32(5):254–63.
24. Whitlock J, Pietrusza C, Purington A. Young adult respondent experiences of disclosing self-injury, suicide-related behavior, and psychological distress in a web-based survey. Arch Suicide Res. 2013;17(1):20–32.
25. Mathias CW, et al. What's the harm in asking about suicidal ideation? Suicide Life Threat Behav. 2012;42(3):341–51.
26. Glenn CR, Nock MK. Improving the short-term prediction of suicidal behavior. Am J Prev Med. 2014;47(3 Suppl 2):S176–80.
27. Franklin JC, et al. Risk factors for suicidal thoughts and behaviors: a meta-analysis of 50 years of research. Psychol Bull. 2017;143(2):187–232.
28. Muehlenkamp JJ, et al. Emotional and behavioral effects of participating in an online study of nonsuicidal self-injury. Clin Psychol Sci. 2014;3(1):26–37.
29. Arbuthnott AE, Lewis SP, Bailey HN. Rumination and emotions in nonsuicidal self-injury and eating disorder behaviors: a preliminary test of the emotional cascade model. J Clin Psychol. 2015;71(1):62–71.
30. Wadman R, et al. A sequence analysis of patterns in self-harm in young people with and without experience of being looked after in care. Br J Clin Psychol. 2017;56:388–407.
31. Lloyd-Richardson EE, et al. Research with adolescents who engage in non-suicidal self-injury: ethical considerations and challenges. Child Adolesc Psychiatry Ment Health. 2015;9:37.
32. Leech NL, Onwuegbuzie AI. Guidelines for conducting and reporting mixed research in the field of counseling and beyond. J Couns Dev. 2010;88(1):61–9.
33. NICE, N.i.f.H.a.C.E. Self-harm in over 8 s: short-term management and prevention of recurrence. London: NICE; 2004.
34. Orlando CM, et al. Nonsuicidal self-injury and suicidal self-injury: a taxometric investigation. Behav Ther. 2015;46(6):824–33.
35. O'Connor RC, et al. Self-harm in adolescents: self-report survey in schools in Scotland. Br J Psychiatry. 2009;194(1):68–72.
36. Wadman R, et al. An interpretative phenomenological analysis of the experience of self-harm repetition and recovery in young adults. J Health Psychol. 2016;22:1631–41.
37. Nittono H, et al. The power of kawaii: viewing cute images promotes a careful behavior and narrows attentional focus. PLoS ONE. 2012;7(9):e46362.
38. Goritz AS. The induction of mood via the WWW. Motiv Emot. 2007;31(1):35–47.
39. Braun V, Clarke V. Using thematic analysis in psychology. Qual Res Psychol. 2006;3(2):77–106.
40. Boyatzis RE. Transforming qualitative information. Thousand Oaks: Sage; 1998.
41. Mckenzie SK, Li C, Jenkin G, Collings S. Ethical considerations in sensitive sucide research reliant on non-clinical researchers. Res Ethics. 2016;13:173–83.
42. Morrison K. Interviewing children in uncomfortable settings: 10 lessons for effective practice. Educ Stud. 2013;39(3):320–37.
43. Morrow V, Richards M. The ethics of social research with children: an overview. Child Soc. 1996;10:90–105.
44. Gallacher L, Gallager M. methodological immaturity in childhood research? Thinking through 'participatory methods'. Childhood. 2008;15(4):499–516.
45. O'Connor RC, Rasmussen S, Hawton K. Predicting deliberate self-harm in adolescents: a six month prospective study. Suicide Life Threat Behav. 2009;39(4):364–75.
46. Jacobs D, et al. Signs of self-injury prevention manual. Wellesley Hills: Screening for Mental Health; 2009.
47. Muehlenkamp JJ, Walsh BW, McDade M. Preventing non-suicidal self-injury in adolescents: the signs of self-injury program. J Youth Adolesc. 2010;39(3):306–14.

18

Deliberate self-harm among adolescent psychiatric outpatients in Singapore: prevalence, nature and risk factors

Michelle Siu Min Lauw*❶, Abishek Mathew Abraham and Cheryl Bee Lock Loh

Abstract

Background: Deliberate self-harm (DSH) is a prominent mental health concern among adolescents. Few studies have examined adolescent DSH in non-Western countries. This study examines the prevalence, types and associated risk factors of DSH in a clinical sample of adolescents in Singapore.

Methods: Using a retrospective review of medical records, demographic and clinical data were obtained from 398 consecutive adolescent psychiatric outpatients (mean age = 17.5 ± 1.4 years, range = 13–19 years) who presented at Changi General Hospital from 2013 to 2015.

Results: 23.1% (n = 92) of adolescents engaged in at least one type of DSH. Cutting was the most common type of DSH reported. Females were three times more likely to engage in DSH than males. DSH was positively associated with female gender (odds ratio [OR] 5.03), depressive disorders (OR 2.45), alcohol use (OR 3.49) and forensic history (OR 3.66), but not with smoking behaviour, living arrangement, parental marital status, past abuse or family history of psychiatric illness.

Conclusion: Interventions targeting adolescent DSH should also alleviate depressive symptoms, alcohol use and delinquent behaviours.

Keywords: Deliberate self-harm, Self-harm, Adolescent outpatients, Prevalence, Risk factors

Background

Deliberate self-harm (DSH) refers to the intentional, self-inflicted destruction of bodily tissue without suicidal intent and for reasons not socially or culturally acceptable [1]. DSH generally begins during early-to-mid-adolescence and commonly includes cutting (with a knife or razor), scratching, biting, burning, or hitting oneself [2]. Most adolescents engage in DSH in order to cope with intense negative emotional states such as depression and anxiety [3]. Adolescents may also engage in DSH as an attempt to punish oneself, generate sensations of excitement or stimulation and/or gain attention from others [4]. Although adolescents engage in DSH without lethal intent, it could lead to fatality.

Varying prevalence rates of adolescent DSH have been reported within Western community samples, ranging from 18 to 38% [5, 6], and rates rise up to about 80% among adolescent psychiatric inpatient [7]. Adolescent DSH has been found to occur alongside a range of psychiatric issues such as mood and anxiety disorders, borderline personality traits, alcohol and drug use, conduct problems and an elevated risk of suicide [8–10] as well as psychosocial issues such as severe illness of a parent, parental divorce and poor family structure [4, 8]. Depression, in particular, has been consistently found to be the most common diagnosis among adolescents with DSH [6, 9, 11, 12]. Using a Canadian sample, Asbridge et al. [13] reported that adolescents with elevated depressive symptoms experienced a 40% increase in the total number of DSH acts occurring within the preceding 6 months.

Research on the gender differences in adolescent DSH has been mixed. Some studies have indicated higher

*Correspondence: michelle_lauw@cgh.com.sg
Department of Psychological Medicine, Changi General Hospital, 2 Simei Street 3, Singapore 529889, Singapore

prevalence rates (up to threefold) in adolescent females compared to males [6, 12, 14–18], while others failed to report this gender difference [19–21]. Some studies have also noted gender over-representations in the type of adolescent DSH reported, with females reporting more cutting behaviours and males reporting more violence-related behaviours such as hitting, burning or aggressive driving [6, 13, 21]. However, other studies failed to replicate these gender patterns in the type of adolescent DSH reported [9].

Few studies have examined adolescent DSH in non-Western samples. Among adolescents in Japan, the reported annual prevalence of DSH was 1.5% among males and 6.9% among females aged 15–18 years old [22]. In Hong Kong, the overall prevalence was found to be 32.7% among adolescents aged 10–18 years old [23]. Consistent with the gender patterns reported in Western samples, adolescent females were also found to have significantly higher rates of DSH than adolescent males in Singapore [18], Japan [22] and Hong Kong [23, 24]. In Singapore, one published study reported that 23.6% of adolescent patients at a psychiatric outpatient clinic engaged in DSH, and DSH was associated with female gender, mood disorders, adjustment disorders and alcohol use [18]. However, the authors did not examine the different types of DSH behaviours engaged and did not account for variables such as history of abuse and forensic history.

Using a sample of adolescent psychiatric outpatients in Singapore, this follow-up study described the prevalence as well as different types of DSH behaviours engaged. We also investigated gender differences in the prevalence and types of DSH and explored whether gender, primary diagnosis, alcohol use, smoking behaviour, living arrangements, parental marital status, family history of psychiatric illness, history of abuse and forensic history were predictive of adolescent DSH. This study expands existing knowledge about the clinical phenomenology of DSH in Singapore and allows us to monitor trends over time.

Methods

Participants and procedures

Data was retrospectively collected from medical records of all new adolescent outpatients referred for psychiatric treatment (ages 13–19) seen at the Psychological Medicine Centre of Changi General Hospital, Singapore, from 2013 to 2015. All data was de-identified and study procedures were approved by the institutional review board at Changi General Hospital.

Each patient's demographic data (e.g., age, gender, employment, living arrangements and parental marital status) and clinical information (e.g., presence and

type of DSH behaviours, primary diagnosis, past abuse, alcohol use, smoking behaviour, family history of psychiatric illness and forensic history) were obtained from routine psychiatric intake interview records. In order to avoid unintentionally assessing treatment effects on DSH behaviours, only data from the intake interview was used. In this study, DSH was defined as the intentional self-inflicted destruction of bodily tissue, without the intention to die and excluding culturally sanctioned procedures. Primary diagnoses were made according to the fourth edition of the Diagnostic and Statistical Manual of Mental Disorders [25].

Statistical analyses

Data were analyzed using IBM SPSS Statistics Version 19.0. Descriptive statistics were used to describe demographic and clinical variables. Pearson's Chi square tests were used to analyze the relations between DSH and categorical variables. A value of $p < 0.05$ was considered statistically significant. Candidate risk factors were screened using univariate logistic regression and variables with a value of $p < 0.2$ were further analysed using multivariate stepwise logistic regression where variables were entered sequentially into the model, and the model with the best fit controlling for confounding variables was selected.

Results

The final sample consisted of 398 adolescents (mean age $= 17.5 \pm 1.4$ years) of whom 203 (51%) were males. Majority of the sample were students (n = 316, 79.4%) who lived with both biological parents (n = 299, 75.1%) and had married parents (n = 309, 77.6%). The most common primary diagnosis was depressive disorders (n = 106, 26.6%), followed by adjustment disorders (n = 104, 26.1%) and anxiety disorders (n = 96, 24.1%). 98 adolescents (24.6%) had at least one first degree relative with a psychiatric disorder. About one-fifth of the sample reported current or past history of smoking behaviour (n = 77, 19.3%) and alcohol use (n = 89, 22.4%). Selected demographic and clinical characteristics of the study sample can be found in Table 1. 23.1% (n = 92) of the sample engaged in at least one type of DSH. The most common type of DSH reported was cutting (n = 78), followed by hitting or punching (n = 8), scratching (n = 1) and multiple methods (n = 5; see Table 1).

Females were significantly (about threefold) more likely than males to engage in DSH, χ^2 (1, n = 393) = 28.3, $p = 0.00$, $\varphi = 0.274$. More females (n = 63) compared to males engaged in cutting (n = 15). Those who engaged in hitting or punching were all males (n = 8).

Among adolescents with DSH, 73.9% were female, 44.6% had a depressive disorder as their primary

Table 1 Sample demographic and clinical characteristics

Characteristic	N (%)
Age (years old)	
13–16	89 (22.5)
17–19	309 (77.7)
Gender	
Male	203 (51)
Female	195 (49)
Employment status	
Student	316 (79.4)
Employed	60 (15.1)
Not working or studying	22 (5.5)
Living arrangements	
Both biological parents	299 (75.1)
Single biological parent	63 (15.8)
Blended families	17 (4.3)
Other biological relatives	10 (2.5)
Others (e.g., student hostel)	9 (2.3)
Parental marital status	
Married	309 (77.6)
Divorced or unmarried or separated	73 (18.3)
Deceased	16 (4.0)
Main diagnosis	
Depressive disorders	106 (26.6)
Adjustment disorders	104 (26.1)
Anxiety disorders	96 (24.1)
Eating disorders	12 (3.0)
Neurodevelopmental disorders	20 (5.0)
Conduct disorders	9 (2.3)
Psychotic disorders	7 (1.8)
Substance disorders	3 (0.8)
No mental illness	25 (6.3)
Family history of psychiatric illness	
At least one first degree relative	98 (24.6)
Other relatives	43 (10.8)
Current or past history	
Smoking	77 (19.3)
Alcohol	89 (22.4)
Physical or sexual abuse	26 (6.6)
Forensic	18 (4.6)
Type of deliberate self-harm	
Cutting	78 (19.8)
Hitting or punching	8 (2)
Scratching	1 (0.3)
Multiple methods	5 (1.3)

diagnosis, 41.3% had a current or past history of alcohol use, 33.7% had a current or past history of smoking, and 32.6% had a positive family history of psychiatric illness. Most patients with DSH lived with their biological

Table 2 Risk factors of adolescent psychiatric outpatients with and without DSH

Factor	N (%)		p-value
	With DSH (n = 92)	Without DSH (n = 301)	
Female gender	68 (73.9)	125 (41.5)	< 0.001
Depressive disorders	41 (44.6)	65 (21.6)	< 0.001
Anxiety disorders	15 (16.3)	81 (26.9)	0.053
Adjustment disorders	22 (23.9)	82 (27.2)	0.618
Eating disorders	0 (0)	11 (3.7)	0.134
Neurodevelopmental disorders	1 (1.1)	19 (6.3)	0.085
Psychotic disorders	0 (0)	7 (2.3)	0.305
Conduct disorders	2 (2.2)	6 (2.0)	1.000
Substance disorders	1 (1.1)	1 (0.3)	0.958
Alcohol use	38 (41.3)	50 (16.6)	< 0.001
Smoking	31 (33.7)	44 (14.6)	< 0.001
Family history of psychiatric illness	30 (32.6)	109 (36.2)	0.614
Married parents	68 (73.9)	237 (78.7)	0.407
Living with both biological parents	66 (71.7)	229 (76.1)	0.481
Past abuse	11 (12.0)	15 (5.0)	0.029
Forensic history	8 (8.7)	10 (3.3)	0.061

parents (71.7%) and 12% had a past or current history of physical or sexual abuse. Table 2 compares the risk factors of adolescents presenting with and without DSH. DSH was found to be significantly associated with female gender, depressive disorders, alcohol use, smoking and past abuse. These five variables were then further analyzed using stepwise logistic regression, where variables were entered sequentially into the model, and Table 3 illustrates the model with the best fit controlling for confounding variables.

DSH was significantly associated with female gender (odds ratio [OR] 5.03), depressive disorders (OR 2.45), alcohol use (OR 3.49) and forensic history (OR 3.66), but not with smoking behaviour, living arrangements, parental marital status, family history of psychiatric illness or history of abuse (Table 3).

Table 3 Multivariate regression analyses of risk factors associated with DSH

Variable	OR (95% CI)	p-value
Female gender	5.03 (2.772–9.130)	0.000
Depressive disorders	2.45 (1.429–4.187)	0.001
Alcohol use	3.49 (1.933–6.305)	0.000
Forensic history	3.66 (1.164–11.527)	0.026

Discussion

DSH is harmful to the body and can result in unintentional death. Adolescents who engage in DSH represent a vulnerable and high-risk population. The main goal of this study was to examine the prevalence, nature and associated risk factors of DSH among Singaporean adolescents in an outpatient setting. This will improve our understanding of the population attending psychiatric services for young people, identify at-risk groups for DSH and design targeted interventions for DSH and its associated risk factors.

The prevalence of DSH in this study (23.1%) was similar to an earlier study in Singapore [18]. The consistency in this finding, in addition to the sizeable number of patients involved and the equal gender proportion in the current sample, contributes to the accuracy in estimating prevalence. Given that DSH can sometimes be a secretive act, the consistency in prevalence across time suggests that DSH continues to be a significant feature of adolescents presenting with psychiatric symptoms.

The prevalence of DSH in this study was lower than that generally reported in Western clinical samples [7], although there were similarities in the nature of presentation and some associated factors. This may be unsurprising given the growing impact of the internet on globalization and exposure to Western media, which may facilitate the gradual homogenizing of how mental illnesses and coping behaviours such as DSH manifest worldwide [26].

Consistent with previous research on gender differences in DSH in both Western [6, 12, 14–17] and Asian studies [22–24], female adolescents in this study were about three times more likely to engage in DSH than males. These gender patterns have been suggested to reflect the higher rates of depression and anxiety in females as well as the differential ways in which males and females respond to emotional distress [21]. Males have been known to have a greater risk-taking propensity and tend to engage in more externalizing coping methods, whereas females tend to engage in more internalizing coping methods. Findings also mirror prior research on the associations between DSH and depression, alcohol use and delinquent behaviours [4, 9, 13, 22, 24]. Alcohol use and delinquent behaviours may be associated with disinhibition and recklessness, which may lead to increased DSH. Heavy alcohol use and depression have also been significantly associated with DSH among Hong Kong adolescents [24] and it has been suggested that alcohol use may independently increase DSH, or depression may drive adolescents to self-medicate using alcohol. Although DSH was positively associated with a forensic history in this study, more research on this association

is needed as the number in this study was small; only 8 patients with DSH had a forensic history.

DSH was not significantly associated with poor family structure (i.e., not living with both biological parents and not having married parents), positive family history of psychiatric disorder and history of abuse, despite these factors being commonly associated with depression and DSH [4, 8]. However, because the current sample was comprised mostly of adolescents who were in school, not smoking, living with both biological parents who were married, had no positive family history of psychiatric disorder, and had no history of drug use and physical or sexual abuse, it is possible that DSH, as a symptom, may be associated with different risk factors when investigated within different socio-demographic profiles. Singaporean adolescents who engaged in DSH have been found to have higher perceived invalidating home environment, despite being from intact families [27]. This finding suggests the need for further research on how the quality of family relationships, rather than the type of family structure, may be implicated in the development of DSH in Singaporean adolescents. Further, the lack of association between DSH and a positive family history of psychiatric disorder may also be attributed to the lack of accurate report from the adolescent patient. Because of the stigma and common misperceptions towards mental illness in Singapore, many individuals cope by withholding information to avoid discrimination [28]; this may mask the presence of mental illness in some families. Future studies would benefit from the use of more sensitive indicators to investigate DSH and its associations with social and familial stressors and supports.

The positive associations between DSH and female gender, depressive disorders, alcohol use and delinquent behaviours suggest that it may be helpful to refine interventions in order to target these factors. For example, developing group therapy programs tailored for adolescent females, including formal screening tools for depressive disorders in patients presenting with DSH as well as addressing alcohol use and delinquent behaviours which may at times be overlooked during discussions about DSH. Because under-aged alcohol use and delinquent behaviours are often socially influenced, consistent social supports provided via individual and family psychoeducation, case management, psychotherapy groups and a supportive familial environment are important in managing these behaviours.

Several limitations warrant consideration. The cross-sectional design of this study precludes causal conclusions. Future prospective longitudinal studies with data on DSH among Singaporean adolescents are needed. Further, because data from this study were drawn from specialist outpatient clinics, the generalizability of our findings to community or primary care settings may be limited.

Conclusions

This study adds to our understanding of the phenomenon of DSH behaviours among Singaporean adolescents. Continued research is needed to expand our understanding of DSH and its associated risk factors and to refine interventions to include the most feasible, culturally-sensitive and cost-effective treatment targets on group and individual levels. In particular, clinicians should not only aim to analyze and modify the antecedents or circumstance around which DSH occurs for the adolescent, but also look to minimize associated risk factors such as low mood, alcohol intake and delinquent behaviours. Furthermore, DSH has been increasingly described within the scientific literature since the 1970s, it would be interesting to see whether and how changes in the affected population and associated factors over time may impact on the meanings, motivations and manifestation of DSH presenting in adolescents.

Abbreviations
DSH: deliberate self-harm; OR: odds ratio.

Authors' contributions
ML conducted statistical analyses, literature review and drafted the manuscript. CL and AA provided feedback and revisions on the literature review and manuscript and facilitated data collection and analyses. All authors read and approved the final manuscript.

Acknowledgements
Not applicable.

Competing interests
All authors declare that they have no competing interests.

Funding
No funding was obtained for this study.

References
1. Pattison EM, Kahan J. The deliberate self-harm syndrome. Am J Psychiatry. 1983;140(7):867–72.
2. Nock MK. Self-injury. Annu Rev Clin Psychol. 2010;6:339–63.
3. Klonsky ED. The functions of deliberate self-harm: a review of the evidence. Clin Psychol Rev. 2007;27:226–39.
4. Klonsky ED, Muehlenkamp JJ, Lewis SP, Walsh B. Non-suicidal self-injury. Cambridge: Hogrefe Publishing; 2011.
5. Muehlenkamp JJ, Claes L, Havertape L, Plener PL. International prevalence of adolescent non-suicidal self-injury and deliberate self-harm. Child Adolesc Psychiat Ment Health. 2012;6(1):10.
6. Brunner R, Kaess M, Parzer P, Fischer G, Carli V, Hoven CW, et al. Life-time prevalence and psychosocial correlates of adolescent direct self-injurious behaviour: a comparative study of findings in 11 European countries. J Child Psychol Psychiatry. 2014;55:337–48.
7. Adrian M, Zeman J, Erdley C, Lisa L, Sim L. Emotional dysregulation and interpersonal difficulties as risk factors for non-suicidal self-injury in adolescent girls. J Abnorm Psych. 2011;39:389–400.
8. Skegg K. Self-harm. Lancet. 2005;366:1471–83.
9. Jacobson CM, Muehlenkamp JJ, Miller AL, Turner JB. Psychiatric impairment among adolescents engaging in different types of deliberate self-harm. J Clin Child Adolesc Psychol. 2008;37:363–75.
10. Lewis SP, Heath NL. Non-suicidal self-injury among youth. J Pediatr. 2015;3(166):526–30.
11. Nock M, Joiner TE, Gorden KH, Lloyd-Richardson E, Prinstein MJ. Non-suicidal self-injury among adolescents: diagnostic correlates and relation to suicide attempts. Psychiatry Res. 2006;144:65–72.
12. Kidger J, Heron J, Lewis G, Evans J, Gunnell D. Adolescent self-harm and suicidal thoughts in the ALSPAC cohort: a self-report survey in England. BMC Psychiatry. 2012;12:69.
13. Asbridge M, Azagba S, Langille DB, Rasic D. Elevated depressive symptoms and adolescent injury: examining associations by injury frequency, injury type, and gender. BMC Public Health. 2014;14(1):190.
14. Madge N, Hewitt A, Hawton K, de Wilde EJ, Corcoran P, Fekete S, van Heeringen K, De Leo D, Ystgaard M. Deliberate self-harm within an international community sample of young people: comparative findings from the Child and Adolescent Self-Harm in Europe (CASE) study. J Child Psychol Psychiatry. 2008;49(6):667–77.
15. O'Connor RC, Rasmussen S, Miles J, Hawton K. Self-harm in adolescents: self-report survey in schools in Scotland. Br J Psychiatry. 2009;194:68–72.
16. Plener PL, Libal G, Keller F, Fegert JM, Muehlenkamp JJ. An international comparison of adolescent non-suicidal self-injury and suicide attempts: Germany and the USA. Psychol Med. 2009;39:1549–58.
17. Giletta M, Scholte RH, Engels RC, Ciairano S, Prinstein MJ. Adolescent non-suicidal self-injury: a cross-national study of community samples from Italy, the Netherlands and the United States. Psychiatry Res. 2012;197:66–72.
18. Loh C, Teo YW, Lim L. Deliberate self-harm in adolescent psychiatric outpatients in Singapore: prevalence and associated risk factors. Singapore Med J. 2013;54(9):491–5.
19. Muehlenkamp JJ, Gutierrez PM. An investigation of differences between self-injurious behaviour and suicide attempts in a sample of adolescents. Suicide Life Threat Behav. 2004;34(1):12–23.
20. Lloyd-Richardson EE, Perrine N, Dierker L, Kelley ML. Characteristics and functions of non-suicidal self-injury in a community sample of adolescents. Psychol Med. 2007;37:1183–92.
21. Hilt LM, Nock MK, Lloyd-Richardson EE, Prinstein MJ. Longitudinal study of non-suicidal self-injury among young adolescents: rates, correlates, and preliminary test of an interpersonal model. J Early Adolesc. 2008;28:455–69.
22. Watanabe N, Nishida A, Shimodera S, Inoue K, Oshima N, Sasaki T, et al. Deliberate self-harm in adolescents aged 12–18: a cross-sectional survey of 18,104 students. Suicide Life Threat Behav. 2012;42(5):550–60.
23. Shek DTL, Lu Y. Self-harm and suicidal behaviours in Hong Kong adolescents: prevalence and psychosocial correlates. Sci World J. 2012;2012:1–14.
24. Cheung YT, Wong PW, Lee AM, Lam TH, Fan YS, Yip PS. Non-suicidal self-injury and suicidal behaviours: prevalence, co-occurrence and correlates of suicide among adolescents in Hong Kong. J Affect Disord. 2012;48:1133–44.
25. American Psychiatric Association. Diagnostic and statistical manual of mental disorders: DSM-IV-TR. Washington, DC: American Psychiatric Association; 2000.
26. Watters E. Crazy like us: the globalization of the American psyche. New York: Free Press; 2010.
27. Tan A, Rehfuss M, Suarez E, Parks-Savage A. Nonsuicidal self-injury in an adolescent population in Singapore. Clin Child Psychol Psychiatry. 2014;19(1):58–76.
28. Lim L, Goh J, Chan YH. Stigma and non-disclosure in psychiatric patients from a Southeast Asian hospital. Open J Psychiatry. 2018;8:80–90.

19

Childhood ADHD and treatment outcome: the role of maternal functioning

Pernille Darling Rasmussen[1,2,3,7*] [iD], Ole Jakob Storebø[1,2,4], Yael Shmueli-Goetz[6], Anders Bo Bojesen[3], Erik Simonsen[2,5] and Niels Bilenberg[3]

Abstract

Background: Relatively little is known about the role of maternal functioning in terms of attention deficit hyperactivity disorder (ADHD) symptoms, attachment style and resilience as predictive factors for treatment outcome when offspring are diagnosed with ADHD.

Objective: To investigate whether maternal functioning is associated with treatment outcome in children with ADHD.

Methods: The study formed part of a larger naturalistic observational study of children with ADHD. A battery of self-report measures was used to assess selected factors in maternal functioning at the point of referral (baseline data); adult ADHD-symptoms, adult attachment style and adult resilience. Associations between these domains and child treatment response were subsequently examined in a 1-year follow up.

Results: Maternal ADHD-symptoms and degree of resilience were significantly correlated to symptom reduction in offspring diagnosed with ADHD. However, the association between maternal attachment style and child treatment response as measured by the ADHD-RS did not reach statistical significance.

Conclusion: To our knowledge, this is the first study to consider potential protective factors along with risk factors in maternal functioning and the impact on child treatment outcome. The study contributes to our knowledge of the potential role of maternal functioning in treatment outcome for children with ADHD.

Keywords: ADHD, Attachment, Resilience, Maternal functioning, Developmental outcome

Background

Attention deficit hyperactivity disorder (ADHD) is the most commonly occurring neurodevelopmental disorder in childhood with a prevalence ranging from 3 to 5% and symptoms often continuing into adulthood [1]. It is characterized by a number of core symptoms including inattention, hyperactivity and impulsivity [2]. Both the DSM-5 and ICD-10 criteria require excessive inattention, hyperactivity, and impulsivity to be inconsistent with the developmental level and to be pervasive [3, 4]. According to the DSM-5 three presentations of ADHD, differentiated on the basis of symptom load, are commonly referred to: combined-type, inattentive-type and hyperactive/impulsive-type. For a formal diagnosis, the symptoms have to be present for at least 6 months and result in impairment in more than one setting before the age of 6 (ICD-10) or 12 (DSM-5) (WHO 1992, [4]).

Maternal ADHD, attachment style, and resilience

The etiology of ADHD is multifactorial, as both genetic and environmental factors have been evidenced in the development of ADHD [5, 6]. For example, a relative with ADHD [7], an increase in Copy Number Variation (CNV, [8]), prematurity [9] and some form of neglect (Thapar et al. 2012) have all been implicated. Moreover, numerous studies have found ADHD to be associated with a poor prognosis (e.g. more divorces, higher rates of substance abuse disorders in adulthood, and increased mortality rate) [11–13]. Furthermore, the prognosis of ADHD worsens in the presence of comorbidity [11, 14].

*Correspondence: pdra@regionsjaelland.dk
[7] Ny Østergade 12, 4000 Roskilde, Denmark
Full list of author information is available at the end of the article

Parent and child ADHD are found to be significantly associated, as well as parent and child conduct problems [15]. However, factors associated with the developmental progression and the long-term prognosis of ADHD are not fully understood [15–17] and hence, a greater focus on the developmental progression of ADHD is required. Whereas studies converge in proposing that parental psychopathology poses a high risk of transmission to offspring, relatively little is known about the role of maternal functioning in terms of attention deficit hyperactivity disorder (ADHD) symptoms, attachment style and resilience as predictive factors for treatment outcome when offspring are diagnosed with ADHD.

Maternal ADHD may be a potential risk factor in the development of offspring ADHD [18–21]. Moreover, in a recent study on associations between parental psychiatric disorders and offspring ADHD, maternal diagnosis showed stronger associations with child ADHD than paternal diagnosis [22]. Despite research establishing a link specifically between parental ADHD and parenting, measured as the level of home chaos, and parenting practices assessed through self-reports [23], to date there have been no studies investigating the role of maternal ADHD symptomatology as a prognostic factor in offspring treatment outcome.

In addition to the contribution of maternal ADHD symptoms to the increased risk of offspring developing ADHD, the quality of the mother–child relationship has also come under scrutiny. Indeed, both ADHD and attachment have been proposed as risk factors [24]. Reviewing the literature on ADHD and attachment, we found a clear association between ADHD and insecure attachment. When one condition was present, this increased the risk of developing the other. This underlines that ADHD and insecure attachment may constitute mutual risk factors [25]. In a recent comprehensive review of parental self-reported attachment style and caregiving, adult attachment security was consistently associated with more positive parenting whereas insecurity was related to more negative parenting [26]. These findings underscore the importance of investigating maternal ADHD-symptoms and attachment style as part of a broad assessment of maternal functioning. Alongside the contribution of adult attachment to maternal functioning, a growing body of research suggests that resilience is also a key factor, with greater resilience associated with psychological adaptation and functioning in the face of adversity [27–29]. Broadly, resilience theory focuses on understanding healthy development in the face of risk, and on strengths as opposed to weaknesses. It has been defined as a "pattern of positive adaptation in the context of past or present adversity" [30]. Critically, resilience does not suggest the absence of adversity or risk, but rather highlights the presence of protective processes leading to healthy adaptation. Whilst definitions and measurement of resilience vary considerably from study to study and the scientific value of the concept generally has been debated and challenged [31] resilience has been found to influence treatment response across different manifestations of adversity. These include chronic illness, psychiatric disorders and school bullying [32, 33].

In this study, the focus is on the significance of maternal resilience for parenting in situations where the child needs extra support.

The current study

The aim of the present study was to examine associations between mothers' functioning and treatment response in their children diagnosed with ADHD who are receiving care as usual.

We hypothesized that maternal self-reported ADHD symptoms; self-reported attachment style and maternal resilience would all be significantly correlated with treatment outcome. More specifically, we anticipated the following; (1) higher maternal ADHD-symptom scores would be associated with lower ADHD symptom reduction in offspring within the first year of treatment. (2) Higher scores for self-reported anxiety or ambivalence on the attachment style questionnaire are associated with lesser symptom reduction in offspring. (3) A higher degree of self-reported maternal resilience is associated with better treatment response in offspring diagnosed with ADHD.

Methods

The current study was part of a naturalistic observational study exploring different aspects of maternal functioning expected to influence treatment response in children diagnosed with ADHD.

Participants

The families participating were recruited from two child psychiatric outpatient clinics in Region Zealand, Denmark. The four interviewers participating were the same at the two sites; two conducting maternal attachment interviews and two conducting child attachment interviews. Sixty-seven (N = 67) child-mother dyads were included in the follow up.

Of the 67 mothers, 64 (95.5%) provided adequate responses on the baseline questionnaires to include for analysis. Three dyads were excluded from the analysis as they had not responded to all the questions. Age, gender distribution and the diagnoses of the children, along with other sample characteristics of parents and children can be seen in Table 1a and b. The mean age was 9.1 years, with children ranging in age from 7 to 12 years. A large

Table 1 (a) Child characteristics, (b) family characteristics

	n	%
a		
Gender		
Male	46	71.88
Female	18	28.13
Age at baseline—mean (SD) = 9.1 (1.3)		
ADHD subtype		
Combined type	50	78.1
Inattentive type	14	21.9
Comorbidity		
None	51	79.7
Oppositional defiance disorder	5	7.8
Autism spectrum	4	6.3
Other	4	6.3
b		
Parent job status		
Unemployed	15	23.4
Employed or student	42	65.6
No information	7	10.9
Household type		
Nuclear family	30	46.9
Split family	34	53.1
Psychiatric history		
No	9	14.1
Yes	54	84.4
No information	1	1.6

proportion of the children came from one-parent households (53%) with the rest living together with both biological parents. Fifty-four (84.4%) responders reported a history of psychiatric illness in parents, siblings or grandparents. The children received *Care as usual* according to national guidelines [34]. At 3 months follow up, 43.8% of the children received medical treatment increasing to 70.3% at 6 months follow up, and 71.9% at 9 and 73.4% 12 months follow up. There were no reports of children dropping out of treatment during the 1-year follow up.

Measures
Maternal measures
Resilience in Adults Scale (RSA; [35, 36])
Maternal resilience was measured by the Resilience in Adults Scale (RSA)—a 33-item self-report scale for measuring resilience in adults. The scale covers six dimensions assessing protective factors at the personal level as well as at a family and a social level. The RSA is based on a seven point semantic differential scale with a positive attribute at the high end of the scale and a negative attribute at the low end of the scale. An example of a positive attribute in Personal Competence is "I know if I continue, I will

succeed". Half of the items are reversed to reduce acquiescence biases. The maximum score achievable is 231 (high resiliency) and the lowest possible score is 33. The scale has been found reliable for distinguishing clinical samples versus the normal population [37–39].

The Adult ADHD Self-Report Scale (ASRS 1.1; [40])
Maternal ADHD symptoms were measured using the Adult ADHD Self-Report Scale (ASRS 1.1, short version of 6 items, two dimensions). The ASRS 1.1 is a 6-item screening version of a longer 18-item scale. It is used to assess ADHD symptoms in the previous 6 months and includes four items on inattention and two on hyperactivity. Symptoms are rated on a 5-point response scale (never—scored 0, rarely—1, sometimes—2, often—3, and very often—4). The total score ranges from 0 to 24. In a convenience subsample of subscribers to a large health plan in the US, the ASRS Screener was administered twice to assess test–retest reliability and then a third time together with a clinical interviewer. The ASRS Screener was found to be in high concordance with clinician diagnoses. Internal consistency reliability was in the 0.63–0.72 range and test–retest reliability (Pearson correlations) in the 0.58–0.77 range [41].

Experiences in Close Relationships Scale—Revised (ECR-R; [42])
Maternal attachment style was measured using the Experiences in Close Relationships Scale—Revised (ECR-R)—36 items in total, 18 items assessing romantic attachment anxiety (model of self) and 18 items assessing romantic attachment avoidance (model of others). The questionnaire is a widely used self-report measure of adult romantic attachment and is based on the theoretical assumption that anxiety and avoidance are the two fundamental dimensions underlying attachment. Items are rated on a 7-point Likert scale ranging from 0 (*strongly disagree*) to 6 (*strongly agree*). In a study by Sibley and colleagues psychometric properties (i.e., the test–retest reliability, convergent, and discriminant validity) of the ECR-R were investigated and documented [43]. For the current study, participating parents were instructed to include previous and current relationship experiences when answering the questions.

Child measures
K-SADS-PL; [44, 45]
The children were screened using the Schedule for Affective Disorders and Schizophrenia for School-aged Children, Present and Lifetime Version (K-Sad-PL).

The interview is a valid and widely established diagnostic measure and it allows clinicians to classify children and adolescents with respect to their psychiatric diagnoses according to DSM-IV systems. In a recent study, the convergent and divergent validity of two diagnostic groups, anxiety disorders and ADHD was investigated. It was concluded that the K-SADS-PL generates valid diagnoses of anxiety and ADHD including the predominately inattentive subtype [46].

ADHD-rating scale (ADHD-RS; [47])

Child ADHD symptoms were measured using the revised ADHD-RS [48, 49] (translated into Danish and validated) to assess the severity of ADHD symptoms in children aged 4–17 years. It consists of 26 items loading on to attention deficit, hyperactivity/impulsivity and behavioral problems. Each item is rated from 0, denoting never/rarely, to 3, denoting very often. The total score ranges from 0 to 78. The schedule can be administered by teachers and parents and has been found to be valid and reliable when measuring symptom load in a clinical population [47, 50].

Procedure

Initial identification was based on referral diagnosis based on ICD-10 (ADHD: combined-type, inattentive-type and hyperactive/impulsive-type) followed by a clinical evaluation in order to establish whether the family met the inclusion criteria.

In order to lower the risk of selection bias, we applied consecutive recruitment, as all the families with children in the appropriate age range presenting the relevant referral diagnosis, were invited to participate.

The data obtained through questionnaires and interviews in the two-stage inclusion process and a 1-year follow up period were analysed using structural equation modeling and mixed effects modeling for repeated measures (Fig. 1).

During the recruitment phase, 203 children were referred with a possible diagnosis of ADHD. Only children in the age range of 7–12 representing middle childhood were subsequently invited to participate in the study. Exclusion criteria further included children who were adopted or living in foster care and children with major handicaps, such as hearing impairment or learning disabilities, preventing them from participating in and completing the interviews. Children who during the inclusion procedure were suspected of psychosis or who had an IQ below 70 were excluded.

Those who met the above criteria were invited to participate and were given further information about the study in a telephone call by the 1st author. The second stage of inclusion involved a formal assessment of ADHD diagnosis, using the Schedule for Affective Disorders and Schizophrenia for School-aged Children, Present and Lifetime Version (K-Sad-PL) [44, 45].

Only patients assigned an ADHD/ADD diagnosis according to DSM-V with ADHD (314.01) or ADD (314.00) in step two were included for follow up. The included families attended both a clinical and a research track separated from each other (Fig. 2).

Apart from exchanging information on treatment initiation, child IQ and in the event of drop out from medical treatment, the research project was separated from the clinical track.

Care as usual

The children included all received *care as usual* consisting of standard medical treatment with methylphenidate as first choice for moderate and severe ADHD. The interventions were standardized and formalized according to national guidelines [34].

In Denmark, clinical guidelines adhere to recommendations from NICE-guidelines [51]. Recommendations are divided into three age groups; pre-school children, school-age children and young people with ADHD and moderate impairment and school-age children and young people with severe ADHD and severe impairment. For the school-aged children/moderate impairment, group-based parent-training/education programs are recommended as first-line treatment. Drug therapy is recommended only for those with "severe symptoms and impairment or for those with moderate levels of impairment who have refused non-drug interventions, or whose symptoms have not responded sufficiently to parent-training/education programs". When the child has severe ADHD/impairment, medical treatment is recommended as the first line. All the participating children in this study were school-aged children. The research project was not involved in choosing treatment, but was informed from the clinical track that no families received additional treatment initiatives than that described in the standard program. The compliance rate was excellent, as there was no reports of dropout from treatment during the 12 months of follow up.

Baseline screening of parents

Mothers were asked to complete questionnaires regarding themselves. The questionnaires screened for ADHD symptoms using the ASRS 1.1, assessed attachment styles as relating to current romantic relationships using the ECR, and measured the degree of resilience using the RSA. All questionnaires were sent as links by e-mail from the online data managing system Easytrial.

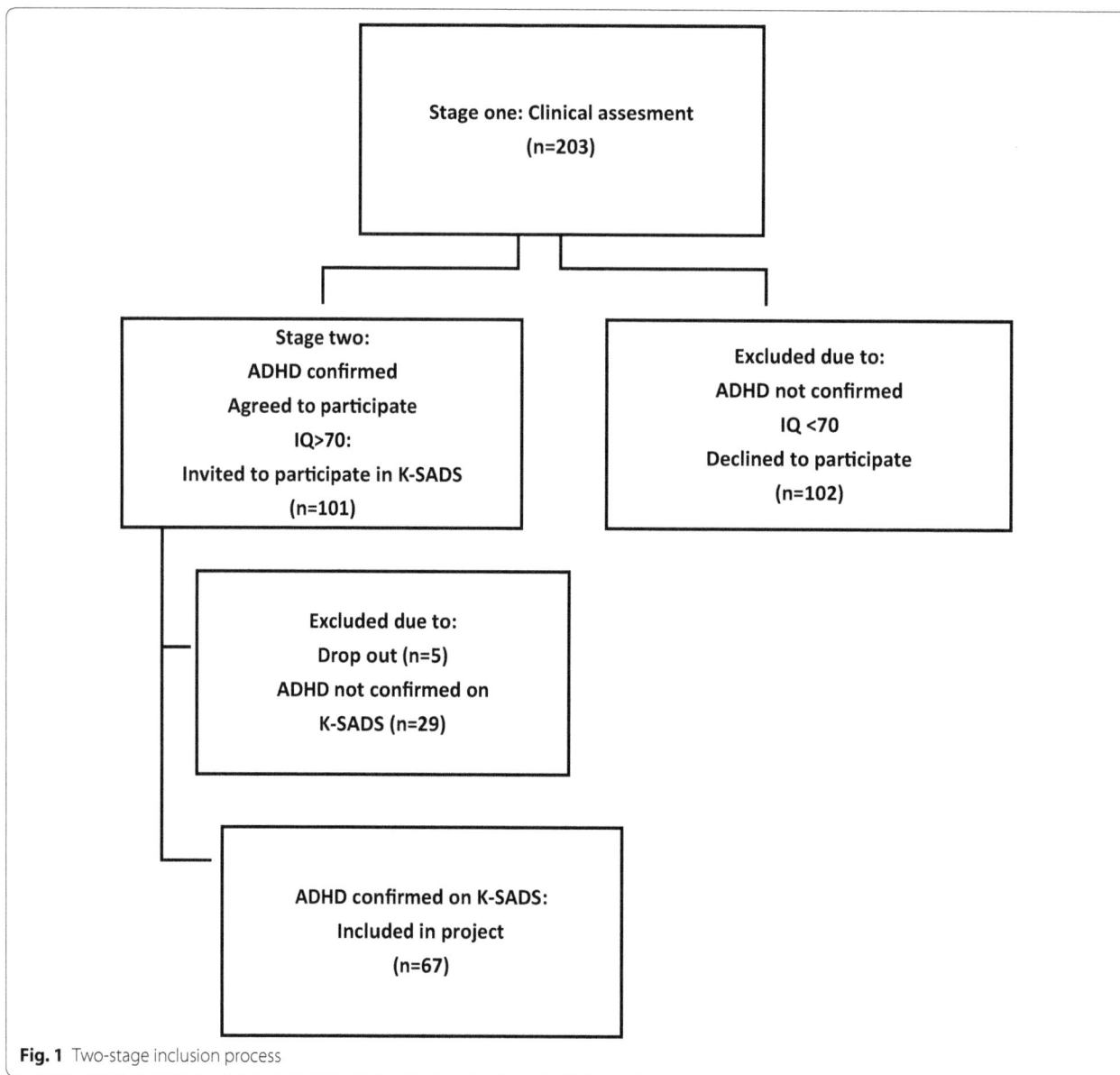

Fig. 1 Two-stage inclusion process

Easytrial ©

In order to obtain a high response rate in the follow-up period, we used the Easytrial© online clinical data management system. All questionnaires from the baseline procedure as well as the follow up sequence were sent out as links to the parents by e-mail. The system provided an opportunity to monitor non-responders and send out 'gentle reminders'. Responses were collected directly in a secured database compliant with good clinical practice (GCP) and database security legislation.

Follow up

The families progressed to the follow up 3 months after the initial assessment (Fig. 3).

This delay was to ensure that the assigned treatment had been initiated. The attachment assessment was conducted at the child psychiatric clinics by four trained interviewers. The interviewers were not involved in treatment and had no prior knowledge of the families. The two interviewers of the mothers were blinded to results of the child assessment and vice versa.

The follow up consisted of four ADHD-symptom screenings completed every third month within the first year of inclusion. The ADHD-RS was sent to the parents

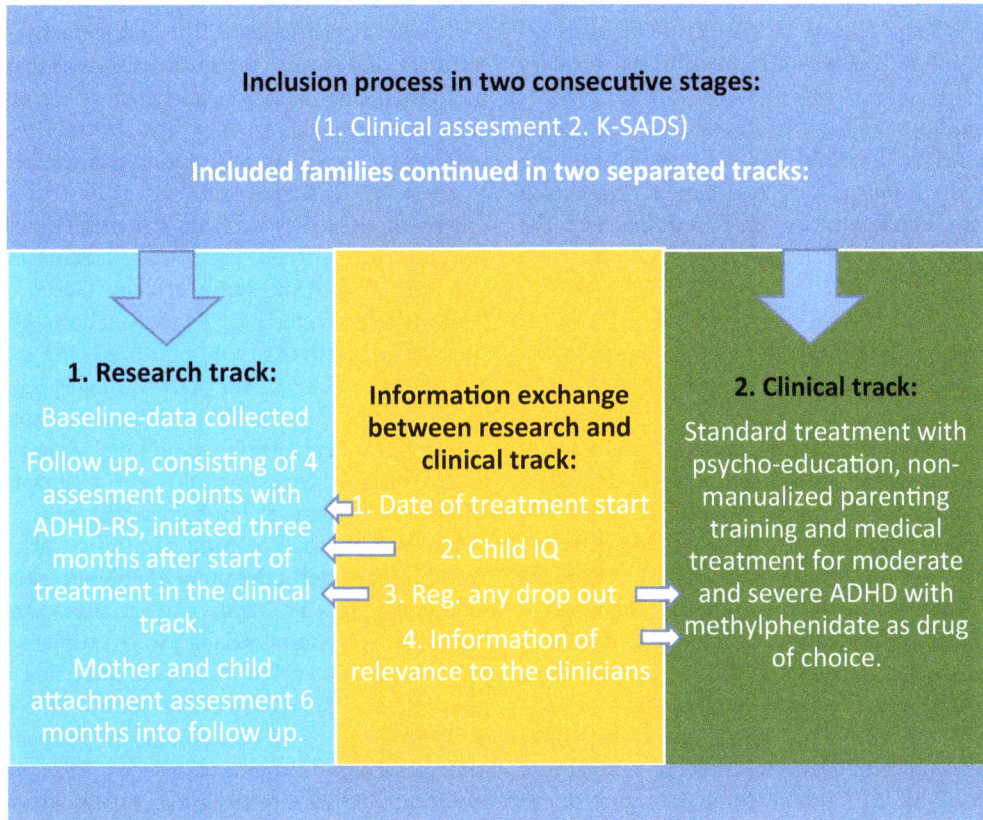

Fig. 2 Overview of clinical and research track

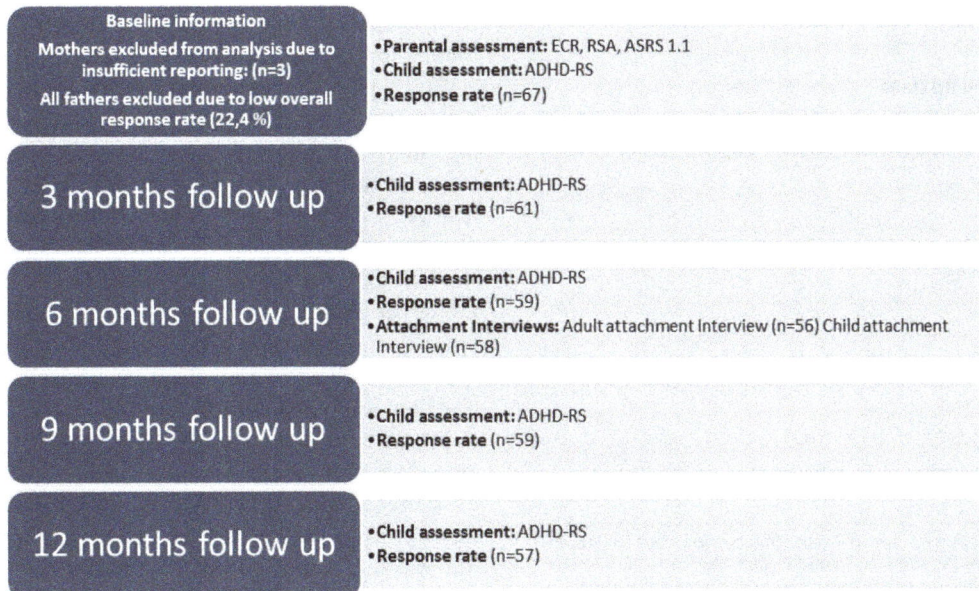

Fig. 3 Details of research track during follow up

for assessment of ADHD-symptom load in their children. The observed change (slope) in ADHD-RS from baseline to the 12 month follow up represents the primary outcome".

In one-parent households, the schedule was sent to the household in which the child was residing. More than half (53%) of the families were one-parent households and only in one family was the child residing with the father.

Data analysis

Treatment response was measured as the change in the ADHD-RS scale over the course of the 12 months of follow up. The change was calculated as the best fitting linear slope for each patient with time as a predictor of ADHD-RS. Due to some missed self-reports, this slope was in some cases based on only two observations in the follow up sequence with the other three missing (baseline and four follow up ADHD-RS measurements). A random effects linear regression was used to predict the slope of ADHD-RS change for each child. This slope is used as a continuous measure of treatment response. For instances of missing baseline measurements, the baseline score was approximated by an intercept estimate based on other measurements available. Data on missed self-reports is provided in Table 2. Random intercepts and slopes were predicted using a random effects linear regression model, with repeated measures (baseline and four follow up ADHD-RS measurements) nested in patients. In a set of linear regression models, each patient's predicted slope (change in ADHD-RS) was regressed on ECR, RSA and ASRS with and without adjustment for gender, age, family type, medical treatment status, familial psychiatric

history and the number of missing data points out the five follow up measurements. This last element is included to estimate and control for any possibly association between non-attendance and treatment effect. Control variables and background variables are summarized using frequency tables, means and standard deviations.

The ECR, RSA and ASRS scores used are latent variable predictions derived from structural equation models. ECR and RSA items are modeled assuming multivariate normality. ASRS items are considered ordinal items and modeled using a logit link function. All three latent variable predictions are standardized with means at 0 and variances fixed to 1. The latent variable approach has the advantage of removing the residual (unexplained by the latent factor) variance for each item when predicting the latent variable. Measurement error associated with psychometric scales is minimized in this way.

Because of some missing data on covariates, we used a full information maximum likelihood estimator implemented in Stata 14. Means and variances as well as covariance for exogenous variables were estimated and used as the basis for corrected regression estimates. Missing data due to non-attendance at the follow up measurements were assumed to be random, i.e. not associated with the unobserved outcome measurement. This assumption was substantiated by a missing data analysis showing no significant association between baseline ADHD-RS score and missing data ($RR = 1.02$, $p = 0.47$) and between the ADHD-RS score preceding (t_{-1}) a missing data incident ($RR = 1.01$, $p = 0.66$). Mixed effects Poisson models were used for the missing data analysis.

Results

In the follow up sequence, 92.2% ($N = 59$) had a maximum of one missed self-report.

Whilst all fathers were invited to participate and all consented to do so, only a minority actually completed the questionnaires (22.4%). Consequently, the paternal response rate was too low to include for further analysis. Complete information from all planned assessments was obtained for 62.5% ($N = 40$) of the children. Two children were only measured twice from baseline to the 12 month follow up. Table 2 presents the descriptive results, including means, standard deviations and number of observations for ECR, RSA and ASRS as well as ADHD-RS at baseline, follow up and the overall ADHD-RS reduction as predicted in a random effects regression. Correlations are provided in Additional file 1: Table S1. ADHD-RS was on average reduced by 12.15 points as predicted in the random effects regression. The mean ADHD-RS at baseline was 43.1 and reduced to 30.25 one year after initiating treatment.

Table 2 Follow up data

	Mean	SD	n
Child measurements			
ADHD-RS reduction	− 12.15	6.46	64
ADHD-RS baseline	43.11	12.53	53
ADHD-RS 3 months	37.36	12.24	61
ADHD-RS 6 months	34.56	13.33	59
ADHD-RS 9 months	31.31	13.45	59
ADHD-RS 12 months	30.25	14.44	57
Parent measurements			
ASRS 1.1	28.05	14.57	59
RSA	146.07	31.12	57
ECR	166.75	40.11	56

The ADHD-RS reduction is a linear prediction from a mixed effects model. This a reflection of the observed average reduction from baseline to the 12 months follow up but allowing for missing data points caused by non-attendance

ADHD-RS ADHD-Rating Scale, ASRS 1.1 Adult ADHD Self-Report Scale, RSA Resilience Scale for Adults, ECR Experiences in Close Relationships

Predicting ADHD-RS reductions

The following demographic variables were included in the analysis: gender, age, family history of mental illness and whether the child is living in a one or two parent household. A binary indicator of medical treatment and the number of non-attendances were also included as covariates. Table 3 show regression estimates for the association between maternal ECR, RSA, ASRS and the change in child ADHD-RS over the 12 months of follow up. Adjusted and unadjusted results are shown. The negative association between RSA and the outcome (b = − 1.76; 95% CI − 3.45, − 0.07) suggests that a higher degree of maternal resilience is associated with larger reductions in child ADHD-RS during treatment. The significant association between maternal ASRS and child ADHD-RS (b = 3.48; 95% CI 1.76,5.20) suggests that children of mothers scoring higher on ADHD symptoms achieved a more modest treatment effect than children of mothers scoring lower on ADHD symptoms. There was no significant association between maternal ECR and the change in child ADHD-RS. The coefficients correspond to the predicted absolute change in ADHD-RS from baseline to 12 months follow up when ECR, RSA or ASRS increase by one standard deviation.

Discussion

The current study was undertaken with the broad aim of attempting to shed further light on the role of maternal functioning in the treatment response of children diagnosed with ADHD. Informed by the literature and existing empirical findings we chose to evaluate three domains of potential importance in maternal

functioning: self-reported ADHD symptoms, self-reported attachment style and degree of resilience. A sample of sixty-seven mother–child dyads with ADHD-diagnosed children was recruited. The children and families received care as usual, and treatment response was evaluated in terms of ADHD symptom-load measured at 3 monthly intervals over a 1-year period. We anticipated that all three maternal functioning factors would correlate with treatment response, independent of treatment strategy.

The findings suggested a significant association between maternal self-reported ADHD symptoms and treatment outcome, measured by a reduction in children's reported ADHD symptoms. Thus, mothers scoring high on ADHD symptoms had children who showed a lower reduction in ADHD symptoms at the 12 months' follow up.

Contrary to expectations, we found no significant correlation between maternal self-reported attachment style on the ECR and child outcome on the ADHD-RS.

Lastly and in line with our prediction, we found a negative association between maternal resilience as measured by the RSA and offspring treatment response on the ADHD-RS. This suggested that a higher degree of resilience in mothers was associated with greater symptom-reduction in their children receiving care as usual.

The correlation between maternal ADHD symptomatology and treatment outcome of children with ADHD may be increased level of conflict in the parent–child relationship and exacerbated negative parenting [52]. Harvey and colleagues found that parental ADHD symptomatology was associated with a number of factors in

Table 3 Overall ADHD-RS reduction predicted by ECR, RSA and ASRS

	Crude		Adjusted	
	b	95% CI	b	95% CI
ECR	− 1.68	[− 3.38, 0.02]	− 1.18	[− 2.91, 0.55]
RSA	− 1.98	[− 3.66, − 0.31]*	− 1.76	[− 3.45, − 0.07]*
ASRS	3.44	[1.78, 5.10]***	3.48	[1.76, 5.20]***
Control variables				
Female (ref. male)			0.30	[− 3.06, 3.66]
Age at baseline			− 0.29	[− 1.55, 0.98]
Split family (ref. nuclear)			0.09	[− 2.88,3.07]
In medical treatment (ref. not)			− 5.32	[− 8.79, − 1.84]**
Psych. disp. (no psych. Disp.)			− 1.21	[− 5.71,3.29]
Missed out follow ups			0.30	[− 1.86,2.46]

N = 64. Linear regression using full information maximum likelihood estimator. ECR, RSA and ASRS are standardized factor scores used only in separate models. Outcome is the reduction in ADHD-RS score during 12 months follow up. It is predicted in a mixed effects regression including all information available. Crude and adjusted estimates are controlled for baseline ADHD-RS

ASRS 1.1 Adult ADHD Self-Report Scale, *RSA* Resilience Scale for Adults, *ECR* Experiences in Close Relationships

* p < 0.05, ** p < 0.01, *** p < 0.001

parenting practices and quality of parent–child interactions. This is supported by the findings of a number of studies, suggesting that maternal psychiatric history is significantly associated with child symptom severity and that there is a need for parental screening and treatment programs developed specifically for families in need [53, 54].

Regarding ADHD and attachment, these have been found to constitute mutual risk factors and show extensive overlap in symptomatology, [55]. However, our results did not support a correlation between maternal attachment style and treatment outcome in offspring ADHD. Notably, the ECR assesses attachment-related thoughts and feelings in adult romantic relationships and belongs to the social psychological tradition, whereas instruments such as the Adult Attachment Interview (AAI) represent the developmental assessment tradition [56]. These alternative traditions in assessing attachment have been found to be only partly overlapping [57]. However, we have assessed the mother–child dyads using the AAI as well, and found that the AAI did not correlate with short-term treatment outcome either [58]. One explanation for this unexpected finding may be that maternal psychopathology is a more important predictor than attachment representations in offspring treatment outcome.

In terms of risk and resilience, numerous studies have documented the relationship between parental risk factors and child development. For example; association between family structure and mental wellbeing of children (rate of readmissions to hospital) were investigated and pointed to the significance of family trauma and family psychiatric history [59]. Further, in a meta-analysis of clinical samples, maternal functioning was found to be more important than factors in the child in shaping the quality of infant-mother attachment relationship [60].

Resilient child development despite adversity and how to promote resilient parenting are topics of increasing interest [61–63]. Surprisingly, however, few studies to date have investigated the potential influence of maternal resilience on treatment outcome in children with psychopathology, and specifically those diagnosed with ADHD. Our findings suggest that maternal resilience may be a significant factor in predicting how the child diagnosed with ADHD responds to treatment. In line with this, a study on parenting practices found the combination of family risk, protection and parenting practices to be highly predictive of child functioning [64]. This underlines the need to consider resources as well as risk factors.

As resilience is generally regarded as a more stable trait than psychiatric symptoms [65] it may prove to be a powerful predictor and a core maternal feature in overall prognosis in children affected by various psychiatric symptoms.

Some studies in ADHD treatment have focused on parenting training and social skills training for children with ADHD. However, the evidence has not been convincing [66–69] which may result from lack of focus on maternal functioning, such as own unmet need for treatment [70]. This omission in the field needs to be addressed by future studies placing greater emphasis on examining the relationship between maternal functioning and child treatment in the prediction of developmental outcomes. This is underlined by the fact that our findings were significant in the domains of maternal ADHD symptoms and resilience regardless of treatment strategy, as not all children received medical treatment. Factors in maternal functioning may potentially provide a basis for more differentiated treatment strategies in the future. This may in turn improve the general prognosis in ADHD.

Methodological considerations

This study is unique in representing the first attempt at exploring the role of maternal functioning in predicting treatment response of children with ADHD; an area which has been lacking in previous studies [15, 16].

The study is, to our knowledge, one of very few studies to address maternal resources as well as risk factors simultaneously and it clearly raises important questions for future research.

Nevertheless, the current study has several limitations.

Our study had a naturalistic design and applied consecutive recruiting in order to include and follow a sample representative of the population we intended to investigate. This was to keep selection bias to a minimum, and hence, we further kept the research track separated from the clinical treatment during the 1-year follow up. However, since a little more than half declined to participate, this then resulted in selection bias. When asked, the participant's main reason for declining to participate was due to the stress of the many appointments entailed by the clinical track.

Further, another limitation relates to the duration of the follow up period. As factors in the parent–child relationship are likely to emerge over time, a longer follow up would have been ideal.

For example, the lack of correlation between maternal self-reported attachment style and child outcome on ADHD-RS may relate to the relatively short follow up period. This is supported by findings from other studies suggesting that the influence of medical treatment tends to wear off, making other factors more influential in long-term treatment strategies [71, 72].

Another limitation concerns the sole reliance on self-reporting in the assessment of various aspects of maternal functioning as socially desirable responding has been shown to affect results in previous research [73]. However, it has been shown that adults provide an accurate assessment of their own ADHD symptoms [74].

Also, maternal ADHD symptomatology was assessed very specifically; other types of maternal psychopathology were not assessed and thus taken into consideration. For example, as maternal depression is known to be a risk factor for symptom severity in offspring ADHD [19], it would have been of interest to gain information on how many mothers were clinically depressed. We did, however, obtain general information on history of mental illness, from preformed protocols collecting psychosocial and demographic data, which was controlled for in the analysis. The same is also true of the assessment of the children, as the degree of impairment in the children was not assessed beyond an assessment of their ADHD symptoms.

Disappointingly, we were not able to draw any conclusions in relation to the role of fathers' functioning in the treatment response of their children diagnosed with ADHD. The response rate of fathers was too low to include in the study. Whilst this is not unique to our study (see for example, [75]), previous findings do suggest a link between child externalizing problems and paternal ADHD symptoms, and this may constitute an area of particular interest for future research [54].

Compared to other reported studies, the rate of comorbidity was very low in our study [76, 77]. However, it would appear that ADHD is a clinical predictor of comorbidities, as ADHD seems to increase the risk of developing comorbidity during childhood and adolescence such as conduct disorder and oppositional defiance disorder, which further increase the risk of antisocial behavior and juvenile delinquency later on ([11, 13, 78, 79].This developmental pathway was also observed in a longitudinal study in which children were included only if they had no comorbidity [12]. Yet, in this study by Klein and colleagues, 84 of 135 participants developed probable or definite conduct disorder during adolescence and a further 25% of these developed antisocial personality disorder in adulthood. The children in our study were included after a first time referral and were in the age range 7–12. Hence, the frequency of comorbid disorders may rise in the years to come.

Conclusion

Taken together, our findings suggest that risk factors as well as protective factors in maternal functioning have an impact on treatment outcome in children with ADHD. This underlines the potential value of a broader assessment of maternal functioning, including screening of mothers for ADHD symptoms. This would permit the identification of parents with unmet needs for treatment and support, which might in turn lead to a better prognosis for their children. On the other hand, a greater focus on protective factors such as maternal resilience may be no less important in differentiating the subgroups of families who are at less of an immediate risk and who may therefore require less support and intervention.

Abbreviations
ADHD: attention deficit hyperactivity disorder; AAI: Adult Attachment Interview; ADHD-RS: ADHD-Rating Scale; ASRS-1.1: Adult ADHD Self-Report Scale; ECR: Experiences in Close Relationships Questionnaire; ECR-R: The Experiences in Close Relationships Scale—Revised; RSA: Resilience Scale for Adults; CT: combined type; IT: inattentive type; ODD: oppositional defiance disorder.

Authors' contributions
The corresponding author, PD, was responsible for data collection and drafting the first manuscript. AB analyzed and interpreted the data in collaboration with PD. All co-authors (AB, OS, ES, YS and NB) made substantial contributions to critical revision of the first draft for key intellectual content, and have given their final approval for the version to be published. All authors read and approved the final manuscript.

Author details
[1] Child and Adolescent Psychiatric Department, Region Zealand, Denmark. [2] Psychiatric Research Unit, Region Zealand, Denmark. [3] Child and Adolescent Psychiatric Department and, Psychiatric Research Unit, University of Southern Denmark, Odense, Denmark. [4] Institute of Psychology, University of Southern Denmark, Odense, Denmark. [5] Department of Clinical Medicine, University of Copenhagen, Copenhagen, Denmark. [6] Anna Freud National Centre for Children and Families, London, UK. [7] Ny Østergade 12, 4000 Roskilde, Denmark.

Acknowledgements
Not applicable.

Competing interests
The authors declare that they have no competing interests.

Funding
The research was funded by Region Zealand Research Foundation, Grant Nb: 15-000342 and Department of Child and Adolescent Psychiatry, Region Zealand.

References

1. Polanczyk G, Zeni C, Genro JP, Guimarães AP, Roman T, Hutz MH, Rohde LA. Association of the adrenergic alpha2A receptor gene with methylphenidate improvement of inattentive symptoms in children and adolescents with attention-deficit/hyperactivity disorder. Arch Gen Psychiatry. 2007;64(2):218–24. https://doi.org/10.1001/archpsyc.64.2.218.

2. Lara C, Fayyad J, de Graaf R, Kessler RC, Aguilar-Gaxiola S, Angermeyer M, Sampson N. Childhood predictors of adult attention-deficit/hyperactivity disorder: results from the World Health Organization World Mental Health Survey Initiative. Biol Psychiatry. 2009;65(1):46–54. https://doi.org/10.1016/j.biopsych.2008.10.005.

3. World Health Organisation. The ICD-10 classification of mental and behavioural disorders. Clinical Descriptions and Diagnostic Guidelines. Geneva: World Health Organisation; 1992.

4. American Psychiatric Association. Diagnostic and statistical manual of mental disorders (DSM-5). Washington, DC: American Psychiatric Association; 2013.

5. Hechtman L. Families of children with attention deficit hyperactivity disorder: a review. Can J Psychiatry. 1996;41(6):350–60.

6. Thapar A, Cooper M, Eyre O, Langley K. Practitioner review: what have we learnt about the causes of ADHD? J Child Psychol Psychiatry. 2013;54(1):3–16. https://doi.org/10.1111/j.1469-7610.2012.02611.x.

7. Faraone SV, Biederman J, Chen WJ, Milberger S, Warburton R, Tsuang MT. Genetic heterogeneity in attention-deficit hyperactivity disorder (ADHD): gender, psychiatric comorbidity, and maternal ADHD. J Abnorm Psychol. 1995;104(2):334–45.

8. Elia J, Gai X, Xie HM, Perin JC, Geiger E, Glessner JT, D'arcy M, Frackelton E, Kim C, Lantieri F, Muganga BM. Rare structural variants found in attention-deficit hyperactivity disorder are preferentially associated with neurodevelopmental genes. Mol Psychiatry. 2010;15:637–46. https://doi.org/10.1038/mp.2009.57.

9. Sucksdorff M, Lehtonen L, Chudal R, Suominen A, Joelsson P. Preterm birth and poor fetal growth as risk factors of attention-deficit/hyperactivity disorder. Pediatrics. 2015;136(3):599–608. https://doi.org/10.1542/peds.2015-1043.

10. Thapar A, Cooper M, Jefferies R, Stergiakouli E. What causes attention deficit hyperactivity disorder? Arch Dis Child 2012;97:260–265. https://doi.org/10.1136/archdischild-2011-300482.

11. Dalsgaard S, Østergaard SD, Leckman JF, Mortensen PB, Pedersen MG. Mortality in children, adolescents, and adults with attention deficit hyperactivity disorder: a nationwide cohort study. Lancet. 2015;385(9983):2190–6. https://doi.org/10.1016/S0140-6736(14)61684-6.

12. Klein RG, Mannuzza S, Olazagasti MA, Roizen E, Hutchison JA, Lashua EC, Castellanos FX. Clinical and functional outcome of childhood attention-deficit/hyperactivity disorder 33 years later. Arch Gen Psychiatry. 2012;69(12):1295–303. https://doi.org/10.1001/archgenpsychiatry.2012.271.

13. Mannuzza S, Klein RG, Bessler A, Malloy P, Lapadula M. Adult psychiatric status of hyperactive boys grown up. Am J Psychiatry. 1998;155(4):493–8. https://doi.org/10.1176/ajp.155.4.493.

14. Caye A, Spadini AV, Karam RG, et al. Predictors of persistence of ADHD into adulthood: a systematic review of the literature and meta-analysis. Eur Child Adolesc Psychiatry. 2016;25:1151. https://doi.org/10.1007/s00787-016-0831-8.

15. Johnston C, Mash EJ. Families of children with attention-deficit/hyperactivity disorder: review and recommendations for future research. Clin Child Fam Psychol Rev. 2001;4(3):183–207. https://doi.org/10.1023/A:1017592030434.

16. Deault LC. A systematic review of parenting in relation to the development of comorbidities and functional impairments in children with attention-deficit/hyperactivity disorder (ADHD). Child Psychiatry Hum Dev. 2010;41(2):168–92. https://doi.org/10.1007/s10578-009-0159-4.

17. Steinberg EA, Drabick DAG. A developmental psychopathology perspective on adhd and comorbid conditions: the role of emotion regulation. Child Psychiatry Hum Dev. 2015;46(6):951–66. https://doi.org/10.1007/s10578-015-0534-2.

18. Chronis AM, Lahey BB, Pelham WE, Kipp HL, Baumann BL, Lee SS. Psychopathology and substance abuse in parents of young children with attention-deficit/hyperactivity disorder. J Am Acad Child Adolesc Psychiatry. 2003;42(12):1424–32. https://doi.org/10.1097/00004583-200312000-00009.

19. Margari F, Craig F, Petruzzelli MG, Lamanna A, Matera E, Margari L. Parents psychopathology of children with attention deficit hyperactivity disorder. Res Dev Disabil. 2013;34(3):1036–43. https://doi.org/10.1016/j.ridd.2012.12.001.

20. Minde K, Eakin L, Hechtman L, Ochs E, Bouffard R, Greenfield B, Looper K. The psychosocial functioning of children and spouses of adults with ADHD. J Child Psychol Psychiatry. 2003;44(4):637–46.

21. Psychogiou L, Daley DM, Thompson MJ, Sonuga-Barke EJS. Do maternal attention-deficit/hyperactivity disorder symptoms exacerbate or ameliorate the negative effect of child attention-deficit/hyperactivity disorder symptoms on parenting? Dev Psychopathol. 2008;20(1):121–37.

22. Joelsson P, Chudal R, Uotila J, Suominen A, Sucksdorff D, Gyllenberg D, Sourander A. Parental psychopathology and offspring attention-deficit/hyperactivity disorder in a nationwide sample. J Psychiatr Res. 2017;94:124–30.

23. Mokrova I, Brien MO, Calkins S, Keane S. Parental ADHD symptomology and ineffective parenting: the connecting link of home. Chaos. 2011;10(2):119–35. https://doi.org/10.1080/15295190903212844.Parental.

24. Roskam I, Stievenart M, Tessier R, Muntean A, Escobar MJ, Santelices MP, Juffer F, Van Ijzendoorn MH, Pierrehumbert B. Another way of thinking about ADHD: the predictive role of early attachment deprivation in adolescents' level of symptoms. Soc Psychiatry Psychiatr Epidemiol. 2014;49(1):133–44. https://doi.org/10.1007/s00127-013-0685-z.

25. Storebø OJ, Darling Rasmussen P, Simonsen E. Association between insecure attachment and ADHD: environmental mediating factors. J Attent Disord. 2013;20(2):187–96. https://doi.org/10.1177/1087054713501079.

26. Jones J, Cassedy J, Shaver PR. Parents' self-reported attachment styles: a review of links with parenting behaviors, emotions, and cognitions. Ratio. 2010;36(3):490–9. https://doi.org/10.1124/dmd.107.016501.CYP3A4-Mediated.

27. Atwool N. Attachment and resilience: implications for children in care. Child Care Pract. 2006;12(4):315–30. https://doi.org/10.1080/13575270600863226.

28. Herrman H, Stewart DE, Diaz-granados N, Berger EL, Beth J. What is resilience? Can J Psychiatry. 2011;56(5):258–65.

29. Windle G. What is resilience? A review and concept analysis. Rev Clin Gerontol. 2011;21(2):152–69. https://doi.org/10.1017/S0959259810000420.

30. Wright MO, Masten AS, Narayan A. Resilience processes in development: four waves of research on positive adaptation in the context of adversity. In: Handbook of Resilience in Children. 2013. p. 15–37.

31. Bodin P, Wiman BLB. Resilience and other stability concepts in ecology: notes on their origin, validity. ESS Bull. 2004;2(2):33–43.

32. Davidson JRT, Payne VM, Connor KM, Foa EB, Rothbaum BO, Hertzberg MA, Weisler RH. Trauma, resilience and saliostasis: effects of treatment in post-traumatic stress disorder. Int Clin Psychopharmacol. 2005;20(1):43–8.

33. Martin AJ, Marsh HW. Academic resilience and academic buoyancy: multidimensional and hierarchical conceptual framing of causes, correlates and cognate constructs. Oxford Rev Educ. 2009;35(3):353–70. https://doi.org/10.1080/03054980902934639.

34. National clinical guideline for the assessment and treatment of ADHD in children and adolescents. Danish Health Authority; 2014. https://www.sst.dk/da/nyheder/2014/~/media/A7931B11333540A184C73465181E29CE.ashx. Accessed 31 May 2018.

35. Friborg O, Hjemdal O. Resilience as a measure of adaptive capacity. J Nor Psychol Assoc. 2004;41:206–8.

36. Friborg O, Hjemdal O, Rosenvinge JH, Martinussen M. A new rating scale for adult resilience: what are the central protective resources behind healthy adjustment? Int J Methods Psychiatr Res. 2003;12(2):65–76. https://doi.org/10.1002/mpr.143.

37. Hjemdal O, Friborg O, Stiles TC, Rosenvinge JH, Martinussen M. Resilience predicting psychiatric symptoms: a prospective study of protective factors and their role in adjustment to stressful life events. Clin Psychol Psychother. 2006;13(3):194–201. https://doi.org/10.1002/cpp.488.

38. Hjemdal O, Roazzi A, Dias M, Friborg O. The cross-cultural validity of the Resilience Scale for Adults: a comparison between Norway and Brazil. BMC Psychol. 2015;3(18):1–9. https://doi.org/10.1186/s40359-015-0076-1.

39. Friborg O, Barlaug D, Martinussen M, Rosenvinge JH, Hjemdal O. Resilience in relation to personality and intelligence. Int J Methods Psychiatr Res. 2005;14(1):29–42. https://doi.org/10.1002/mpr.15.

40. Kessler RC, Adler L, Ames M, Demler O, Faraone S, Hiripi E, Howes MJ, Jin R, Secnik K, Spencer T, Ustun TB, Walters EE. The World Health Organization Adult ADHD Self-Report Scale (ASRS): a short screening scale for use in the general population. Psychol Med. 2005;35(2):245–56. https://doi.org/10.1017/S0033291704002892.

41. Kessler RC, Adler LA, Gruber MJ, Sarawate CA, Spencer T, Van Brunt DL. Validity of the World Health Organization Adult ADHD Self-Report Scale (ASRS) Screener in a representative sample of health plan members. Int J Methods Psychiatr Res. 2007;16(2):52–65. https://doi.org/10.1002/mpr.208.

42. Chris R, Waller NG, Brennan KA. An item response theory analysis of self-report measures of adult attachment. J Pers Soc Psychol. 2000;78(2):350–65. https://doi.org/10.1037/0022-3514.78.2.350.

43. Sibley C, Fischer R, Liu J. Reliability and validity of the revised experiences in close relationships (ECR-R) self-report measure of adult romantic attachment. Pers Soc Psychol Bull. 2005;31(11):1524–36.

44. Birmaher B, Ehmann M, Axelson DA, Goldstein BI, Monk K, Kalas C, Brent DA. Schedule for affective disorders and schizophrenia for school-age children (K-SADS-PL) for the assessment of preschool children—a preliminary psychometric study. J Psychiatr Res. 2009;43(7):680–6. https://doi.org/10.1016/j.jpsychires.2008.10.003.

45. Kaufman J, Birmaher B, Brent D, Rao U, Flynn C, Moreci P, Williamson D, Ryan ND. Schedule for affective disorders and schizophrenia for school-age children-present and lifetime version (K-SADS-PL): initial reliability and validity data. J Am Acad Child Adolesc Psychiatry. 1997;36(7):980–8. https://doi.org/10.1097/00004583-199707000-00021.

46. Villabø MA, Oerbeck B, Skirbekk B, Hansen BH, Kristensen H. Convergent and divergent validity of K-SADS-PL anxiety and attention deficit hyperactivity disorder diagnoses in a clinical sample of school-aged children. Nord J Psychiatry. 2016;70(5):358–64.

47. DuPaul GJ, Power TJ, Anastopoulos AD, Reid R. ADHD rating scale-IV. New York: Guilford; 1998.

48. Barkley RA, Robin AL. Defiant teens: a clinician's manual for assessment and family intervention. New York: Guilford Publications; 2014.

49. Dahmen B, Pütz V, Herpertz-Dahlmann B, Konrad K. Early pathogenic care and the development of ADHD-like symptoms. J Neural Transm. 2012;119(9):1023–36. https://doi.org/10.1007/s00702-012-0809-8.

50. Szomlaiski N, Dyrborg J, Rasmussen H, Schumann T, Koch SV, Bilenberg N. Validity and clinical feasibility of the ADHD rating scale (ADHD-RS) a Danish Nationwide Multicenter Study. Acta Paediatr. 2009;98(2):397–402. https://doi.org/10.1111/j.1651-2227.2008.01025.x.

51. Kendall T, Taylor E, Perez A, Taylor C. Diagnosis and management of attention-deficit/hyperactivity disorder in children, young people, and adults: summary of NICE guidance. BMJ. 2008;337:751–3. https://doi.org/10.1136/bmj.a1239.

52. Harvey E, Danforth JS, McKee TE, Ulaszek WR, Friedman JL. Parenting of children with attention-deficit/hyperactivity disorder (ADHD): the role of parental ADHD symptomatology. J Atten Disord. 2003;7(1):31–42. https://doi.org/10.1177/108705470300700104.

53. López Seco F, Aguado-Gracia J, Mundo-Cid P, Acosta-García S, Martí-Serrano S, Gaviria AM, Vilella E, Masana-Marín A. Maternal psychiatric history is associated with the symptom severity of ADHD in offspring. Psychiatry Res. 2015;226(2–3):507–12. https://doi.org/10.1016/j.psychres.2015.02.010.

54. Middeldorp CM, Wesseldijk LW, Hudziak JJ, Verhulst FC, Lindauer RJL, Dieleman GC. Parents of children with psychopathology: psychiatric problems and the association with their child's problems. Eur Child Adolesc Psychiatry. 2016;25(8):919–27. https://doi.org/10.1007/s00787-015-0813-2.

55. Clarke L, Ungerer J, Johnson S, Stiefel I. Attention deficit hyperactivity disorder is associated with attachment insecurity. Clin Child Psychol Psychiatry. 2002;7(200204):179–98. https://doi.org/10.1177/1359104502007002006.

56. George C, Kaplan N, Main M. The adult attachment interview (Unpublished protocol). Berkeley: Department of Psychology, University of California; 1985.

57. Shaver P, Belsky J, Brennan K. The adult attachment interview and self-reports of romantic attachment: associations across domains and methods. Pers Relationsh. 2000;7:25–43. https://doi.org/10.1111/j.1475-6811.2000.tb00002.x.

58. Rasmussen PD, Bilenberg N, Shmueli-Goetz Y, Simonsen E, Bojesen A, Storebø O. Maternal and child attachment and attention deficit hyperactivity disorder in middle childhood: associations with treatment outcome. 2018. (Unpublished material—in process).

59. Behere AP, Basnet P, Campbell P. Effects of family structure on mental health of children: a preliminary study. Indian J Psychol Med. 2017;39(4):457–63. https://doi.org/10.4103/0253-7176.211767.

60. van IJzendoorn MH, Goldberg S, Kroonenberg PM, Frenkel OJ. The relative effects of maternal and child problems on the quality of attachment: a meta-analysis of attachment in clinical samples. Child Dev. 1992;63(4):840–58.

61. Osofsky JD, Chartrand LCMM. Military children from birth to five years. Future Child. 2013;23(2):61–77. https://doi.org/10.1353/foc.2013.0011.

62. Savage-McGlynn E, Redshaw M, Heron J, Stein A, Quigley MA, Evans J, Ramchandani P, Gray R. Mechanisms of resilience in children of mothers who self-report with depressive symptoms in the first postnatal year. PLoS ONE. 2015;10(11):1–16. https://doi.org/10.1371/journal.pone.0142898.

63. Travis WJ, Combs-Orme T. Resilient parenting: overcoming poor parental bonding. Soc Work Res. 2007;31(3):135–49. https://doi.org/10.1093/swr/31.3.135.

64. Prevatt FF. The contribution of parenting practices in a risk and resiliency model of children's adjustment. Br J Dev Psychol. 2003;21:469–80. https://doi.org/10.1348/026151003322535174.

65. Luthar SS. Developmental psychopathology: perspectives on adjustment, risk, and disorder. Cambridge: Cambridge University Press; 1997.

66. Storebø OJ, Skoog M, Damm D, Thomsen PH, Simonsen E, Gluud C. Social skills training for attention deficit hyperactivity disorder (ADHD) in children aged 5 to 18 years (Review). Cochrane Database Syst Rev Online. 2011;12:CD008223. https://doi.org/10.1002/14651858.CD003018.pub3. Copyright.

67. Zwi M, Jones H, Thorgaard C, York A, Dennis JA. Parent training interventions for attention deficit hyperactivity disorder (ADHD) in children aged 5 to 18 years. Cochrane Database Syst Rev. 2011;12:CD003018. https://doi.org/10.1002/14651858.CD003018.pub3.

68. Punja S, Shamseer L, Hartling L, Urichuk L, Vandermeer B, Nikles J, Vohra S. Amphetamines for attention deficit hyperactivity disorder (ADHD) in children and adolescents. Cochrane Database of Syst Rev. 2016;2:CD009996. https://doi.org/10.1002/14651858.cd009996.pub2.

69. Storebø OJ, Ramstad E, Krogh BH, Nilausen TD, Skoog M, Holmskov M, Gluud C. Methylphenidate for children and adolescents with attention deficit hyperactivity disorder (ADHD). Cochrane Database Syst Rev. 2015. https://doi.org/10.1002/14651858.CD009885.pub2.

70. Shameem S, Stanley A. Are parental ADHD problems associated with a more severe clinical presentation and greater family adversity in children with ADHD. Eur Child Adolesc Psychiatry. 2013;22:369–377. https://doi.org/10.1007/s00787-013-0378-x.

71. Molina BS, Hinshaw SP, Swanson JM, Arnold LE, Vitiello B, Jensen PS, Houck PR. The MTA at 8 years: prospective follow-up of children treated for combined-type ADHD in a multisite study. J Am Acad Child Adolesc Psychiatry. 2009;48(5):484–500. https://doi.org/10.1097/CHI.0b013e31819c23d0.

72. Swanson JM, Arnold LE, Molina BSG, Sibley MH, Hechtman LT, Hinshaw SP, Kraemer HC. Young adult outcomes in the follow-up of the multimodal treatment study of attention-deficit/hyperactivity disorder: symptom persistence, source discrepancy, and height suppression. J Child Psychol Psychiatry. 2017. https://doi.org/10.1111/jcpp.12684.

73. van de Mortel TF. Faking it: social desirability response bias in self-report research report research. Sci Hum. 2008;25(4):40–8.

74. Murphy P, Schachar R. Use of self-ratings in the assessment of symptoms of attention deficit hyperactivity disorder in adults. Am J Psychiatry. 2000;157(7):1156–9. https://doi.org/10.1176/appi.ajp.157.7.1156.

75. Lahey BB, Piacenti JC, McBurnett K, Stone P, Pii S, Hartdagen S, Hynd G. Psychopathology in the parents of children with conduct disorder and hyperactivity. J Am Acad Child Adolesc Psychiatry. 1988;27(2):163–70. https://doi.org/10.1097/00004583-198803000-00005.

76. Barkley R. Attention deficit hyperactivity disorder: a handbook for diagnosis and treatment. 2nd ed. New York: Guilford; 1998.

77. Reale L, Bartoli B, Cartabia M, et al. Comorbidity prevalence and treatment outcome in children and adolescents with ADHD. Eur Child Adolesc Psychiatry. 2017;26(12):1443–57.

Validation of the Child Post-Traumatic Cognitions Inventory in Korean survivors of sexual violence

Han Byul Lee[1], Kyoung Min Shin[2], Young Ki Chung[1,3,4], Namhee Kim[3,4], Yee Jin Shin[5], Un-Sun Chung[6], Seung Min Bae[7], Minha Hong[8] and Hyoung Yoon Chang[1,3,4]*[iD]

Abstract

Background: Dysfunctional cognitions related to trauma is an important factor in the development and maintenance of post-traumatic stress disorder symptoms in children and adolescents. The Child Post-traumatic Cognitions Inventory (CPTCI) assesses such cognitions about trauma. We investigated the psychometric properties of the Korean version of CPTCI and its short form by surveying child and adolescent survivors of sexual violence.

Methods: Children and adolescents aged 7–16 years ($N = 237$, $M_{age} = 12.6$, $SD = 2.3$, 222 [93.7%] were female) who were exposed to sexual violence were included in this survey. We assessed the factor structure, internal consistency, and validity of the CPTCI and its short form through data analysis.

Results: Confirmatory factor analysis results supported the two-factor model presented in the original study. The total scale, its subscales, and the short form had good internal consistency (Cronbach's $\alpha = .96$ for total scale and .91–.95 for the other scales). The CPTCI showed high correlations with scales measuring post-traumatic stress symptoms ($r = .77–.80$), anxiety ($r = .69–.71$), and depression ($r = .74–.77$); the correlation with post-traumatic stress symptoms was the highest. The differences in CPTCI scores per post-traumatic stress symptom levels were significant (all $p < .001$) Sex differences in CPTCI scores were not significant ($p > .05$ for all comparisons); however, the scores exhibited differences per age group (all $p < .001$).

Conclusions: The results indicate that the Korean version of the CPTCI is a valid and reliable scale; therefore, it may be a valuable tool for assessing maladaptive cognitions related to trauma in research and clinical settings.

Keywords: Child Post-traumatic Cognitions Inventory, Post-traumatic cognitions, Child sexual abuse, Sexual violence, Psychometry

Background

Recently, researchers have shown an increased interest in individual differences in how people respond to trauma [1, 2]. Some people experience minimal emotional distress and show only minor and transient disruptions in their ability to function, while others suffer from more intense pain that lasts longer [1]. Researchers have addressed post-traumatic cognitions as one of the factors influencing the severity and persistence of pathological responses to trauma [3–6]. Traumatic events significantly alter survivors' cognitions and beliefs about themselves, the world, and their future, possibly leading to negative emotional responses and maladaptive actions, which in turn contributes to the development and maintenance of PTSD [4, 5]. The importance of such trauma-related cognitions is reflected in the fifth edition of the Diagnostic and Statistical Manual of Mental Disorders' [7] (DSM-5; American Psychiatric Association 2013) revised diagnostic criteria for PTSD. One of the symptom clusters listed among the DSM-5's diagnostic criteria for PTSD

*Correspondence: hyoungyoon@ajou.ac.kr
[3] Department of Psychiatry and Behavioral Sciences, Ajou University School of Medicine, 164 World Cup-ro, Yeongtong-gu, Suwon, Suwon-si 16409, Republic of Korea
Full list of author information is available at the end of the article

is "negative alterations in cognitions and mood," which includes criterion D2 ("persistent and exaggerated negative beliefs or expectations about oneself, others, or the world [e.g., 'I am bad' and 'no one can be trusted'])" and D3("persistent, distorted cognitions about the cause or consequences of the traumatic event(s) that lead the individual to blame himself/herself or others.") (p. 272). Such changes in diagnostic criteria emphasize the importance of assessment of trauma-related cognitions.

Considering the need for a valid and reliable instrument to assess trauma-related cognitions, Foa et al. [6] developed the Post-traumatic Cognitions Inventory (PTCI). This inventory consists of 33 items that comprise three factors: "negative cognitions about the self," "negative cognitions about the world," and "self-blame." The inventory was translated and tested on diverse samples in countries such as Germany [8], the Netherlands [9], Korea [10], and Taiwan [11], where its factor structure was repeatedly verified, and its reliability and validity were confirmed. In these studies, it was reported that certain characteristics like sex, type of trauma experienced, and cultural background could affect PTCI scores and its psychometric properties.

Various studies have shown that cognitive models of PTSD can be extended to children and adolescents; however, they have also indicated the need to consider developmental aspects [12–14]. Therefore, Meiser-Stedman et al. [15] developed the Child Post-traumatic Cognitions Inventory (CPTCI) to assess the post-traumatic cognitions of children and adolescents. They made age-appropriate modifications to the PTCI items, and added some items based on a cognitive model of PTSD to construct an initial 41-item questionnaire that was used with a community sample comprised 223 children and adolescents. Based on the survey results, the researchers performed item reduction to arrive at the final 25-item questionnaire and validate it in two other sets of samples. Unlike the adult version, the CPTCI comprises only two subscales. First, the "permanent and disturbing change" subscale (CPTCI-PC) comprises 13 items and focuses on the negative effects that a frightening event has on a child and the child's perception of the future. Second, the "fragile person in a scary world" subscale (CPTCI-SW) comprises 12 items and assesses the child's sense of vulnerability and perception of the world and other people as threatening. One of the factors of the PTCI, "self-blame," is not included in the CPTCI.

The CPTCI turns out to be a valid and reliable measure regarding multiple criteria, benefits from being standardized within a large population of children and adolescents [15]. Based on the theoretical model of PTSD, it has been proposed that the cognitive therapy of PTSD should target post-traumatic cognitions, and studies treating

post-traumatic cognitions as a mediator of therapeutic change are being conducted using CPTCI [16–20]. Furthermore, a recently published study updated the CPTCI and evaluated its utility and psychometric properties, providing additional information on the test–retest reliability of CPTCI, as well as suggesting a short form of CPTCI and cutoff points in CPTCI scores for clinical use [21].

The CPTCI has been translated into several languages, and different versions have been validated and their psychometric properties have been reported in Germany [22], the Netherlands [17], Brazil [23] and Taiwan [24]. Previous studies generally report adequate levels of reliability and validity. Moreover, in all these samples the two-factor structure emerged as the best solution. These studies, however, showed that the original two-factor structure of CPTCI exhibits unsatisfactory model fit indices that do not meet the widely accepted criteria [17, 21, 22, 24, 25]. Authors attribute these discrepancies to sample characteristics and cultural differences. In the original study, most of the participants were exposed to traumatic events that did not last for longer than a few minutes and affected few people (e.g., motor vehicle accidents). In contrast, Taiwanese sample predominantly comprises natural disaster survivors. Meanwhile, the majority of children participated in the Brazilian CPTCI study experienced multiple traumas, such as ongoing physical or sexual abuse. The Dutch version and The German version of the CPTCI were also validated in the samples including survivors of interpersonal violence.

To address the issue, the Brazilian version used an exploratory factor analysis to derive a new two-factor model with items that were different from those of the extant two-factor model [23]. In the Chinese version of the CPTCI developed in Taiwan, researchers revised the original PTCI by deleting five items based on the results of confirmatory factor analysis (CFA). Both methods result in theoretically less sound models because the models were modified based on the results of the analysis. The models neither have enough empirical grounds. Therefore, the models need to replicate, in new sets of samples [26].

Sexual violence is a type of trauma that leads to severe psychological aftereffects. Sexual assault and sexual violence jointly make up the second largest share of traumas causing PTSD worldwide [27]. Especially, Child sexual abuse is associated with numerous adverse sequelae during childhood including depression, anxiety, behavioral problems, and post-traumatic stress disorder (PTSD), and is also correlated with an increased risk for mental health problems in adulthood [28, 29]. Several studies have shown that post-traumatic cognitions in survivors of sexual violence play a significant role in how they adapt afterwards [30, 31]. Some studies utilizing PTCI reported that a higher proportion of sexual violence survivors had maladaptive post-traumatic cognitions and beliefs as compared to survivors of other types of trauma [6, 11]. Moreover, since it is now well established that child sexual abuse survivors benefit from TF-CBT targeting maladaptive post-traumatic cognitions, assessment of post-traumatic cognitions in these populations is crucial for intervention [32, 33]. To date, however, the CPTCI has not been tested on a sample consisting solely of sexual violence survivors to determine its psychometric properties.

Consequently, this study has the following goals. First, we aimed to verify the factor structure of the CPTCI regarding child and adolescent survivors of sexual violence in Korea. Specifically, we sought to determine whether the original two-factor structure derived in the process of developing the scale could be used without adapting it for cultural differences or types of trauma. Second, we aimed to determine the convergent validity and discriminant validity of the CPTCI in comparison with scales that measure the severity of trauma symptoms, anxiety, and depression. Third, we examined the

factor structure, reliability, and validity of the short form of the CPTCI (CPTCI-S) [21].

Methods

Participants

Children and adolescents ($N=237$) aged 7–16 years who visited support centers for sexual assault survivors to receive medical, investigative, and counseling support after being exposed to sexual violence were included in the analysis. The sample was collected from four sexual assault victim support centers located across Korea from 2014 to 2016. Demographic variables and trauma-related information are shown in Table 1.

Procedure

Questionnaire results were obtained with the consent of the survivors themselves and their guardians who provided consent for the collection and use of the data for research purposes. The questionnaire was completed with paper and pencil by the survivors and included the CPTCI, CRIES, TSCC, CDI, and RCMAS. The questionnaires that were submitted at each of the support centers were collected at a single center along

Table 1 Demographic characteristics and trauma-related Information

Variable	Total sample (N=237) n (%)	CPTCI total m	sd	CRIES m	sd	TSCC-PT m	sd	CDI m	sd	RCMAS m	sd
Sex											
Male	15 (6.3)	52.73	17.64	31.87	12.36	12.57	8.17	18.33	10.33	16.07	8.40
Female	222 (93.7)	52.14	19.62	32.18	17.23	11,70	8.23	17.62	9.61	20.98	8.41
Age groups											
8–11	76 (32.1)	45.17	17.84	27.08	16.09	9.72	7,49	13.83	8.62	17.76	9.27
12–14	106 (44.7)	53.16	18.82	33.49	16.66	12.43	8.59	18.80	9.11	22.08	7.64
15–16	55 (23.1)	59.96	19.81	36.53	17.19	13.37	8.00	20.73	10.43	21.96	7.97
Type of trauma											
Rape	94 (39.7)	56.31	19.22	33.78	16.25	12.63	8.40	20.32	9.20	21.90	7.96
Sexual abuse other than rape	143 (60.3)	49.46	19.21	31.10	17.35	11.21	8.07	15.94	9.56	19.85	8.73
Time since trauma											
Less than 1 week	98 (41.4)	51.28	19.13	32.28	17.65	11.66	8.29	18.19	10.35	20.82	8.24
1 week–1 month	40 (16.9)	56.25	20.46	35.90	16.91	13.23	8.62	18.65	10.22	21.78	8.76
1–3 months	20 (8.4)	48.90	16.51	27.75	14.94	10.63	7.07	15.75	8.47	19.25	8.07
3 months or more	72 (30.4)	52.58	19.82	31.40	16.30	11.25	8.16	16.83	8.50	20.28	8.89
Unspecified	7 (3.0)	50.17	23.84	34.33	16.17	13.00	9.72	19.00	12.43	21.17	8.80
Region											
Suwon	164 (69.2)	51.66	19.70	32.96	16.71	11.92	8.19	17.64	9.92	20.71	8.61
Seongnam	28 (11.8)	54.46	19.49	34.43	16.75	12.57	8.09	17.57	8.02	20.68	8.30
Goyang	27 (11.4)	55.67	17.03	32.38	14.30	12.81	8.44	19.23	9.25	21.00	7.52
Jeju	18 (7.6)	48.06	21.09	21.06	20.00	7.33	7.39	15.83	10.20	19.78	9.47

CPTCI total Total Score of Korean version of Child Post-Traumatic Cognitions Inventory, *CRIES* Children's Revised Impact of Event Scale, *TSCC-PT* Post-traumatic stress Subscale of the Traumatic Symptom Checklist for Children, *CAPS* Children's Attributions and Perceptions Scale, *CDI* Children's Depression Inventory, *RCMAS* Revised Children's Manifest Anxiety Scale with basic information on the survivors and details about the traumatic incidents they had experienced. All the procedures conducted by this study were reported to and approved by the Institutional Review Board of the Ajou University Medical Center (IRB number: SBR-SUR-17-041).

Measures
CPTCI

The CPTCI is a self-report questionnaire consisting of 25 items that is designed to assess dysfunctional trauma-related cognitions in children and adolescents [15]. Each item is rated on a four-point Likert scale: "*do not agree at all*" (1 point), "*do not agree a bit*" (2 points), "*agree a bit*" (3 points), and "*agree a lot*" (4 points). Two factors were confirmed in the process of developing the scale: CPTCI-PC and CPTCI-SW. CPTCI-PC has 13 items and CPTCI-SW has 12 items; the scores each are calculated along with the total score. A higher score indicates greater dysfunction in trauma-related cognitions. The reliability and the validity of the CPTCI total score and its subscales were reported to be adequate in the original paper. In 2016, the researchers of the original paper developed the CPTCI-S [21]. The short form comprises 6 items from the CPTCI-PC subscale and 4 items from the CPTCI-SW subscale. Items were selected on the basis of factor loadings and relationships with the CPTCI total score as well as a PTSD diagnosis. The 2016 study found that the CPTCI-S had excellent psychometric properties. As for the Korean version of the CPTCI, the second author of this study (KMS) received permission from one of the CPTCI authors (i.e. Meiser-Stedman, R.), to translate the CPTCI items into Korean. Then, the corresponding author (HYC), a child and adolescent psychiatrist and bilingual speaker of Korean and English, reviewed the translated items. Total score of the CPTCI ranges 25–100.

Children's Revised Impact of Event Scale (CRIES)

The CRIES is used to assess children who have been exposed to traumatic events and are at risk of suffering from PTSD [34]. The CRIES comprises 13 items measuring various PTSD symptoms like intrusion, avoidance, and hyperarousal. Each item is rated on a four-point Likert scale (0 = "*not at all*," 1 = "*rarely*," 3 = "*sometimes*," and 5 = "*often*"). The score for each item is summed to yield a total score; higher scores indicate greater severity of children's post-traumatic stress response. We used the Korean version of the CRIES in this study [35]. The Korean version of the CRIES exhibited adequate levels of internal consistency (Cronbach's α = .93 for the total

scale) and both convergent and discriminant validity. The study proposed a cutoff of 26 to screen PTSD in children and adolescent. Total score of CRIES ranges 0–65.

Trauma Symptom Checklist for Children (TSCC)

The TSCC is a self-report assessment scale that was designed by Briere [36]. It includes two validity scales measuring under-response and hyper-response, along with six clinical scales measuring anxiety, depression, anger, post-traumatic stress symptoms, dissociation (two subscales on overt dissociation and fantasy), and sexual concerns (two subscales on sexual preoccupation and sexual distress). In this study, we use post-traumatic stress subscale to measure post-traumatic symptoms severity. Post-traumatic stress subscale comprises 10 items rated on a four-point scale ranging from 0 ("*never*") to 3 ("*almost all of the time*"). We used a version of the scale translated by Son and colleagues (2007), which reported an internal consistency of α = .97.

Revised Children's Manifest Anxiety Scale (RCMAS)

The RCMAS was developed by Castenada, McCandlless, and Palermo (1956) to measure the manifest anxiety of children and adolescents, and revised and supplemented by Reynolds and Richmond [37]. It consists of 37 items addressing anxiety, asking the child to answer *yes/no* on how the child thinks and feels about oneself. We used the Korean version of the RCMAS, which was translated by Choe et al. [38] and has an adequate level of internal consistency (α = .81). Total score of the RCMAS ranges from 0 to 37.

Children's Depression Inventory (CDI)

To test the convergent validity of the CPTCI, we used the CDI, which measures depression in children. The CDI was devised by Kovacs [39] to assess the depression of school-aged children and adolescents. It comprises 27 items, and each item consists of three statements. The statement that most closely matches their mood over the past 2 weeks is chosen by respondents. Total score of the CDI ranges from 0 to 54. The Korean version of the CDI has adequate reliability and validity (i.e., α = .76.).

Statistical analysis

The data were analyzed as follows. First, a confirmatory factor analysis was performed on the sample using AMOS 18.0 to assess the factor structure of the Korean version of the CPTCI [40]. To determine the valid factor structure through model comparisons, three models of the full scale were tested. The first model is the two-factor one presented in the original paper using the CPTCI-PC and CPTCI-SW subscales, and each item was restricted to load on just one fixed factor. The modified two-factor model for the Brazilian version of CPTCI was presented in Lobo et al. [23]; like the original model, it consists of two factors: CPTCI-PC and CPTCI-SW. However, these factors comprise 14 and 11 items, respectively in the Brazilian model, and the items included in each factor are also different from those in the original model. In the one-factor model, all 25 items were made to load on one factor.

Besides, we tested 20-item model which Taiwanese researchers have proposed. Removed items are item number 3, 8, 12, 14 and 25. Other items are loaded onto the same factor as the original version.

Aside from these factor models, we also tested the factor structure of the 10-item CPTCI-S. In the CPTCI-S, six items load on the CPTCI-PC and four items load on the CPTCI-SW. To compare different models of the CPTCI-S, a one-factor model that accounts for all items for one factor was tested here as well.

The χ^2 test results and fit indices for each model were compared. χ^2 index is very sensitive to sample size, making it highly likely to commit the error of dismissing the null hypothesis. Therefore, it is necessary to consider the χ^2 index in conjunction with other goodness-of-fit indices [25]. Based on the criteria proposed in earlier studies, we set the root mean square error of approximation (RMSEA) < .08 and comparative fit index (CFI) and Tucker–Lewis index (TLI) at > .90 as the criteria for judging goodness of model fit [25, 41]. Because the scores were not normally distributed, the method of maximum-likelihood estimation was applied using the Bollen-Stine bootstrap procedure. To assess the internal consistency of the scale, Cronbach's α values were computed for the full scale, the two subscales, and the CPTCI-S. Next, to assess convergent validity, Pearson correlation coefficients were calculated for the CPTCI, PTSD, anxiety,

and depression scales. Then, to determine discriminant validity, we conducted an independent samples t test comparing a high PTSD-risk group and a low PTSD-risk group with respect to their CPTCI total scores and scores for the two subscales and the short form. The high PTSD-risk group and the low PTSD-risk group were classified based on the cutoff point of the CRIES (i.e., a score of 26 points) [35]. For differences in CPTCI scores that depend on demographic variables, we performed t-tests and an analysis of variance (ANOVA) per sex and three age groups (8–11-year-olds, 12–14-year-olds, and 15–16-year-olds). All statistical analyses were conducted using SPSS 18.0 [42] and AMOS 18.0 [40].

Results

Confirmatory factor analysis

A confirmatory factor analysis revealed a significant disparity between the model and the observed data regarding the original two-factor model for the full scale: $\chi^2(274, N=237)=878.2$, $p<.001$. Excluding the SRMR, the values indicate that the model's goodness of fit falls short of the criteria set earlier (see Table 2). Lobo et al. (2015) two-factor model exhibited somewhat poorer fit in comparison with the original two-factor model, $\chi^2(274, N=237)=908.0$, as did the one-factor model, $\chi^2(275, N=237)=981.8$. Moreover, when the χ^2 test was used to compare the one-factor model with the original two-factor model, it was found that $\Delta\chi^2=103.6$ with a significance level of $p=.01$. Liu and Chen's (2015) 20-item two-factor model yielded better fit indices in CFI, TLI, RMSEA, and SRMR than the original 25-item model did. $\chi^2(169, N=237)=528.1$. The fit indices for the two-factor model of CPTCI-S ($\chi^2(34, N=237)=106.7$) revealed that all the fit indices except RMSEA showed good model fit; and the two-factor model fared much better than the one-factor model (Table 2). Although goodness-of-fit

Table 2 Summary of results from confirmatory factor analyses

Model	χ^2	df	CFI	TLI	RMSEA	90% CI	SRMR	Removed items
Cut-off criteria of the GoF	–	–	> .90	> .90	< .08		< .08	
CPTCI original 25-item version								
1. Original two-factor [15]	878.2	274	.858	.844	.097	.090–.104	.057	None
2. Modified two-factor [23]	908.0	274	.851	.837	.099	.092–.106	.058	None
3. One-factor	981.8	275	.834	.819	.104	.097–.111	.060	None
CPTCI 20-item version [24]	528.1	169	.896	.884	.095	.086–.104	.051	3, 8, 12, 14, 25
CPTCI-S [21]								
1. Original two-factor	106.7	34	.950	.933	.095	.075–.116	.038	1, 2, 3, 89, 11, 12, 13, 17, 18, 20, 22, 23, 24, 25
2. One-factor	114.0	35	.945	.929	.098	.078–.118	.039	

GoF goodness-of-Fi, *CFI* comparative fit index, *TLI* Tucker–Lewis index, *RMSEA* root mean square error of approximation, *CI* confidence interval, *SRMR* standardized root mean square error of approximation, *CPTCI* Child Post-traumatic Cognitions Inventory, *CPTCI-S* short form of the CPTCI indices indicate that Liu and Chen's (2015) 20-item model fits better the data than the original 25-item model, we agreed that there are several issues need to be addressed to use the 20-item model and decided to retain the all 25 items and use the data of full version of the CPTCI in the rest of the article. Backgrounds for the decision is discussed in the discussion section. The factor coefficients analyzed using the original two-factor model are shown in Table 3.

Reliability

The Cronbach's α for CPTCI was .96, showing that the scale was highly reliable. The internal consistency of the two subscales were .95 for CPTCI-PC and .91 for CPTCI-SW. The internal consistency of the CPTCI-S was .93. The correlations among the CPTCI total score and the scores for the two subscales as well as the short form were significant and strong (range = .85 to .98). The correlations are provided in Table 4.

Validity

To assess the convergent validity of the CPTCI, we computed its Pearson correlations with other self-report scales. The CPTCI exhibited significant correlations in all the measured values at the level of $p < .001$ with two scales for measuring post-traumatic stress symptoms: the CRIES and TSCC. The CPTCI's total score, the scores for the two subscales, and the scores for the short form showed correlations ranging from .77 to .80 with the CRIES, and ranging from .74 to .78 with the TSCC-PT. Correlations between CPTCI scores and the CDI were high at .76 to .77, and correlations with the RCMAS were also higher than .7. However, these correlations were relatively low compared to those between the CPTCI and the two scales measuring PTSD symptoms. To verify that the correlations between CPTCI and PTSD symptoms are not an artifact arising from the correlations among trauma-related cognitions and depression and anxiety, partial correlations between CPTCI and PTSD scales were computed while controlling for CDI

Table 3 Factor Loadings of Korean CPTCI

	Item	CPTCI-PC		CPTI-SW	
		Original	CPTCI-S	Original	CPTCI-S
4.	My reactions since the frightening event mean I have changed for the worse	.764	.857		
6.	My reactions since the frightening event mean something is seriously wrong with me	.823	.887		
8.	Not being able to get over all my fears means that I am a failure	.750			
13.	My reactions since the frightening event mean I will never get over it	.729			
14.	I used to be a happy person but now I am always sad	.707	.753		
16.	I will never be able to have normal feelings again	.771	.800		
17.	I'm scared that I'll get so angry that I'll break something or hurt someone	.740			
19.	My life has been destroyed by the frightening event	.796	.819		
20.	I feel like I am a different person since the frightening event	.768			
21.	My reactions since the frightening event show that I must be going crazy	.836	.838		
22.	Nothing good can happen to me anymore	.814			
23.	Something terrible will happen if I do not try to control my thoughts about the frightening event	.762			
24.	The frightening event has changed me forever	.792			
1.	Anyone could hurt me			.531	
2.	Everyone lets me down			.679	
3.	I am a coward			.565	
5.	I don't trust people			.696	.776
7.	I am no good			.780	.808
9.	Small things upset me			.683	
10.	I can't cope when things get tough			.758	.776
11.	I can't stop bad things from happening to me			.792	
12.	I have to watch out for danger all the time			.458	
15.	Bad things always happen			.749	.778
18.	Life is not fair			.807	
25.	I have to be really careful because something bad could happen			.553	

CPTCI Child Post-traumatic Cognitions Inventory, *CPTCI-PC* permanent and disturbing change subscale of the CPTCI, *CPTCI-SW* fragile person in a scary world subscale of the CPTCI, *Original* original form of the CPTCI, *CPTCI-S* short form of the CPTCI

Table 4 Correlations among the CPTCI and other study measures

		CPTCI total	CPTCI-PC	CPTCI-SW	CPTCI-S
1.	CPTCI total	–	.97	.96	.98
2.	CPTCI-PC		–	.85	.96
3.	CPTCI-SW			–	.91
4.	CPTCI-S				–
5.	CRIES				
	r	.80	.77	.78	.79
	rp	.61	.57	.50	.56
6.	TSCC-PT				
	r	.78	.74	.78	.77
	rp	.54	.48	.51	.51
7.	CDI	.76	.77	.77	.74
8.	RCMAS	.71	.73	.73	.69

r correlation coefficient, *rp* partial correlation coefficients between the CPTCI and other study measures controlling for CDI and RCMAS, *CPTCI total* Total Score of Korean version of Child Post-Traumatic Cognitions Inventory, *CPTCI-PC* Permanent and disturbing Change subscale of the CPTCI, *CPTCI-SW* fragile person in a scary world subscale of the CPTCI, *CPTCI-S* Short form of the CPTCI, *CRIES* Children's Revised Impact of Event Scale, *TSCC-PT* post-traumatic stress subscale of the Traumatic Symptom Checklist for Children, *CAPS* Children's Attributions and Perceptions Scale, *CDI* Children's Depression Inventory, *RCMAS* Revised Children's Manifest Anxiety Scale. All correlations $p < .001$

and RCMAS scores. The results showed that the correlations among CPTCI total score, CPTCI-PC, and CPTCI-SW remained strong. The partial correlation coefficients between CPTCI and CRIES scores ranged from .50 to .61, and those between CPTCI and TSCC-PT scores ranged from .48 to .54 (Table 4).When comparing CPTCI scores and PTSD symptoms severity by age groups, similar correlations were observed between CPTCI scores and PTSD symptom severity (.68–.85). Though the correlations coefficients tend to be the stronger in the older group(15–16 years old), they did not differed significantly per age group.

Discriminant validity

Table 5 shows the results of comparing two groups considering differences in their CPTCI total score and scores for the subscales and the short form corresponding to differences in the severity of PTSD symptoms. The high PTSD-risk group ($n = 152$) and the low PTSD-risk group (n = 85) showed significant differences in various CPTCI scores (Table 5). All between groups differences were very large (all d's > 1.92).

Differences by age group, phase and type of trauma

CPTCI scores by age group, phase following traumatic stressor and type of trauma are listed in Table 5. Based on the PTSD diagnostic criteria, acute/chronic groups were divided on a monthly basis. All the indices show that there were no significant differences in CPTCI scores between acute and chronic group; however, there were significant differences in CPTCI scores per age group as shown in the results of the ANOVA, CPTCI total score: $F(2,234) = 10.19$, $p < .001$; CPTCI-PC: $F(2,234) = 8.95$, $p < .001$; CPTCI-SW: $F(2,234) = 9.38$, $p < .001$; and CPTCI-S: $F(2,234) = 9.38$, $p < .001$. Scheffé's post hoc test results showed that there were significant differences in all the scores except those for CPTCI-PC at the p = .05 level between 8 and 11-year-olds and 12- to 14-year-olds and between 8 and 11-year-olds and 15- to 16-year-olds. As for CPTCI-PC scores, the difference between 8 and 11-year-olds and 15- to 16-year-olds was significant. In all indices, an older age was accompanied by higher scores. Individuals were classified into two subgroups regarding types of sexual trauma they experienced. These subgroups differed on the CPTCI index scores, CPTCI total score: $t = 2.69$, $p = .008$; CPTCI-PC: $t = 2.73$, $p = .007$; CPTCI-SW: $t = 2.31$, $p = .022$; CPTCI-S: $t = 2.83$, $p = .005$; (Table 5).

Discussion

We investigated the psychometric properties of the Korean version of the CPTCI by examining child and adolescent survivors of sexual violence in Korea. This study is the first to validate the CPTCI among Koreans and the first to apply the scale in a sample of survivors exposed to one specific type of trauma (i.e., sexual violence).

Our confirmatory factor analysis revealed that the original two-factor model has the best fit to data among the 25-item models subjected to comparison. Additionally, each of the two factors is loaded on all the items at appropriate levels in the factor matrix, which seems to support the two-factor model. Moreover, model comparison via the χ^2 test showed that the original two-factor model was superior to the one-factor model [23]. Nevertheless, it was revealed that some model fit values for the original two-factor model fell short of the criteria set based on earlier studies.

The 20-item Chinese version showed better fit indices than the original version. This finding may have significant implications for understanding cultural effects on response to trauma. In this model, the items 3 (I am a coward), 12 (I have to watch out for danger all the time), and 25 (I have to be really careful because something bad could happen) were deleted because their standardized factor loadings were insufficient [24]. Researchers inferred that in Chinese culture, such cognitions of preparing for dangers are common in parenting and are internalized in children's self-discipline. It is interesting to note that the current study also found that Item 3,

Table 5 Comparison of Korean CPTCI scores by sample characteristics

	CPTCI total					CPTCI-PC				CPTCI-SW				CPTCI-S			
	n	m	sd	t or F	d or ε²	m	sd	t or F	d or ε²	m	sd	t or F	d or ε²	m	sd	t or F	d or ε²
				F	ε²			F	ε²			F	ε²			F	ε²
Age groups[a]																	
8–11 (1)	76	45.17	17.84	10.19**	.087	21.03	9.08	8.95**	.077	24.42	9.36	9.38**	.080	17.04	7.18	10.35**	.089
12–14 (2)	106	53.16	18.82			24.53	10.53			28.63	9.16			20.39	8.30		
15–16 (3)	55	59.96	19.81			28.69	11.03			31.27	9.24			23.40	8.25		
				t	d			t	d			t	d			t	d
Type of trauma																	
Rape	94	56.31	19.22	2.69*	.35	26.66	10.54	2.73*	.36	29.65	9.30	2.31	.32	21.85	8.04	2.83*	.38
Sexual abuse other than rape	143	49.46	19.21			22.88	10.33			26.74	9.60			18.79	8.21		
				t	d			t	d			t	d			t	d
Time since trauma																	
Less than 1 month	138	52.72	19.58	.36	.05	24.63	10.85	.43	.06	28.09	9.47	.25	.03	20.22	8.45	.37	.05
More than 1 month	99	51.78	19.12			24.02	10.31			27.76	9.55			19.80	8.11		
				t	d			t	d			t	d			t	d
PTSD symptoms																	
Higher	152	62.03	16.74	14.14**	2.07	29.41	9.72	15.99**	1.92	32.61	8.03	15.05**	1.92	24.06	7.32	13.37**	1.98
Lower	85	34.56	8.44			15.29	3.64			19.46	5.38			12.73	3.49		

CPTCI Child Post-traumatic Cognitions Inventory, *CPTCI-PC* permanent and disturbing change subscale of the CPTCI, *CPTCI-SW* fragile person in a scary world subscale of the CPTCI, *CPTCI-S* Short form of the CPTCI

* $p < .01$, ** $p < .001$

[a] Comparisons of the three groups by Sheffe post-test

12 and 25 yielded relatively low factor loadings in CFA. A possible explanation for this similarity might be that Confucianism-based societal norms that East Asian societies have in common.

Nevertheless, we did not adopt the model for following reasons. First, although goodness-of-fit values of the model are better than those of the original model, they still fell short of the criteria set based on earlier studies, and are inferior to those of the CPTCI-S. Second, the version does not include one of the items which consist the CPTCI-S, making it difficult used along with the short form. Third, the item selection was based on the results of CFA in the study which it originates, which can be methodologically problematic. Last, utilizing the version which comprises different items from the original one would not allow the opportunity to compare research on the CPTCI across the regions.

The repetitive failures of different versions of the CPTCI to replicate the original factor structure seems to be related to the characteristic of different sample. In the original study, Researchers have raised the possibility that being at different stages of post-traumatic reactions may have an impact on factor structure and factor loadings. The participants in this study, in many cases, completed the questionnaire when they had visited the support center to receive crisis intervention immediately after their exposure to sexual violence. It is believed that trauma-related cognitions exhibited during the acute phase of traumatic stress may differ in kind and degree from cognitions exhibited after some passage of time when they have naturally recovered or become negatively distorted and consolidated [15, 43, 44].

Furthermore, the type of trauma experienced by the sample group in this study differs from that experienced by the samples in the original study. The original study used its scale on children who were exposed to a single traumatic event; more specifically, a traffic accident or a violent incident, and derived its factor structure from this basis. Therefore, negative cognitions related to physical injury and internal vulnerability could have become more salient. In contrast, this study was conducted with child and adolescent survivors of sexual violence, representing a mix of single, multiple, or complex trauma survivors. Other studies that have translated and validated the CPTCI, unlike the original study, included many participants who were exposed to continuous trauma like sexual violence and abuse. These studies have likewise reported that they could not confirm a good enough model fit for the original two-factor structure [17, 22, 23].

The CPTCI was shown to be highly correlated with scales measuring PTSD symptoms, depression, and anxiety. This may be due to the fact that PTSD symptoms are frequently accompanied by depression and anxiety, and

it is consistent with findings from previous studies that showed high correlations between post-traumatic cognitions and depression and anxiety symptoms in children and adolescents [15, 17, 22, 45]. PTSD symptoms and CPTCI scores were significantly correlated even when depression and anxiety scores were controlled for, indicating that the correlation between these two sets of variables is not merely an artifact due to depression or anxiety, but rather due to cognitions and responses specific to traumatic experiences that are shared between the two sets of variables. Traumatic experiences are associated not only with PTSD, but also with various types of psychopathology, and it seems possible to examine post-traumatic cognitions as a transdiagnostic target of therapy and intervention [17, 19, 46, 47].

Earlier studies found that there were no significant differences in CPTCI results per age [15, 17]. However, we revealed the opposite. However, the sample characteristics may have affected our results. Previous studies reported that adolescent survivors of sexual violence are closely associated with more violent and severe assault characteristics like penetrative sexual assault, paid sex, brokering, and exhibit more serious and extensive psychological aftereffects than do child survivors [48, 49]. The adolescents included in the sample of this study also had a higher rate of exposure to rape rather than non-penetrative sexual harassment when compared to children, and their experiences were frequently accompanied by physical violence, multiple assailants, and so on. Other reasons for the CPTCI score differences per age may be related to cognitive and emotional development. In adolescence, more elaborate and complex emotions develop, and there is also the maturing of one's self-concept and self-consciousness. Accordingly, one's post-traumatic cognitions concerning threats to oneself, which are also one's higher cognitions mediating secondary emotions, tend to become negatively distorted and exaggerated [48, 50–52]. Therefore, it is necessary to consider such age characteristics when interpreting the CPTCI results. In addition, future studies need to investigate whether CPTCI reveals any differences per age in the severity and persistence of maladaptation and psychological distress resulting from exposure to sexual violence. As for sex differences, which were not evident, the sample included few male survivors; therefore, it is difficult to interpret and generalize the research findings in this respect.

We also sought to verify the reliability and validity of the CPTCI-S. It was confirmed that the internal consistency, convergent validity, and discriminant validity of the CPTCI-S were similar to those of the CPTCI's total score. Moreover, our confirmatory factor analysis showed that CPTCI-S had better overall model fit than the original 25-item scale, which was consistent with previous findings [21]. Among the fit indices for the CPTCI-S, the RMSEA did not have a good fit; however, this may be because the index in question has the property of yielding poor fit when there are only a few items or measurement variables and consequently few degrees of freedom [53]. When other indices such as the CFI, TLI, and SRMR were considered, they support the two-factor structure. Consequently, the CPTCI-S is expected to be useful in clinical practice and its subscales seem amenable to interpretation.

This study had some limitations. First, instead of using structured interviews with clinicians to perform PTSD diagnoses, the cutoff point for the self-report CRIES was used to distinguish the high PTSD-risk group and the low PTSD-risk group. The Korean version of the CRIES was found to have high sensitivity (.88) and specificity (.85; [35]); therefore, we felt it could be used to diagnose PTSD with relative accuracy. However, it is necessary to confirm the validity of the CPTCI through more precise criteria in the future. Second, formal backward translation has not been done. Third, this study was conducted only on survivors of sexual violence; therefore, it is difficult to generalize our results to groups exposed to other types of trauma. However, it must be made clear that this limitation is at the same time a strength of this study. Previous studies have shown that CPTCI scores and its factor structure may vary per type of trauma [15]. For this reason, the original CPTCI paper mentioned the need to apply the scale to various types of samples. Until now, however, no studies had confirmed the psychometric properties of CPTCI as applied solely to survivors of sexual violence. Another limitation is gross underrepresentation of males in the sample. Due to nature of the sexual violence, the sample consists mostly of females. Further study is needed to identify the characteristics of male survivors of the sexual assault.

Despite these limitations, this study is the first to use the CPTCI on child and adolescent survivors of sexual violence, thereby adding new evidence on the scale's applicability. The present study may extend our understanding of the CPTCI by validating the scale in a different cultural context to previous studies, and in a homogenous sample regarding types of trauma. Further research should be undertaken to investigate the utility of the CPTCI and distinct response patterns considering types of trauma, the phases of response to trauma, and cultural differences.

Conclusion

This study investigated the psychometric properties of the CPTCI among child and adolescent survivors of sexual violence in Korea. In general, the scale was found to be a valid instrument for measuring dysfunctional trauma-related cognitions. Moreover, the CPTCI-S was also confirmed to have excellent psychometric properties. Therefore, the Korean versions of the CPTCI and CPTCI-S are valuable tools that can be used in clinical and research settings to better understand the psychological mechanisms behind the responses of children and adolescents who have been exposed to trauma.

Abbreviations
CPTCI: Child Post-Traumatic Cognitions Inventory; PTSD: post-traumatic stress disorder; CRIES: Children's Revised Impact of Event Scale; TSCC: Traumatic Symptom Checklist for Children; CAPS: Children's Attributions and Perceptions Scale; CDI: Children's Depression Inventory; RCMAS: Revised Children's Manifest Anxiety Scale; CPTCI-PC: permanent and disturbing change subscale of the CPTCI; CPTCI-SW: fragile person in a scary world subscale of the CPTCI; CFI: comparative fit index; TLI: Tucker–Lewis index; RMSEA: root mean square error of approximation; CI: confidence interval; SRMR: standardized root mean square error of approximation.

Authors' contributions
HYC and KMS designed the study. HYC and HBL wrote the draft of the paper. YKC, YJS oversaw the whole process and provided critical comments. KMS, HBL and MH collected and organized the data from the Sexual Assault Center. USC, SMB and NK helped the statistical analysis and validation process. All authors read and approved the final manuscript.

Author details
[1] Sunflower Center of Southern Gyeonggi for Women and Children Victims of Violence, Suwon, Republic of Korea. [2] Hanyang Cyber University, Seoul, Republic of Korea. [3] Department of Psychiatry and Behavioral Sciences, Ajou University School of Medicine, 164 World Cup-ro, Yeongtong-gu, Suwon, Suwon-si 16409, Republic of Korea. [4] Center for Traumatic Stress, Ajou University Medical Center, Suwon, Republic of Korea. [5] Yonsei University College of Medicine, Seoul, Republic of Korea. [6] Kyungpook National University Hospital, Daegu, Republic of Korea. [7] Gil Hospital, Gachon University College of Medicine, Incheon, Republic of Korea. [8] Myongji Hospital, Seonam University College of Medicine, Goyang, Republic of Korea.

Acknowledgements
This work was supported by Ministry of Gender Equality and Family, Republic of Korea. The sponsor did not play a role in the design of the study, the collection, analysis, and interpretation of the data, the writing of this manuscript, or the decision to submit the article for publication.

Competing interests
The authors declare that they have no competing interests.

Funding
Not applicable.

References

1. Bonanno GA. Loss, trauma, and human resilience: have we underestimated the human capacity to thrive after extremely aversive events? Am Psychol. 2004;59(1):20.
2. Layne CM, Warren JS, Watson PJ, Shalev AY. Risk, vulnerability, resistance, and resilience: toward an integrative conceptualization of posttraumatic adaptation. In: Friedman MJ, Keane TM, Resick PA, editors. Handbook of PTSD: science and practice. New York: Guilford Press; 2007. p. 497–520.
3. Dalgleish T. Cognitive approaches to posttraumatic stress disorder: the evolution of multirepresentational theorizing. Psychol Bull. 2004;130(2):228–60.
4. Dalgleish T, Meiser-Stedman R, Smith P. Cognitive aspects of posttraumatic stress reactions and their treatment in children and adolescents: an empirical review and some recommendations. Behav Cogn Psychother. 2005;33(04):459–86.
5. Ehlers A, Clark DM. A cognitive model of posttraumatic stress disorder. Behav Res Ther. 2000;38(4):319–45.
6. Foa EB, Ehlers A, Clark DM, Tolin DF, Orsillo SM. The posttraumatic cognitions inventory (PTCI): development and validation. Psychol Assess. 1999;11(3):303.
7. American Psychiatric Association. Diagnostic and statistical manual of mental disorders (DSM-5®). Philadelphia: American Psychiatric Pub; 2013.
8. Müller J, Wessa M, Flor H, Rabe S, Dörfel D, Knaevelsrud C, Maercker A, Karl A. Psychometric properties of the Posttraumatic Cognitions Inventory (PTCI) in a German sample of individuals with a history of trauma. Psychol Trauma. 2010;2(2):116–25.
9. van Emmerik AA, Schoorl M, Emmelkamp PM, Kamphuis JH. Psychometric evaluation of the Dutch version of the posttraumatic cognitions inventory (PTCI). Behav Res Ther. 2006;44(7):1053–65.
10. Shin KM, Chung YK, Kim NH, Kim KA, Chang HY. Factor structure and reliability of the Posttraumatic Cognitions Inventory (PTCI) in Korean female victims of sexual violence. J Interpers Violence. In press.
11. Su YJ, Chen SH. The posttraumatic cognitions inventory-Chinese revised: validation and refinement with a traumatized college sample in Taiwan. J Anxiety Disord. 2008;22(7):1110–9.
12. Ehlers A, Mayou RA, Bryant B. Cognitive predictors of posttraumatic stress disorder in children: results of a prospective longitudinal study. Behav Res Ther. 2003;41(1):1–10.
13. Meiser-Stedman R. Towards a cognitive–behavioral model of PTSD in children and adolescents. Clin Child Fam Psychol Rev. 2002;5(4):217–32.
14. Stallard P. A retrospective analysis to explore the applicability of the Ehlers and Clark (2000) cognitive model to explain PTSD in children. Behav Cogn Psychother. 2003;31(3):337–45.
15. Meiser-Stedman R, Smith P, Bryant R, Salmon K, Yule W, Dalgleish T, Nixon RD. Development and validation of the Child Post-Traumatic Cognitions Inventory (CPTCI). J Child Psychol Psychiatry. 2009;50(4):432–40.
16. Pfeiffer E, Sachser C, de Haan A, Tutus D, Goldbeck L. Dysfunctional posttraumatic cognitions as a mediator of symptom reduction in Trauma-Focused Cognitive Behavioral Therapy with children and adolescents: results of a randomized controlled trial. Behav Res Ther. 2017;97:178–82.
17. Diehle J, de Roos C, Meiser-Stedman R, Boer F, Lindauer RJ. The Dutch version of the Child Posttraumatic Cognitions Inventory: validation in a clinical sample and a school sample. Eur J Psychotraumatol. 2015;6:26362.
18. Nixon RD, Sterk J, Pearce A, Weber N. A randomized trial of cognitive behavior therapy and cognitive therapy for children with posttraumatic stress disorder following single-incident trauma: predictors and outcome at 1-year follow-up. Psychol Trauma. 2016;9(4):471–8.
19. Smith P, Yule W, Perrin S, Tranah T, Dalgleish T, Clark DM. Cognitive-behavioral therapy for PTSD in children and adolescents: a preliminary randomized controlled trial. J Am Acad Child Adolesc Psychiatry. 2007;46(8):1051–61.
20. Meiser-Stedman R, Smith P, McKinnon A, Dixon C, Trickey D, Ehlers A, Clark DM, Boyle A, Watson P, Goodyer I. Cognitive therapy as an early treatment for post-traumatic stress disorder in children and adolescents: a randomized controlled trial addressing preliminary efficacy and mechanisms of action. J Child Psychol Psychiatry. 2017;58(5):623–33.
21. McKinnon A, Smith P, Bryant R, Salmon K, Yule W, Dalgleish T, Dixon C, Nixon RD, Meiser-Stedman R. An update on the clinical utility of the Children's Post-Traumatic Cognitions Inventory. J Trauma Stress. 2016;29(3):253–8.
22. de Haan A, Petermann F, Meiser-Stedman R, Goldbeck L. Psychometric properties of the German version of the Child Post-Traumatic Cognitions Inventory (CPTCI-GER). Child Psychiatry Hum Dev. 2016;47(1):151–8.
23. Lobo BO, Brunnet AE, Ecker KK, Schaefer LS, Arteche AX, Gauer G, Kristensen CH. Psychometric properties of the Child Posttraumatic Cognitions Inventory in a sample of Brazilian children. J Aggress Maltreat Trauma. 2015;24(8):863–75.
24. Liu S-T, Chen S-H. A community study on the relationship of posttraumatic cognitions to internalizing and externalizing psychopathology in Taiwanese children and adolescents. J Abnorm Child Psychol. 2015;43(8):1475–84.
25. Browne MW, Cudeck R, Bollen KA, Long JS. Alternative ways of assessing model fit. Sage Focus Editions. 1993;154:136.
26. Hurley AE, Scandura TA, Schriesheim CA, Brannick MT, Seers A, Vandenberg RJ, Williams LJ. Exploratory and confirmatory factor analysis: guidelines, issues, and alternatives. J Organ Behav. 1997;18(6):667–83.
27. Kessler RC, Rose S, Koenen KC, Karam EG, Stang PE, Stein DJ, Heeringa SG, Hill ED, Liberzon I, McLaughlin KA, et al. How well can post-traumatic stress disorder be predicted from pre-trauma risk factors? An exploratory study in the WHO World Mental Health Surveys. World Psychiatry. 2014;13(3):265–74.
28. Finkelhor D. Early and long-term effects of child sexual abuse: an update. Prof Psychol Res Pract. 1990;21(5):325.
29. Saywitz KJ, Mannarino AP, Berliner L, Cohen JA. Treatment of sexually abused children and adolescents. Am Psychol. 2000;55(9):1040.
30. Shin KM, Cho SM, Lee SH, Chung YK. A pilot prospective study of the relationship among cognitive factors, shame, and guilt proneness on posttraumatic stress disorder symptoms in female victims of sexual violence. J Korean Med Sci. 2014;29(6):831–6.
31. Startup M, Makgekgenene L, Webster R. The role of self-blame for trauma as assessed by the Posttraumatic Cognitions Inventory (PTCI): a self-protective cognition? Behav Res Ther. 2007;45(2):395–403.
32. Cohen JA, Mannarino AP, Knudsen K. Treating sexually abused children: 1 year follow-up of a randomized controlled trial. Child Abuse Negl. 2005;29(2):135–45.
33. Harvey ST, Taylor JE. A meta-analysis of the effects of psychotherapy with sexually abused children and adolescents. Clin Psychol Rev. 2010;30(5):517–35.
34. Smith P, Perrin S, Dyregrov A, Yule W. Principal components analysis of the impact of event scale with children in war. Pers Individ Differ. 2003;34(2):315–22.
35. Oh EA, Park EJ, Lee SH, Bae SM. Validation of the Korean version of the Children's Revised Impact of Event Scale. Clin Psychopharmacol Neurosci. 2014;12(2):149–56.
36. Briere J. Trauma symptom checklist for children. Odessa: Psychological Assessment Resources; 1996.
37. Reynolds CR, Richmond BO. Revised children's manifest anxiety scale. Los Angeles: Western Psychological Services; 1985.
38. Choi JS, Cho SC. Assessment of anxiety in children-reliability and validity of revised Children's Manifest Anxiety Scale. 신경정신의학 (Neuropsychology). 1990;29(3):691–702.
39. Kovacs M. Children's depression inventory: manual. North Tonawanda: Multi-Health Systems; 1992.
40. Arbuckle JL. Amos 18 user's guide. Crawfordville: Amos Development Corporation; 2007.
41. Lt Hu. Bentler PM: cutoff criteria for fit indexes in covariance structure analysis: Conventional criteria versus new alternatives. Struct Equ Model Multidiscip J. 1999;6(1):1–55.
42. Spss I. PASW statistics 18. Chicago: SPSS Inc; 2009.
43. Dalgleish T, Meiser-Stedman R, Kassam-Adams N, Ehlers A, Winston F, Smith P, Bryant B, Mayou RA, Yule W. Predictive validity of acute stress disorder in children and adolescents. Br J Psychiatry. 2008;192(5):392–3.
44. Meiser-Stedman R, McKinnon A, Dixon C, Boyle A, Smith P, Dalgleish T. Acute stress disorder and the transition to posttraumatic stress disorder in children and adolescents: prevalence, course, prognosis, diagnostic suitability, and risk markers. Depress Anxiety. 2017;34:348–55.

45. Hyland P, Murphy J, Shevlin M, Murphy S, Egan A, Boduszek D. Psychometric properties of the Posttraumatic Cognition Inventory within a Northern Ireland adolescent sample. Br J Clin Psychol. 2015;54(4):435–49.
46. Kleim B, Grey N, Wild J, Nussbeck FW, Stott R, Hackmann A, Clark DM, Ehlers A. Cognitive change predicts symptom reduction with cognitive therapy for posttraumatic stress disorder. J Consult Clin Psychol. 2013;81(3):383–93.
47. Meiser-Stedman R, Smith P, McKinnon A, Dixon C, Trickey D, Ehlers A, Clark DM, Boyle A, Watson P, Goodyer I et al. Cognitive therapy as an early treatment for post-traumatic stress disorder in children and adolescents: a randomized controlled trial addressing preliminary efficacy and mechanisms of action. J Child Psychol Psychiatry. 2016.
48. Feiring C, Taska L, Lewis M. Age and gender differences in children's and adolescents' adaptation to sexual abuse. Child Abuse Negl. 1999;23(2):115–28.

49. Yoon D-K, Lee M, Chang M, Joo J-S, Song H-J. Analysis of sex crime trends against children and the youth in 2015: with focus on sex offenders registered in 2014. Seoul: Ministry of Gender Equality and Family, Korea; 2015.
50. Finkelhor D. The victimization of children: a developmental perspective. Am J Orthopsychiatry. 1995;65(2):177–93.
51. Fletcher KE. Understanding and assessing traumatic responses of guilt, shame, and anger among children, adolescents, and young adults. J Child Adolesc Trauma. 2011;4(4):339–60.
52. Wolfe DA, Sas L, Wekerle C. Factors associated with the development of posttraumatic stress disorder among child victims of sexual abuse. Child Abuse Negl. 1994;18(1):37–50.
53. Kenny DA, Kaniskan B, McCoach DB. The performance of RMSEA in models with small degrees of freedom. Sociol Methods Res. 2015;44(3):486–507.

Effectiveness of a cognitive behavioural therapy-based anxiety prevention programme at an elementary school in Japan: a quasi-experimental study

Yuko Urao[1]* , Michiko Yoshida[2], Takako Koshiba[5], Yasunori Sato[3], Shin-ichi Ishikawa[4] and Eiji Shimizu[1,2]

Abstract

Background: The efficacy of cognitive behavioural therapy (CBT) for anxiety related problems in children is empirically supported. In addition, universal anxiety prevention programmes based on CBT have been demonstrated in recent years. The purpose of this study was to verify the effectiveness of a CBT based original programme 'Journey of the Brave,' aiming to prevent anxiety disorders and anxiety-related problems for Japanese children aged 10–12 years old.

Methods: Intervention groups from two classes of 5th grade elementary students ($n = 41$) received ten 45-min programme sessions. The control group was drawn from one class of 5th grade children ($n = 31$) from a nearby school. All participants completed the Spence Children's Anxiety Scale (SCAS) at pre, post, and 3 months follow-up. Mixed-effects model for repeated measures analysis was conducted.

Results: The mean anxiety score on the SCAS for the intervention group was significantly reduced at both post intervention and 3 months follow-up compared with the control group. The group differences on the SCAS from baseline to post-test were -5.321 (95% CI -10.12 to -0.523, $p = 0.030$), and at the 3-month follow-up were -7.104 (95% CI -11.90 to -2.306, $p = 0.004$).

Conclusions: The effectiveness of the anxiety prevention programme 'Journey of the Brave' was verified though this study using a quasi-experimental design on a small sample.

Keywords: Anxiety, Prevention, Cognitive behavioural therapy, Elementary school, Universal, Japan

Background

Anxiety disorders are the most common mental health problem in children and adolescents [1] with lifetime prevalence rates averaging between 8 and 27% [2]. Despite the high prevalence rates, many children and adolescents remain undiagnosed and untreated [3].

Children and adolescents with anxiety symptoms and disorders suffer from considerable adverse effects on their psychosocial functioning [4]. For example, many studies report that anxiety symptoms in childhood significantly interfere with children's interpersonal functioning, self-esteem, social competencies, and academic achievement [1, 5, 6]. Moreover, comorbidity between anxiety and other psychological disorders is common, and there is evidence suggesting that anxiety disorders may precede the onset of other psychological disorders including depression [7–9].

Because of the high prevalence rates and considerable adverse effects of anxiety symptoms and disorders, the

*Correspondence: yurao@faculty.chiba-u.jp
[1] Research Centre for Child Mental Development, Chiba University
Graduate School of Medicine, 1-8-1 Inohana, Chuo-ku, Chiba 260-8670,
Japan
Full list of author information is available at the end of the article

need to prevent anxiety disorders in children is paramount. The application of prevention science to reduce anxiety disorders, however, is in its infancy [10].

There are three approaches to addressing mental disorders of children: (1) universal approach, (2) selective approach, and (3) indicated approach [11]. The universal approach works with all children, including those who have no disorder symptoms, while the selective approach targets children with specific risks and the indicated approach is for those with subclinical signs or symptoms [12]. In 2000, Offord summarized the advantages of universal programmes as avoiding participants' stigma, such as the labelling effects of being singled out, and reaching those with a wide range of risk factors rather than those with a limited number of factors [13].

Studies attempting to verify the effectiveness of anxiety prevention programmes for children have been gradually increasing since 2000. Several studies have systematically reviewed the effectiveness of various preventive programmes and suggested that many universal, selected, and indicated approach programmes demonstrate effectiveness with small to medium effect sizes [3, 4, 14, 15].

Cognitive behavioural therapy (CBT) is a psychological treatment method which has been verified to be effective against anxiety disorders in children in many studies in both individual [16, 17] and group formats [18, 19]. Currently, it is suggested that CBT is one of the evidence-based treatments for anxiety disorders in children [20, 21]. The FRIENDS programme has been verified to be effective not only for treatment of children with anxiety disorders but also as a preventive intervention. FRIENDS was originally developed by modifying the Coping Cat programme [22] which was developed by Kendall in the USA for the treatment of children's anxiety disorders. The effectiveness of the FRIENDS programme conducted with the universal approach has been verified in various random block design studies from the early 2000's [23–26]. Effectiveness trials of the FRIENDS programme have been conducted in several countries and are ongoing [27–29]. Moreover, a new trend is emerging. Specifically, country-adapted programs which are designed to be suitable for children in specific countries are being developed and examined. For example, Collins and colleagues [30] studied the effects of a universal school-based mental health intervention in schools in Scotland and reported significant anxiety reduction and improved coping at post-intervention and again at a 6-month follow-up compared with a comparison group who received regular personal and social education (PSE) sessions [30]. In a randomized controlled trial, Calear and colleagues in Australia randomly assigned children from three schools to intervention and control groups, and although children in the intervention group only undertook an online

CBT based anxiety prevention programme, there were no significant score differences between groups on anxiety, depression, and other measures of mental wellbeing at post programme and follow-up timepoints [31].

While evidence of the effectiveness of CBT based anxiety prevention programmes has been compiled overseas, the progress of research and implementation is very slow and there is little mental health education targeting anxiety prevention in Japan. In this country, anxiety issues are handled in the mental health sessions of Physical Education classes of 5th grade elementary school children with remarks such as 'In order to deal with anxiety issues, there are options such as to consult, to play, and to exercise'. Furthermore, only three 45-min sessions of class time are allocated [32] and there is no systematic education based on psychiatry or psychology.

Under these circumstances, adapting an anxiety prevention programme proven effective in western countries to Japanese school classes is promising. However, there are many potential obstacles such as time requirements (ten sessions plus a booster session of 60–120 min/session), personnel and financial costs (teacher training and workbook), and introduction methods (group work format, parent/facilitator participation desired, etc.). It has been pointed out that 'the programme which turned out to be effective in preceding studies in other countries is not always successful in this country' [33]. Therefore, it is necessary to develop an adapted programme and examine its effectiveness in Japanese schools.

We developed a new CBT based anxiety disorder prevention programme, 'Journey of the Brave,' for Japanese children [34]. The pilot study indicated a significant improvement in anxiety scores on parents' evaluation at 3 months compared with the control group, although there was no significant improvement in children's reports. In addition, equal or better effect sizes were found in both children's ($d = 0.72$) and parents' ($d = 0.65$) ratings in comparison with the sizes shown by previous research [3, 14]. Therefore, effectiveness and feasibility of the 'Journey of the Brave' programme were partially demonstrated, although its feasibility and effectiveness should be addressed in more robust future research, especially in regular Japanese school classrooms. As such, this study examined the effectiveness of the programme for anxiety symptoms in children when implemented in a regular school class as part of the school curriculum.

Methods

Study design and participants

This was a universal quasi-experimental study with an intervention and a control group. Intervention group participants received the anxiety prevention programme and control group participants received no intervention.

The intervention group consisted of 41 5th grade children (10–11 years old, two classes) attending an elementary school in City A adjacent to Tokyo. The control group consisted of one class with 31 children of the same age at another nearby elementary school in the same city. The control group school was selected based on the nomination from the principal of the intervention group school.

The research design for this study involved measuring children's anxiety levels across three time points during the school year. Data were collected at pre-test (Time 1; week 0), post-test (Time 2; month 6), and follow-up (FU; Time 3; 3-months following post-test).

Intervention—Journey of the Brave

The following is a summary of the 'Journey of the Brave' programme.

This programme consists of ten 45-min sessions and the contents are taught according to a workbook and teacher's manual (Table 1). The first half of the programme is dedicated to the development of anxiety stairs and the experience of exposure, while the second half mainly concerns cognitive restructuring. More precisely, after psychological education regarding anxious feelings (i.e., anxiety is a natural feeling everybody has and plays an important role in protecting you from danger, but if excessive anxiety persists, it may lead to disturbances in life, etc.), each child is encouraged to establish his or her own goal throughout the program such as to make a presentation in front of all the children, to remain alone in a dark room, and so on. In stage 3, relaxation skills such as breathing methods and muscle relaxation are taught. In stage 4, children develop the anxiety stairs table to reach the goal set in stage 2. Stages 5, 6, and 7 encompass the process of gradually learning the cognitive model (the relationship between cognition, behaviour, emotion, and body reaction) as well as cognitive restructuring. At the

Table 1 Contents of 'Journey of the Brave' by session

Session	Content of Journey of the Brave
1	Understanding of four basic feelings
2	Monitoring feelings of anxiety and setting goals
3	Body reactions and relaxation
4	Anxiety level stages and stair step exposure
5	Anxiety cognition model
6	Identify cognitive distortions and coping with rumination
7	Cognitive restructuring when anxious
8	Assertiveness skills to reduce social stress
9	Review
10	Summary

same time, gradual exposure homework to address anxiety proceeds in accordance with the anxiety stairs table developed in stage 4. Assertion skills to reduce interpersonal anxiety are taught in stage 8, stage 9 is the overall review session, and stage 10 is the summary and graduation ceremony.

In the workbook used by the children, actual examples of many anxiety-provoking moments in their daily life are raised so that they can deepen their understanding of anxious feelings and CBT.

Procedure

The 45-min 'Journey of the Brave' programme sessions were conducted in the intervention group over 6 months from October 2013 to March 2014 at a pace of twice a month, although no sessions were held during winter holidays.

Each session started with a PowerPoint presentation and workbook and homework sheets were distributed. Homework to consolidate the content learned was given at the end of each session to be worked on at home and returned by the next session.

The actual intervention was conducted by TK who is an expert (MA) in education psychology. She met with the programme author YU prior to each session to discuss facilitation. In addition, YU supported the facilitator in the class during the session and the teacher in charge of the class was also present providing partial support.

Children in the control group followed the regular school curriculum led by the classroom teacher.

Each of the 45-min sessions were conducted with the intervention group children in regular classes. The programme contents were supervised by a MD/PhD university professor who is a CBT expert.

Measurements

Primary-outcome measure

SCAS: Spence Children's Anxiety Scale   The primary outcome measure was the Spence Children's Anxiety Scale (SCAS) which is one of the most valid self-reported measures for assessing child anxiety meeting diagnostic standards for 8- to 15-year-old children [35]. Reliability and validity of the SCAS Japanese version has been confirmed [36]. The SCAS includes 38 items regarding children's anxiety symptoms divided into six subcategories: separation anxiety, social phobia, panic disorder/agoraphobia, generalized anxiety disorder, physical injury fears, and obsessive–compulsive disorder. The SCAS item scores range between 0 (never) and 3 (always) and the maximum possible score is 114. According to a previous study, the average SCAS score of 7 to 12-year old children was 20.51 (SD = 14.20) and the cut-off point was 42 [37].

Furthermore, one additional question was added as the 39th question—'Are any of the items severely negatively affecting your daily life?'—to be answered in the same 0–3 scale to evaluate the degree of severity of the anxiety symptoms affecting the child's daily life.

Secondary-outcome measure

SDQ: Strengths and Difficulties Questionnaire   The secondary outcome measure was the self-report version of the Goodman Strengths and Difficulties Questionnaire (SDQ) [38]. The SDQ includes 25 items, each scored 0 (not true), 1 (somewhat true), or 2 (certainly true) according to the perceived severity of the symptom. The items are divided into five subcategories: emotional symptoms, behaviour problems, hyperactivity/inattention, peer relationship problems, and pro-social behaviour. A total difficulty score is computed by summing scores of the first four sub categories and the maximum possible score is 40.

Statistical analysis

The statistical analysis and reporting of this trial were conducted in accordance with the CONSORT guidelines, with the primary analyses based on the intent-to-treat principle. For baseline variables, summary statistics were constructed using frequencies and proportions for categorical data and means and SDs for continuous variables.

The participant characteristics were compared using Chi squared tests for gender differences and t tests for baseline score differences between the intervention and control group.

Primary analysis was performed with the mixed-effects model for repeated measures (MMRM) with treatment group, time, and interactions between treatment group and time as fixed effects; an unstructured covariate was used to model the covariance of within-subject variability. MMRM analysis assumes that any missing data occur randomly. The secondary analysis was performed in the same manner as the primary analysis. All comparisons were planned and all p-values were two-sided. A p-value < 0.05 was considered statistically significant. All statistical analyses were performed using the SAS software program, version 9.4 (SAS Institute, Cary, NC, U.S.A.) and SPSS Version 22.0 (IBM, Armonk, New York, USA).

Results

Gender-based differences in participant characteristics were examined with Chi square tests between the 41 intervention group (male = 21, female = 20) and 31 control group (male = 16, female = 15) children at pre-test. There were no significant differences ($p = 0.974$). Next,

to compare the group differences at baseline, t tests were conducted of the pre-test SCAS and SDQ scores. The intervention group demonstrated significantly higher scores on the two measures than the control group (SCAS: $p < 0.01$, SDQ: $p < 0.01$).

All ten sessions were held in the classroom of the intervention group during regular school class time. There were no dropouts since all the children who were present participated in the programme. Self-reported questionnaires were distributed to the children from the teacher in charge of each class and all the children in the class (41 intervention group and 31 control group) answered. In the process, the teachers assisted the children by orally reading out the questions. The data count was reduced only by one at post-test and at follow up because one child from each group left school (Fig. 1).

After 6 months (the post-test), the adjusted means of the SCAS were 19.60 (95% CI 14.98–24.22) in the intervention group and 14.93 (95% CI 9.60–20.26) in the control group. At 3-months following post-test, the adjusted means of the SCAS were 17.48 (95% CI 13.07–21.88) and 14.63 (95% CI 9.55–19.72), respectively (Table 2 and Fig. 2). In primary analysis, the group difference from baseline SCAS scores by the MMRM analysis at the post-test were -5.321 (95% CI -10.12 to -0.523, $p = 0.030$) and at the 3-month FU were -7.104 (95% CI -11.90 to -2.306, $p = 0.004$).

Showing the same pattern, the adjusted means of the SDQ were 11.39 (95% CI 10.00–12.77) in the intervention group and 9.53 (95% CI 7.85–11.22) in the control group. At 3-months following the post-test, the adjusted means of the SDQ were 11.51 (95% CI 10.11–12.91) and 10.87 (95% CI 9.27–12.46), respectively (Table 2 and Fig. 3). The group difference from baseline SDQ scores by MMRM analysis at the post-test were -1.975 (95% CI -3.989 to 0.038, $p = 0.054$) and at the 3-month FU were -3.284 (95% CI -5.297 to -1.270, $p = 0.002$).

To visually confirm the score change of each child in the intervention and control group, scatter plot charts were developed using the SCAS at pre-test, post-test, and FU, assigning scores of each group by sex vertically and children's ID horizontally (Fig. 4).

In the plot chart, a baseline T-score of 50 (male = 24, female = 31–32) and T-score of 60 (male = 40–41, female = 50–51), based on the SCAS web site, were drawn as a standard line, and changes in the number of children above a T-score of 50 were counted (Table 3). The results indicated that the number of children with T-scores above 50 were reduced to about half in the intervention group, while the number stayed the same or increased in the control group.

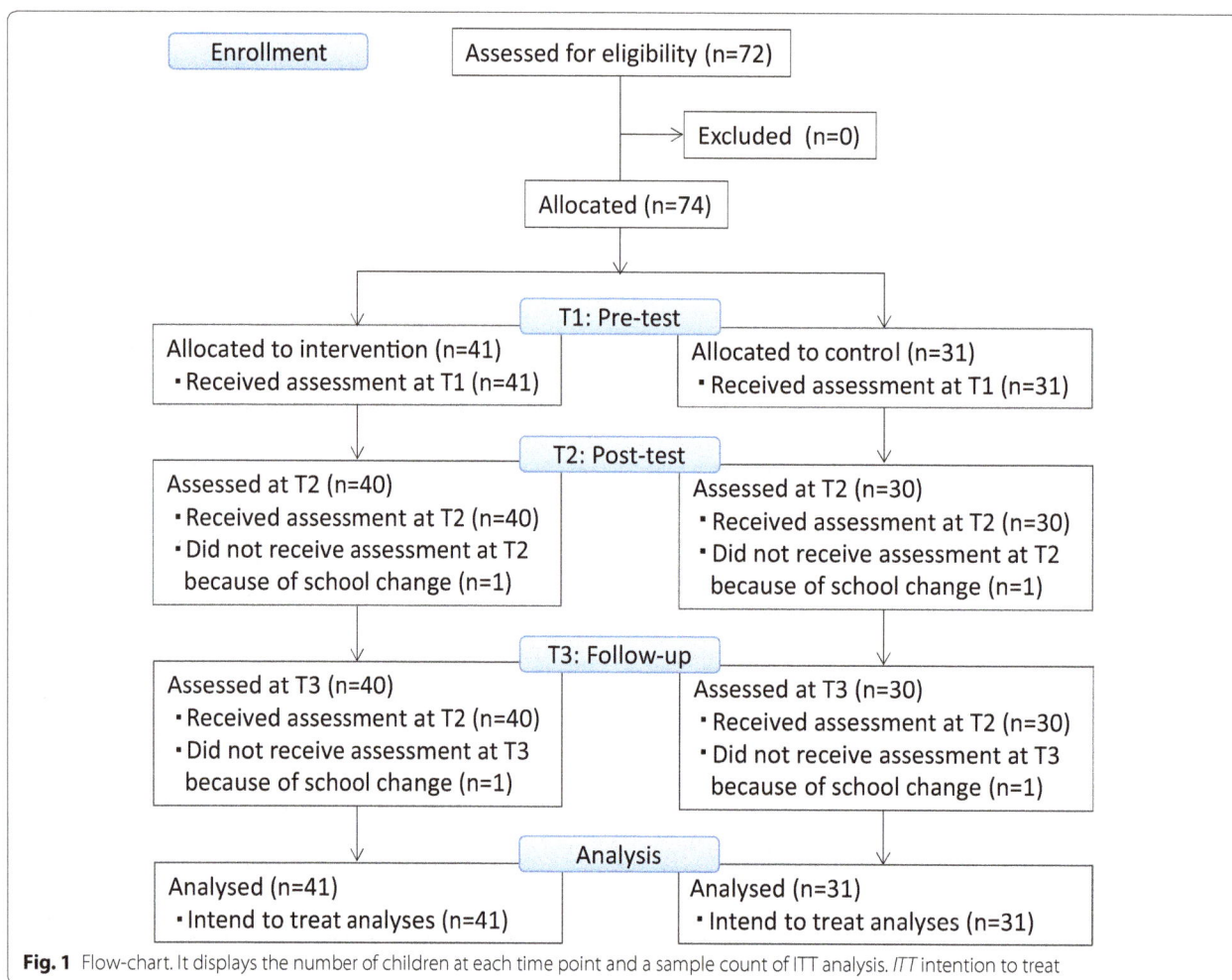

Fig. 1 Flow-chart. It displays the number of children at each time point and a sample count of ITT analysis. *ITT* intention to treat

Table 2 Estimated values and changes from baseline at each visit in SCAS and SDQ by MMRM

Score	Visit	IG (n = 40) Estimated mean (95% CI)	CG (n = 30) Estimated mean (95% CI)	Between group difference for baseline change	p value
SCAS	Pre	26.42 (21.74–31.11)	16.23 (10.83–21.64)	NA	
	Post	19.60 (14.98–24.22)	14.93 (9.60–20.26)	− 5.321 (− 10.12 to − 0.523)	0.030
	FU	17.48 (13.07–21.88)	14.63 (9.55–19.72)	− 7.104 (− 11.90 to − 2.306)	0.004
SDQ	Pre	13.10 (11.63–14.58)	9.53 (7.85–11.22)	NA	
	Post	11.39 (10.00–12.77)	9.53 (7.96–11.12)	− 1.975 (− 3.989 to 0.038)	0.054
	FU	11.51 (10.11–12.91)	10.87 (9.27–12.46)	− 3.284 (− 5.297 to − 1.270)	0.002

SCAS Spence Children's Anxiety Scale, *SDQ* Strengths and Difficulties Questionnaire, *IG* Intervention Group, *CG* Control Group, *FU* follow-up, *NA* not available

Discussion

The purpose of this study was to verify the feasibility and effectiveness of the CBT based 'Journey of the Brave' programme with a universal approach in a Japanese school class. The results of this study indicated that the SCAS and SDQ scores of the intervention group children were significantly reduced compared with the control group children. Therefore, the feasibility and effectiveness of this programme using a universal approach were supported in line with the previous pilot trial [32].

Currently, several programmes for the prevention of depression and anxiety are being developed based on the universal approach in school classes; however, it has been pointed out that although the effectiveness of anxiety

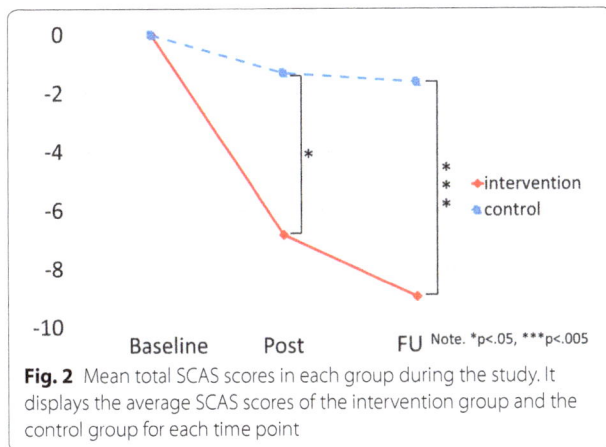

Fig. 2 Mean total SCAS scores in each group during the study. It displays the average SCAS scores of the intervention group and the control group for each time point

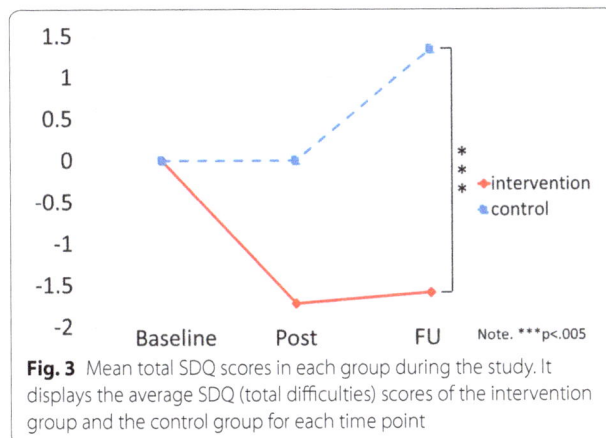

Fig. 3 Mean total SDQ scores in each group during the study. It displays the average SDQ (total difficulties) scores of the intervention group and the control group for each time point

and junior high schools is already fully occupied by the government-controlled curriculum and it was practically impossible to keep up with the originally planned pace. For this reason, we had to extend the interval between sessions to accommodate the request of the school. Initially we were concerned about a potential negative impact on children's learning, but this study did not find noticeable negative effects; rather, significant reduction in the anxiety scores of the intervention group children was found. Thus, in implementing a CBT programme as a school based preventive education initiative, flexible session scheduling might be applicable according to the situation of each school, as opposed to strictly following the once a week guideline. Moreover, this extended period may enable children enough learning time to complete the homework, apply what was learned to their behaviour change, and consolidate the programme content.

The second major difference was that the programme was implemented in a universal setting in a school class. Our pilot study was originally designed as a universal programme, but could be suitable as a targeted level programme because we had to use only a limited number of recruited children from the community as participants. The effect size of this study could be smaller because targeted level studies tend to result in higher effect sizes [4]. However, the SCAS score of the intervention group was significantly reduced in this study, whereas the pilot study failed to find clear differences. Therefore, the effectiveness and feasibility of our 'Journey of the Brave' programme as a universal approach was verified. In addition, a scatter plot chart comparing intervention and control group children by sex was conducted. The result confirmed the reduction of children's anxiety in the intervention group with T-scores above 50 from the post program period to 3-months after. A preventive programme basically targets healthy children; therefore, the anxiety scores of children whose initial score was low from the beginning did not require further reduction and are likely to show only a small reduction. However, at the same time, there are a limited number of children with high anxiety scores in each school and they are regarded as the high-risk group. Thus, children with T scores above 50 were treated as the high-risk group in this study, and their anxiety score changes were closely monitored. The results indicated that the number of children with T scores above 50 was reduced in both males and females after the programme intervention. This result suggests that this programme could possibly serve a role in early intervention for high-risk children.

The third difference is the usage of the SDQ as a secondary outcome measure to evaluate children's behavioural problems. Considering the focus of the program, the SDQ score might demonstrate no positive results

prevention programmes has been proven to a degree, the effectiveness of depression prevention programmes is questionable. For example, Werner-Seidler conducted a systematic review in 2017 on school-based depression and anxiety prevention programmes for young people and reported that universal depression prevention programs had smaller effect sizes at post-test relative to targeted programmes. On the other hand, for anxiety, effect sizes were comparable for universal and targeted programmes [39]. The 'Journey of the Brave' programme was designed as a universal approach focusing on children's anxiety problems based on a CBT model for the treatment of children's anxiety disorders, and the positive results demonstrated in this study are in line with the result of Werner-Seidler's study.

There are three major differences of this study compared with the aforementioned pilot study. The first is the reduction in frequency of programme sessions from once a week in the pilot study to twice a month in the current study. Usually, CBT treatment is conducted at a pace of once a week, and the pilot study adhered to this common interval. However, the class time of Japanese elementary

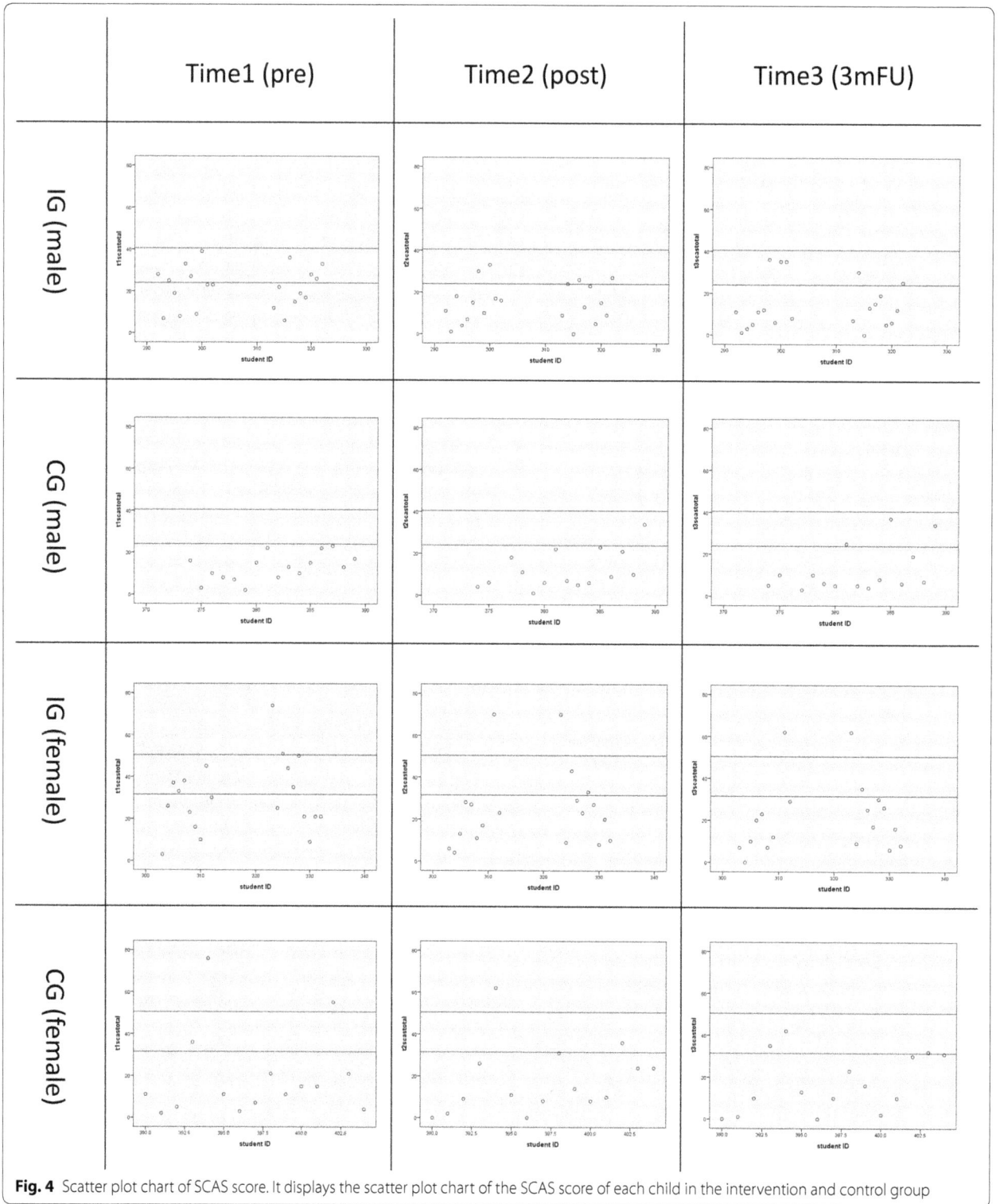

Fig. 4 Scatter plot chart of SCAS score. It displays the scatter plot chart of the SCAS score of each child in the intervention and control group

even if the SCAS score reduced significantly. However, the results of this study indicated equally positive outcomes on the SDQ compared with the control condition. The results indicate that the improvement in the children's anxiety problems may have a positive influence on their behavioural problems.

In other countries, several evidence-based programmes addressing prevention of children's anxiety are being

Table 3 Change in child count in excess of T-score 50 (60)

	Pre	Post	FU
IG (male)	9 (0)	5 (0)	5 (0)
CG (male)	0 (0)	1 (0)	3 (0)
IG (female)	9 (2)	4 (2)	3 (2)
CG (female)	3 (2)	2 (1)	3 (0)

IG Intervention Group, *CG* Control Group, *FU* follow-up

developed and implemented in school classes with the assistance of local authorities and/or the national government. On the contrary, in Japan, although the necessity of prevention and measures to address children's mental health problems are recognized, almost no time is dedicated to this issue in the school curriculum and there are limited class activities based on scientific evidence of psychosocial interventions. Thus, in a practical sense, it is up to each teacher to deal with mental health problems of children. With these considerations, we believe that it is quite a meaningful first step to show a new direction in children's mental health problem prevention in Japan by demonstrating the feasibility and effectiveness of a universal prevention programme for anxiety symptoms in school classes as part of the regular session.

Limitations and future prospects

We acknowledge several limitations in this study.

Firstly, a random assignment method was not applied to both intervention and control groups. When pre-programme scores are compared, the intervention group children showed significantly higher scores on both the SCAS and SDQ. While the average SCAS score as the primary outcome is reported to be 23.50 in Japanese children aged 7–11 [36], intervention group children in this study had an average score that was higher by 3 points and the control group children's score was 7 points lower. This reflected the same tendency as the pilot study [34]. The reason for this imbalance is not clear, but it surely resulted from not using a random assignment method. Because of the utilization of the MMRM method to analyse the change of each score from baseline, results are displayed without considering the intergroup difference; to present the results in a more stringent manner, it would be better to randomize the sample before the intervention and start the statistical analysis from an equalized baseline.

It is reported that in the evaluation of prevention programme effectiveness, many studies have certain shortcomings in their research design and it is difficult to confirm that enough positive evidence has been demonstrated [40]. In this study, a quasi-experimental design was applied to judge the feasibility of implementing this programme at a universal level; to confirm its effectiveness, it is necessary to increase the number of participating schools to 10–20 and apply a cluster randomization method.

The second limitation of this study is the fact that this programme was facilitated by the first author herself who developed this programme and one of the authors who had knowledge of educational psychology. 'Journey of the Brave' is a programme developed for universal level execution in Japanese schools conducted by the classroom teacher. However, a preceding study pointed out that more positive results are likely to occur when it is facilitated by specialists [27, 28]. On the other hand, there are reports of studies with no significant differences in effectiveness, whether they were teacher-led or health care specialist-led [30]. With these considerations, to establish and spread this program as evidence-based, it would be necessary to verify its effectiveness even if the programme is facilitated by the class teacher. In addition, a thorough consideration of quality assurance such as holding a facilitator seminar is required at the stage of making this programme widespread so that the understanding of CBT theory is deepened.

The third limitation relates to the measurement scales. Our programme used the SCAS and SDQ, which essentially are symptom scales to measure anxiety score improvement. However, the purpose of 'Journey of the Brave' is to prevent anxiety related problems and in verifying programme effectiveness, it is essential not only to compare pre- and post-programme scores, but to observe the process of improvement of children and conduct longitudinal studies such as those addressing the prevalence of anxiety disorders and the number of children with school refusal problems.

To evaluate the effectiveness of this preventive programme, it would be advisable not only to apply an RCT design, but also to continuously confirm its long-term effectiveness with longitudinal studies in Japan.

Conclusions

The results of this study confirmed the feasibility and effectiveness of a CBT based anxiety prevention programme, 'Journey of the Brave', when conducted at a Japanese school. In this study, we believe it is quite important that this preventive CBT program was implemented in actual school classes as a part of regular sessions. However, at the same time, there are several limitations in the study design and it is necessary to apply cluster randomization methods and to verify its preventive effects in a vertically integrated manner in the future.

Abbreviations
CBT: cognitive behaviour therapy; CI: confidence interval; FU: follow-up; SCAS: Spence Children's Anxiety Scale; SDQ: Strengths and Difficulties Questionnaire; ITT: intention to treat; MMRM: mixed-effect model for repeated measures.

Authors' contributions
YU designed and managed the study, performed the statistical analyses, and drafted the manuscript. MY and SI participated in the design of the study. TK assisted in programme sessions. YS assisted in the statistical analysis. ES administered and supervised the programme and overall conduct of the study. All authors critically revised the final manuscript. All authors read and approved the final manuscript.

Author details
[1] Research Centre for Child Mental Development, Chiba University Graduate School of Medicine, 1-8-1 Inohana, Chuo-ku, Chiba 260-8670, Japan. [2] Department of Cognitive Behavioural Physiology, Chiba University Graduate School of Medicine, 1-8-1 Inohana, Chuo-ku, Chiba 260-8670, Japan. [3] Department of Global Clinical Research, Chiba University Graduate School of Medicine, 1-8-1 Inohana, Chuo-ku, Chiba 260-8670, Japan. [4] Department of Psychology, Doshisha University, 1-3 Tatara Miyakodani, Kyotanabe, Kyoto 610-0394, Japan. [5] Department of International Communication, Kanda University of International Studies, 1-4-1 Wakaba Mihama-ku, Chiba 261-0014, Japan.

Acknowledgements
Not applicable.

Competing interests
The authors declare that they have no competing interests.

Funding
This work was supported by JSPS KAKENHI Grant Number 15K21267.

References
1. Albano AM, Chorpita BF, Barlow DH. Childhood anxiety disorders. In: Mash EJ, Barkley RA, editors. Childhood psychopathology. 2nd ed. New York: Guilford Press; 2003. p. 279–329.
2. Costello EJ, Egger HL, Angold A. The developmental epidemiology of anxiety disorders: phenomenology, prevalence, and comorbidity. Child Adolesc Psychiatr Clin N Am. 2005;14:631–48.
3. Neil AL, Christensen H. Efficacy and effectiveness of school-based prevention and early intervention programs for anxiety. Clin Psychol Rev. 2009;29:208–15.
4. Teubert D, Pinquart M. A meta-analytic review on the prevention of symptoms of anxiety in children and adolescents. J Anxiety Disord. 2011;25:1046–59.
5. Strauss CC, Frame CL, Forehand R. Psychosocial impairment associated with anxiety in children. J Clin Child Psychol. 1987;16:235–9.
6. McLoone J, Hudson JL, Rapee RM. Treating anxiety disorders in a school setting. Educ Treat Children. 2006;29:219–42.
7. Garber J, Weersing VR. Comorbidity of anxiety and depression in youth: implications for treatment and prevention. Clin Psychol. 2010;17:293–306. https://doi.org/10.1111/j.1468-2850.2010.01221.x.
8. Cole DA, Peeke LG, Martin JM, Truglio R, Seroczynski AD. A longitudinal look at the relation between depression and anxiety in children and adolescents. J Consult Clin Psychol. 1998;66:451–60.
9. Craske MG, Zucker BG. Prevention of anxiety disorders: a model for intervention. Appl Prev Psychol. 2002;10:155–75.
10. Ginsburg GS. The child anxiety prevention study intervention model and primary outcomes. J Consult Clin Psychol. 2009;77:580–7.
11. Mrazek PJ, Haggerty RJ. Reducing risks for mental disorders: frontiers for preventive research. Washington, DC: National Academy Press; 1994.
12. Horowitz JL, Garber J. The prevention of depressive symptoms in children and adolescents: a meta-analytic review. J Consult Clin Psychol. 2006;74:401–15.
13. Offord DR. Selection of levels of prevention. Addict Behav. 2000;25:833–42.
14. Fisak BJ Jr, Richard D, Mann A. The prevention of child and adolescent anxiety: a meta-analytic review. Prev Sci. 2011;12:255–68.
15. Stockings EA, Degenhardt L, Dobbins T, Lee YY, Erskine HE, Whiteford HA, Patton G. Preventing depression and anxiety in young people: a review of the joint efficacy of universal, selective and indicated prevention. Psychol Med. 2016;46:11–26.
16. Kendall PC. Treating anxiety disorders in children: results of a randomized clinical trial. J Consult Clin Psychol. 1994;62:100–10.
17. Kendall PC, Flannery-Schroeder E, Panichelli-Mindel SM, Southam-Gerow M, Henin A, Warman M. Therapy for youths with anxiety disorders: a second randomized clinical trial. J Consult Clin Psychol. 1997;65:366–80.
18. Dadds MR, Spence SH, Holland DE, Barrett PM, Laurens KR. Prevention and early intervention for anxiety disorders: a controlled trial. J Consult Clin Psychol. 1997;65:627–35.
19. Silverman WK, Kurtines WM, Ginsburg GS, Weems CF, Lumpkin PW, Carmichael DH. Treating anxiety disorders in children with group cognitive-behavioural therapy: a randomized clinical trial. J Consult Clin Psychol. 1999;67:995–1003.
20. Silverman WK, Hinshaw SP. The second special issue on evidence-based psychosocial treatments for children and adolescents: a 10-year update. J Clin Child Adolesc. 2008;37:1–7. https://doi.org/10.1080/1537441070 1817725.
21. Walkup JT, Albano AM, Piacentini J, Birmaher B, Compton SN, Sherrill JT, Ginsburg GS, Rynn MA, McCracken J, Waslick B, Iyengar S, March JS, Kendall PC. Cognitive behavioural therapy, sertraline, or a combination in childhood anxiety. New Engl J Med. 2008;359:2753–66.
22. Kendall PC, Hedtke KA. Cognitive behavioural therapy for anxious children: therapist manual. 3rd ed. Ardmore: Workbook Publishing; 2006.
23. Barrett P, Turner C. Prevention of anxiety symptoms in primary school children: preliminary results from a universal school-based trial. Br J Clin Psychol. 2001;40:399–410.
24. Lowry-Webster HM, Barrett PM, Dadds MR. A universal prevention trial of anxiety and depressive symptomatology in childhood: preliminary data from an Australian study. Behav Change. 2001;18:36–50.
25. Lowry-Webster HM, Barrett PM, Lock S. A universal prevention trial of anxiety symptomology during childhood: results at 1-year follow-up. Behav Change. 2003;20:25–43.
26. Barrett PM, Farrell LJ, Ollendick TH, Dadds M. Long-term outcomes of an Australian universal prevention trial of anxiety and depression symptoms in children and youth: an evaluation of the FRIENDS program. J Clin Child Adolesc Psychol. 2006;35:403–11.
27. Skryabina E, Taylor G, Sallard P. Effect of a universal anxiety prevention programme (FRIENDS) on children's academic performance: results from a randomised controlled trial. J Child Psychol Psychiatry. 2016;57:1297–307.
28. Stallard P, Skryabina E, Taylor G, Phillips R, Daniels H, Anderson R, Simpson N. Classroom-based cognitive behaviour therapy (FRIENDS): a cluster

randomized controlled trial to Prevent Anxiety in Children through Education in Schools (PACES). Lancet Psychiatry. 2014;1:185–92.

29. Matsumoto Y, Shimizu E. The FRIENDS cognitive behavioral Program in Japanese schools: an examination of the treatment effect. Sch Psychol Int. 2016;37:397–409.

30. Collins S, Woolfson LM, Durkin K. Effects on coping skills and anxiety of a universal school-based mental health intervention delivered in Scottish primary schools. Sch Psychol Int. 2014;35:85–100.

31. Calear AL, Christensen H, Brewer J, Mackinnon A, Griffiths KM. A pilot randomized controlled trial of the e-couch anxiety and worry program in schools. Internet Interv. 2016;6:1–5.

32. Ministry of Education in Japan. Elementary school curriculum guidelines; 2008. http://www.mext.go.jp/component/a_menu/education/micro _detail/__icsFiles/afieldfile/2010/11/29/syo.pdf. Accessed 2 Apr 2017.

33. Ishikawa S, Togasaki Y, Sato S, Sato Y. Prevention programs for depression in children and adolescents: a review. Jpn J Educ Psychol. 2006;54:572–84.

34. Urao Y, Yoshinaga N, Asano K, Ishikawa R, Tano A, Sato Y, Shimizu E. Effectiveness of a cognitive behavioural therapy-based anxiety prevention programme for children: a preliminary quasi-experimental study in Japan.

Child Adolesc Psychiatry Ment Health. 2016. https://doi.org/10.1186/s13034-016-0091-x.

35. Spence SH. A measure of anxiety symptoms among children. Behav Res Ther. 1998;36:545–66.

36. Ishikawa S, Sato H, Sasagawa S. Anxiety disorder symptoms in Japanese children and adolescents. J Anxiety Disord. 2009;23:104–11.

37. Muris P, Schmidt H, Merckelbach H. Correlations among two self-report questionnaires for measuring DSM-defined anxiety disorder symptoms in children: the screen for child anxiety related emotional disorders and the Spence Children's Anxiety Scale. Pers Individ Differ. 2000;28:333–46.

38. Goodman R, Meltzer H, Bailey V. The Strengths and Difficulties Questionnaire: a pilot study on the validity of the self-report version. Eur Child Adolesc Psychiatry. 1998;7:125–30.

39. Werner Seidler A, Perry Y, Calear AL, Newby JM, Christensen H. School-based depression and anxiety prevention programs for young people: a systematic review and meta-analysis. Clin Psychol Rev. 2017;51:30–47.

40. Corrieri S, Heider D, Conrad I, Blume A, Konig H, Riedel-Hellier SG. School-based prevention programs for depression and anxiety in adolescence: a systematic review. Health Promot Int. 2013;29:427–41.

Internet addiction detection rate among college students in the People's Republic of China: a meta-analysis

Yao-jun Shao, Tong Zheng, Yan-qiu Wang, Ling Liu, Yan Chen and Ying-shui Yao[*]

Abstract

Background: With the development of economy and technology, the Internet is becoming more and more popular. Internet addiction has gradually become a serious issue in public health worldwide. The number of Internet users in China has reached 731 million, with an estimated 24 million adolescents determined as having Internet addiction. In this meta-analysis, we attempted to estimate the prevalence of Internet addiction among College Students in the People's Republic of China in order to improve the mental health level of college students and provide evidence for the prevention of Internet addiction.

Methods: Eligible articles about the prevalence of Internet addiction among college students in China published between 2006 and 2017 were retrieved from online Chinese periodicals, the full-text databases of Wan Fang, VIP, and the Chinese National Knowledge Infrastructure, as well as PubMed. Stata 11.0 was used to perform the analyses.

Results: A total of 26 papers were included in the analyses. The overall sample size was 38,245, with 4573 diagnosed with Internet addiction. The pooled detection rate of Internet addiction was 11% (95% confidence interval [CI] 9–13%) among college students in China. The detection rate was higher in male students (16%) than female students (8%). The Internet addiction detection rate was 11% (95% CI 8–14%) in southern areas, 11% (95% CI 7–14%) in northern areas, 13% (95% CI 8–18%) in eastern areas and 9% (95% CI 8–11%) in the mid-western areas. According to different scales, the Internet addiction detection rate was 11% (95% CI 8–15%) using the Young scale and 9% (95% CI 6–11%) using the Chen scale respectively. Cumulative meta analysis showed that the detection rate had a slight upward trend and gradually stabilized in the last 3 years.

Conclusion: The pooled Internet addiction detection rate of Chinese college students in out study was 11%, which is higher than in some other countries and strongly demonstrates a worrisome situation. Effective measures should be taken to prevent further Internet addiction and improve the current situation.

Keywords: China, College students, Internet addiction, Meta-analysis, Prevalence

Background

Internet addiction can be defined as overuse of the Internet leading to impairment of an individual's psychological state (both mental and emotional), as well as their scholastic or occupational and social interactions [1]. Its symptoms generally include preoccupation, loss of control, high tolerance, withdrawal, craving, impairment of function and a reduction in the ability to make decision [2]. The prevalence of Internet addiction in American college students is 12% and the Internet addiction rate of Iranian medical students is 10.8% [3, 4]. Worse yet, studies have shown that the rate of Internet addiction in Serbian schoolchildren is 18.7% [5]. In China, as well as worldwide, Internet addiction is a significant growing health problem in college students which is harmful to their physical and mental health. According to a survey conducted by the China Internet Network Information Center, the number of Internet users in China has

*Correspondence: yingshuiyao@163.com
Faculty of Epidemiology and Statistics, School of Public Health, Wannan Medical College, 22 Wenchang West Road, Yijiang District, Wuhu 241002, Anhui, People's Republic of China

reached 731 million, which equals the total population in Europe. There is no doubt that the Internet has brought us a lot of benefits. The Internet provides young people with good conditions for learning and strengthen the communication between young people. It is necessary for students to learn how to use the Internet. Internet tools can be effectively applied in school education, specifically in areas of lectures, assignments, real-time procedure demonstration, class discussion, and interaction with teachers. Internet can also realize the sharing of learning resources. So it is useful to integrate this learning modality with the traditional mode of teaching through a well thought out curriculum modification [6]. Besides, Internet has changed the way people socialize and it has become a medium for disease prevention and health promotion. Because young people are able to participate in a growing numbers of online communities providing support and advice for health care. A study of disturbed adolescents found that computer-mediated communication diminished certain traditional gender differences in group communication [7, 8]. However, the disadvantages caused by the Internet cannot be ignored. Internet addiction brings a lot of risks to society. Firstly, it makes people spend more time on Internet games and reduce normal social activities [9]. Secondly, there is a lot of unhealthy information on the Internet, such as pornography, violence and so on, which can affect people's mental health. The current findings suggest that adolescents with Internet addiction seem to have more aggressive dispositions than non-Internet addicted adolescents [10]. Finally, Internet addiction leads to lack of sleep, vision disturbances and decline in work efficiency, which are detrimental to our physical health [11]. Therefore, it is crucial for us to investigate the prevalence of Internet addiction among Chinese college students in order to provide epidemiological information to better understand and tackle this problem.

To the best of our knowledge, currently there is no consensus on the standard for the diagnosis and identification of Internet addiction disorder. Young's Internet Addiction Diagnostic Questionnaire (YDQ) was compiled in 1983. A respondent who answers yes to five or more of the eight questions is diagnosed as addiction Internet user. This questionnaire was further developed in 1998 by Young in order to incorporate the DSM-IV pathologic gambling criteria [12]. This 20-item scale, with its score ranging from 0 to 100, is widely used in diagnosing Internet addiction. Respondent with the total score ranging from 50 to 79 is considered moderate Internet user and 80–100 as severe Internet user with serious problems in Internet use. Previous studies have demonstrated that the scale has a high reliability and validity [12]. To take group differences into account, the Chen Internet Addiction Scale (CIAS) is used to measure the extent of Internet addiction. There are 26 items in the CIAS, and an individual with a score of 68 or more is assessed as Internet addiction [13]. A revision of the CIAS with 19 questions was assembled by Bai in 2005, which divides Internet addiction into three level: normal (from 19 to 45), moderate (from 46 to 53) and excessive (above 53). These scales have been gradually used in Internet addiction research in China.

A lot of in-depth research on drug addiction has been explored, such as the epigenetic mechanisms of drug addiction. Unlike drug addiction, the influence of Internet addiction has been underestimated and few studies explore the mechanisms of it [14]. With the Internet addiction becoming more and more serious, relevant government departments begin to pay more attention to the effects of Internet addiction on teenagers and college students. Since their physical and mental development is not yet mature, their abilities of self regulation and control remain to be improved [15, 16]. In this meta-analysis, we attempted to investigate the prevalence of Internet addiction among college students in the People's Republic of China in order to provide epidemiological evidence for the prevention of Internet addiction and finally improve the mental health level of college students.

Methods
Search strategy
Articles related to Internet addiction between 2006 and 2017 were retrieved from the Chinese periodical databases of Chinese National Knowledge Infrastructure, VIP and WanFang and from PubMed. We searched the following keywords: "Internet addition", "college students/ university students", "detection rate" and "China". Languages were restricted to English and Chinese. In addition, relevant articles were manually searched.

Selection criteria
Inclusion criteria included: the research objects are fulltime Chinese college students or vocational college students who are 18–25 years old; published between 2006 and 2017; using random sampling method; discussion of the Internet addiction detection rate in Chinese college students with reliable and clear statistics; Internet addiction is defined clearly and Internet addiction related questionnaire was adopted. CIAS has a Cronbach's alpha of 0.95, and YDQ has a Cronbach's alpha of 0.93 as well as a good test–retest reliability ($r = 0.85$) [3, 13]; high quality articles have priority among the same subjects (For articles in which the same subjects were included in different publications, only the most recent or complete study was included). Exclusion criteria consisted of: articles unrelated to the purpose of the study; valid data cannot be

extracted from the study; data is incomplete or repeated publication.

Literature screening and quality assessment

According to selection criteria, data extraction was completed independently by two researchers. Disagreements were solved by discussion or a third reviewer. For missing information, we contacted the correspondent authors for completed data. The following information was extracted from the literature: first author, year of publication, investigation time and area, sampling method, sample size, gender composition, and the scale used for Internet addition. Evaluation tools recommended by Agency for Healthcare Research and Quality (AHRQ) were used to measure the quality of research [17].

Statistical analysis

Stata 11.0 software was used for the analysis. According to the results of heterogeneity test, the random effects model was used. Subgroup analyses, cumulative meta-analysis and chart description were also performed. Begg's and Egger's test were applied to examine publication bias [18].

Results

Basic information and quality assessment

A total of 2551 articles were initially retrieved from the online Chinese periodical full-text Chinese National Knowledge Infrastructure (n = 2033), VIP (n = 214), Wan Fang (n = 107) databases, and from PubMed (n = 197). By reading the title 1653 articles were eliminated since the object of study was not college students or vocational college students, most of these articles instead are devoted to the study of middle school students. After quality evaluation, 765 articles were further excluded. Of these, 157 articles did not mention sampling method and 319 articles did not use random sampling method. Another 289 articles had no explicit standard of Internet addiction or a clear definition of Internet addiction. In addition, 107 articles were removed after reading the full text because of lacking necessary data or containing incomplete data. Finally, 26 articles were included. Figure 1 shows the literature search process. The total sample size was 38,245 college students, the largest sample was 4866, and the smallest was 434. 4573 students were diagnosed as Internet addiction. Main characteristics of the included 26 eligible articles are shown in Table 1.

Meta-analysis of Internet addiction detection rates in college students in the People's Republic of China

A total of 26 articles reported Internet addiction detection rate among college students in China. Heterogeneity test showed a result of $I^2 = 0.983$, indicating

heterogeneous among studies. Therefore random-effects model was chosen. The pooled prevalence of Internet addiction in Chinese college students was 11% (95% confidence interval [CI] 9–13%), the result is shown by the forest plots in Fig. 2.

Subgroup analyses

In order to find the source of heterogeneity, subgroup analysis was performed according to stratum of gender, region, and scale. The result of subgroup analyses were presented in Table 2. There is a statistically significant difference of the Internet addiction detection rates between male students and female students (P < 0.05). The mean prevalence of Internet addiction was 16% (95% CI 13–19%) for male students and 8% (95% CI 5–10%) for female students respectively (Fig. 3). The Internet addiction detection rate was 11% (95% CI 8–14%) in southern areas, 11% (95% CI 7–14%) in northern areas, 13% (95% CI 8–18%) in eastern areas and 9% (95% CI 8–11%) in the mid-western areas. According to different scales, the Internet addiction detection rate was 11% (95% CI 8–15%) using the Young scale and 9% (95% CI 6–11%) using the Chen scale.

Cumulative meta-analysis

Cumulative meta-analysis was carried out for the detection rate based on year and sample size. The detection rate had a slight upward trend and gradually stabilized around 12% in the past 3 years as shown in Fig. 4. As for sample size, the detection rate grew more stable with the increase of sample size, also reaching 12%.

Publication bias

Publication bias was assessed using the funnel plots (Fig. 5) [19]. Begg (z = 0.44, P = 0.659) and Egger test (t = −0.31, P = 0.761) results suggested a low possibility of publication bias.

Discussion

The Internet has become an indispensable part of our lives, providing us more convenience. We rely heavily on the Internet, which also brings serious negative effects, such as game addiction. The influence of Internet addiction on college students as a special group has become a hot issue in public health. In this meta-analysis, 26 articles related to Internet addiction published between 2006 and 2017 were retrieved from databases based on our strict inclusion and exclusion criteria. As shown in Table 1, Internet addiction detection rates among college students in China varied widely from 4 to 43.9%, possibly due to the sample sizes, economic development differences and time of investigation. Economic is more developed in eastern coastal areas of China than that in

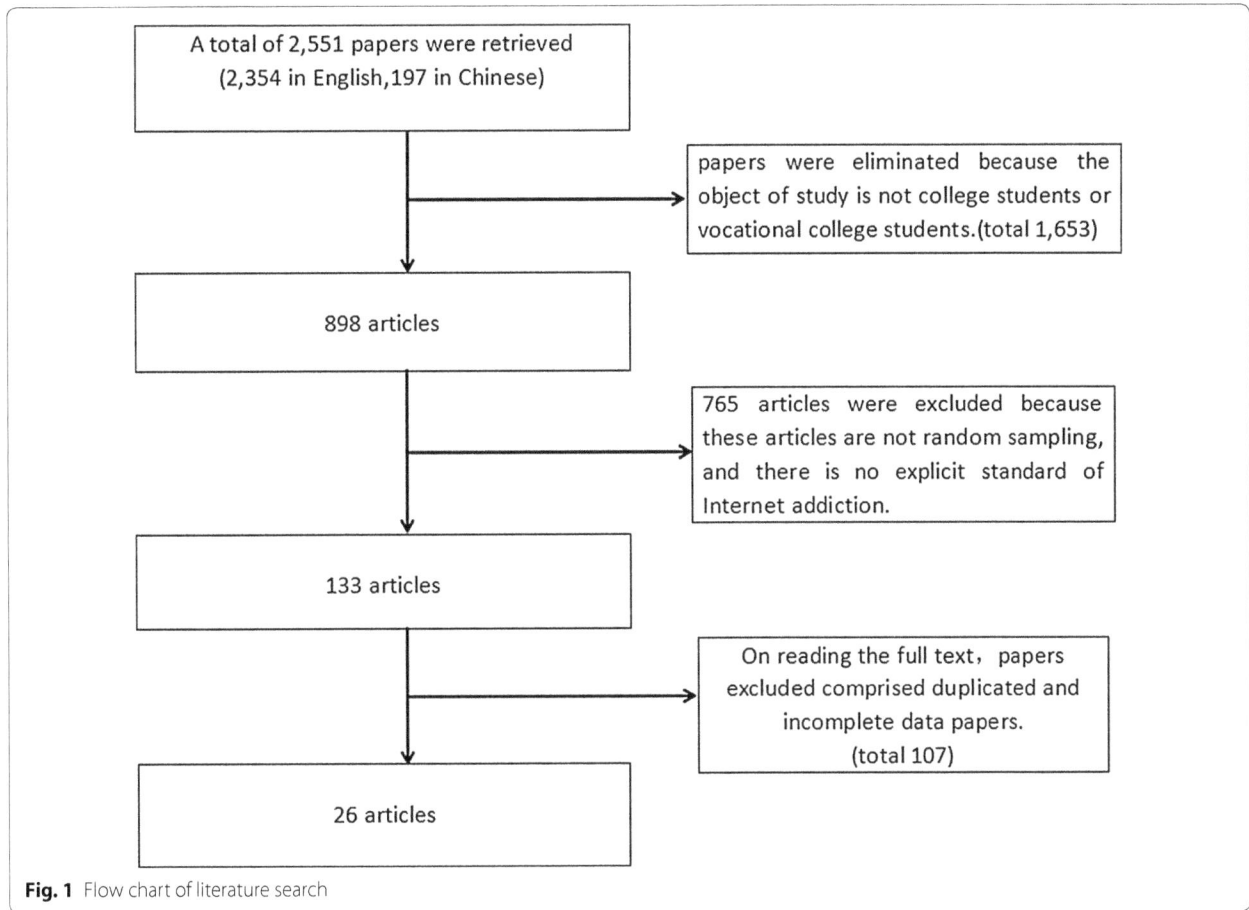

Fig. 1 Flow chart of literature search

other areas, which results in earlier Internet touching among young people in east China. Currently, Internet has gradually become popular in east China. Since few people have been in contact with computer decades ago, low rate of Internet addiction was reported at that time. Our study reflects the general characteristics of Internet addiction prevalence among Chinese college students. A previous study proved that the rate of Internet addiction among teenagers in the world is 10% [20]. In our study, the pooled prevalence of Internet addiction in Chinese college students is 11% (95% CI 9–13%), which is similar to many studies conducted in China but different from studies conducted abroad. Compared with other countries, the detection rate in China is higher than Japan [21] (3.7%) and Italy [2] (4.3%), but similar to Pakistan [22] (16.7%), Chile [12] (11.5%) and Turkey [23] (9.7%).

After subgroup analyses, we find that Internet addiction has different effects on male and female students, with higher detection rates in male students (16%) than in female students (8%). It may be explained by the differences in coping styles when facing life stress or negative life events. Male students tend to solve problems on their own and are reluctant to communicate with others or ask

for help, leading to the low utilization of social support [24]. Some studies report that males are more sensitive to the Internet than females [25]. Compared with females, online games are more attractive to males who have a greater breadth of Internet use and more time surfing on Internet [26]. The above factors may contribute to a higher detection rate in male students. In terms of the regional factor, the Internet addiction detection rate was 11% in northern and southern areas in China. A higher detection rate was seen in the eastern areas as compared with mid-west. The regional difference could be caused by uneven economic development between eastern and mid-west areas, with more popularity of the Internet in the eastern areas attracting more college students. Our findings show that the Internet addiction detection rate using the Young scale was higher than that using the Chen scale. These two scales are widely used in the measurement of Internet addiction, and further research should be made to compare and evaluate the two scales.

According to the results of cumulative meta-analysis, the Internet addiction detection rate of Chinese college students has increased slowly since 2008 and gradually stabilized around 12% in the past 3 years. This shows that

Table 1 Main characteristics of studies showing Internet addiction detection rates among college students in China

References	Years	District	Prevalence of Internet addiction (%)			Scale	Subject
			Total (IA/sample size)	Male (IA/sample size)	Female (IA/sample size)		
Yao et al. [34]	2006	Wuhu	12.9 (260/2010)	16.1 (229/1427)	5.3 (31/583)	Young scale	College student
Feng et al. [35]	2007	Guizhou	8.4 (126/1497)	11.1 (75/675)	6.2 (51/822)	Young scale	College student
Wang et al. [36]	2007	Dalian	7.3 (70/954)			Young scale	College student
Chen and Fan [37]	2008	Hefei	4 (28/705)	6 (22/364)	1.8 (6/341)	Young scale	College student
Gao et al. [38]	2008	Changchun	7.8 (96/1227)	12.7 (51/403)	5.5 (45/824)	Young scale	College student
Zhang et al. [39]	2009	Ningbo	11.7 (119/1014)	18.1 (108/597)	2.6 (11/417)	Young scale	College student
Liu et al. [40]	2009	Wuhan	4.6 (20/434)	7.3 (15/207)	2.2 (5/227)	Young scale	College student
Gao and Ma [41]	2009	Hangzhou	11.9 (81/683)	16.7 (51/306)	8 (30/377)	Young scale	College student
Ju-Yu Yen et al. [42]	2009	Taiwan	12.3 (246/1992)	19.1 (111/581)	9.6 (135/1411)	CIAS	College student
Zhou et al. [43]	2010	Daqing	10.8 (85/787)	18.6 (44/237)	7.5 (41/500)	Young scale	College student
Zhang et al. [44]	2011	Dali	10.4 (100/965)	13.6 (46/338)	8.6 (54/627)	Young scale	College student
Zhao et al. [45]	2012	Lanzhou	11.1 (200/1807)	13.5 (125/926)	8.5 (75/881)	Young scale	College student
Chen et al. [46]	2012	Wuhan	6.8 (32/470)	11.1 (20/181)	4.2 (12/289)	CIAS	College student
Zhang et al. [47]	2013	Jinan	5.5 (52/853)	11.4 (32/280)	3.5 (20/573)	CIAS	College student
Luo et al. [25]	2014	Shandong	4.5 (46/1026)	8.1 (31/384)	2.3 (15/642)	Young scale	College student
Zhang [48]	2014	Xinjiang	8.7 (90/1037)			CIAS	College student
Zhou et al. [49]	2014	Wuxi	12.8 (621/4866)	15.9 (338/2122)	10.3 (283/2744)	Young scale	College student
Luo and Zhu [50]	2015	Jiangxi	7.2 (39/545)	16 (19/119)	4.7 (20/426)	Young scale	College student
Wang et al. [51]	2015	Hainan	33.4 (781/2341)	38.4 (312/812)	30.7 (469/1529)	Young scale	College student
Zhang et al. [52]	2015	Nantong	10.8 (450/4168)	12.2 (185/1515)	10 (265/2653)	CDC standard	College student
Zhou et al. [24]	2015	Yan'an	19.5 (117/601)	27.6 (48/174)	16.2 (69/427)	Young scale	College student
Cong et al. [53]	2016	Yantai	43.9 (249/567)	55.2 (95/172)	39 (154/395)	Young scale	College student
Chi et al. [54]	2016	Hefei	15.2 (178/1173)			Young scale	College student
Chen et al. [55]	2016	Hebei	9.6 (234/2451)	13.5 (162/1204)	5.8 (72/1247)	CIAS	College student
Wu et al. [56]	2017	Taishan	6.7 (93/1385)	9.1 (36/394)	5.8 (57/991)	Young scale	College student
Li et al. [57]	2017	Henan	6 (160/2687)	8.6 (93/1087)	4.2 (67/1600)	Young scale	College student

CDC Chinese Center for Disease Control and Prevention, *CIAS* Chen Internet Addiction Scale, *IA* Internet addiction, *Young* Young Internet Addiction Scale

the Internet addiction has become an increasingly serious problem which can lead to many negative effects on college students, including physical and mental health. Internet addicts are more obvious in obsessive-compulsion, interpersonal sensitivity, depression, anxiety, hostility and other problems. Their mental health level is lower because they are addicted to the Internet for a long time which results in the lack of interpersonal communication, which in itself is a risk factor for mental illness [24]. Furthermore, Internet addiction can also cause many somatic diseases such as neurasthenia, decreased vision, lack of concentration, and sleep disorder. Worst of all, Internet addiction can cause conduct disorder, inducing teenagers to play truant even crime. This study still has limitations: the diagnosis of Internet addiction is only measured by self report, with no clinical assessment of disability or other sources of information. It may have an impact on the integrity of the information collection and

the results accuracy. Thus, we increase the assessment of other information in further research.

Conclusion

According to the research, the mean prevalence of Internet addiction in Chinese college students was 11%. Boys (16%) have a higher rate of Internet addiction than girls (8%). Given the rising Internet addiction rates among college students in China, effective and practical intervention measures should be taken. On one hand, government should strengthen the supervision of the Internet and provide legal protection in order to reduce the harm to college students. For example, no Internet cafes is allowed to be open within 200 meters in school, the opening hours of Internet cafes must be limited to between 8 a.m. and midnight, and an anti-addiction system should be established to limit the time spending on online games [27]. On the other hand, the university should encourage students to participate in

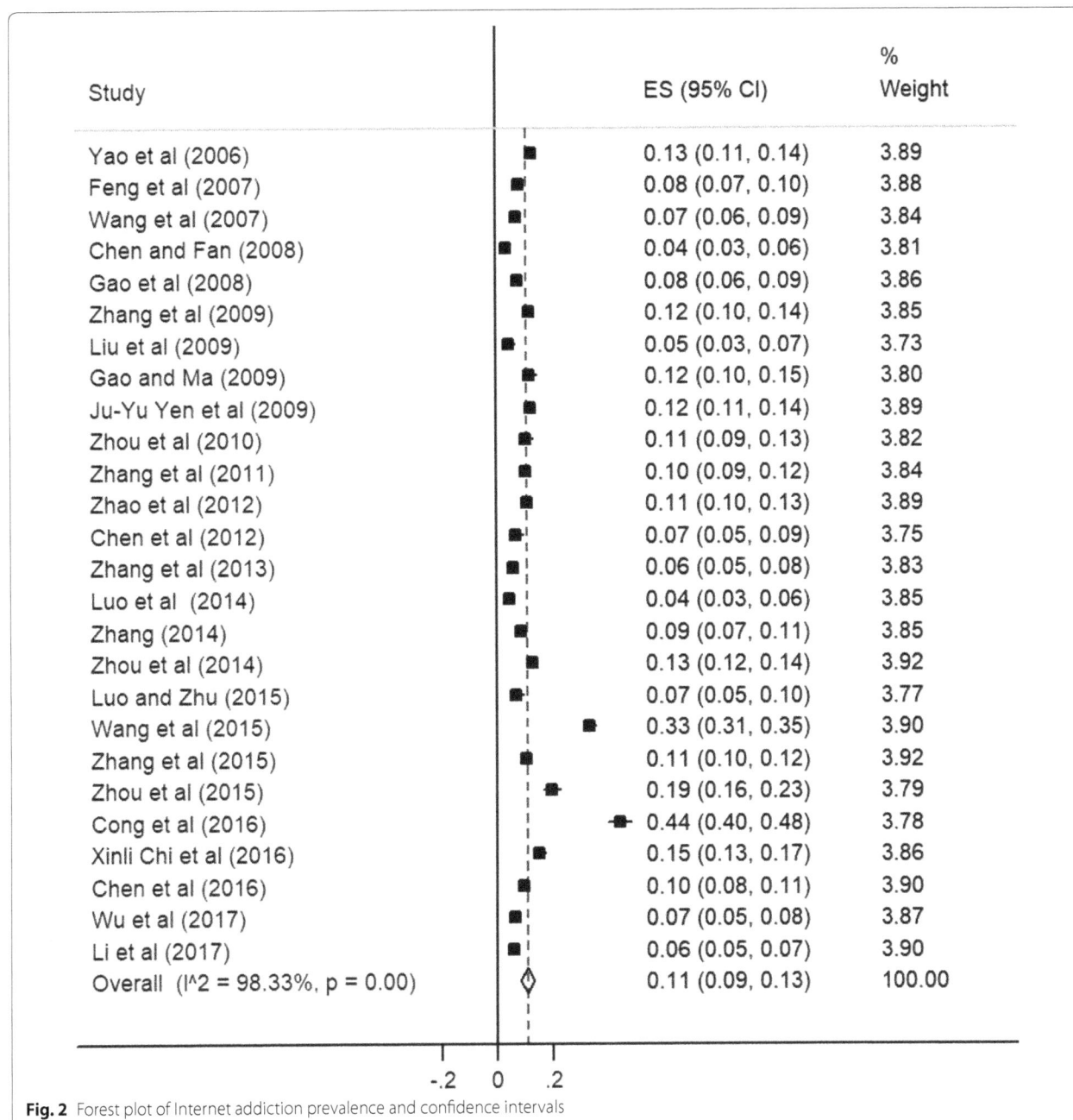

Study	ES (95% CI)	% Weight
Yao et al (2006)	0.13 (0.11, 0.14)	3.89
Feng et al (2007)	0.08 (0.07, 0.10)	3.88
Wang et al (2007)	0.07 (0.06, 0.09)	3.84
Chen and Fan (2008)	0.04 (0.03, 0.06)	3.81
Gao et al (2008)	0.08 (0.06, 0.09)	3.86
Zhang et al (2009)	0.12 (0.10, 0.14)	3.85
Liu et al (2009)	0.05 (0.03, 0.07)	3.73
Gao and Ma (2009)	0.12 (0.10, 0.15)	3.80
Ju-Yu Yen et al (2009)	0.12 (0.11, 0.14)	3.89
Zhou et al (2010)	0.11 (0.09, 0.13)	3.82
Zhang et al (2011)	0.10 (0.09, 0.12)	3.84
Zhao et al (2012)	0.11 (0.10, 0.13)	3.89
Chen et al (2012)	0.07 (0.05, 0.09)	3.75
Zhang et al (2013)	0.06 (0.05, 0.08)	3.83
Luo et al (2014)	0.04 (0.03, 0.06)	3.85
Zhang (2014)	0.09 (0.07, 0.11)	3.85
Zhou et al (2014)	0.13 (0.12, 0.14)	3.92
Luo and Zhu (2015)	0.07 (0.05, 0.10)	3.77
Wang et al (2015)	0.33 (0.31, 0.35)	3.90
Zhang et al (2015)	0.11 (0.10, 0.12)	3.92
Zhou et al (2015)	0.19 (0.16, 0.23)	3.79
Cong et al (2016)	0.44 (0.40, 0.48)	3.78
Xinli Chi et al (2016)	0.15 (0.13, 0.17)	3.86
Chen et al (2016)	0.10 (0.08, 0.11)	3.90
Wu et al (2017)	0.07 (0.05, 0.08)	3.87
Li et al (2017)	0.06 (0.05, 0.07)	3.90
Overall (I^2 = 98.33%, p = 0.00)	0.11 (0.09, 0.13)	100.00

Fig. 2 Forest plot of Internet addiction prevalence and confidence intervals

Table 2 Mean prevalence of Internet addiction among college students in different subgroups

	Gender		District distribution				Scale	
	Male	Female	South	North	East	Mid-west	Young	CIAS
Study number	23	23	14	12	11	15	20	5
Prevalence (%)	16	8	11	11	13	9	11	9
95% CI (%)	13–19	5–10	8–14	7–14	8–18	8–11	8–15	6–11
Heterogeneity (I^2)	0.961	0.979	0.984	0.981	0.991	0.939	0.987	0.902

North and South are divided by Qinling Mountains–Huaihe River Line. East and mid-west are divided by economic development level. One paper which uses CDC standard do not sort by scale

CI confidence interval, *CIAS* Chen Internet Addiction Scale, *Young* Young Internet Addiction Scale

Study	ES (95% CI)	% Weight
male		
Yao et al	0.16 (0.14, 0.18)	2.23
Feng et al	0.11 (0.09, 0.14)	2.20
Chen and Fan	0.06 (0.04, 0.09)	2.16
Gao et al	0.13 (0.10, 0.16)	2.16
Zhang et al	0.18 (0.15, 0.21)	2.19
Liu et al	0.07 (0.04, 0.12)	2.08
Gao and Ma	0.17 (0.13, 0.21)	2.14
Ju-Yu Yen et al	0.19 (0.16, 0.23)	2.19
Zhou et al	0.19 (0.14, 0.24)	2.10
Zhang et al	0.14 (0.10, 0.18)	2.15
Zhao et al	0.13 (0.11, 0.16)	2.22
Chen et al	0.11 (0.07, 0.17)	2.06
Zhang et al	0.11 (0.08, 0.16)	2.13
Luo et al	0.08 (0.06, 0.11)	2.16
Zhou et al	0.16 (0.14, 0.18)	2.24
Luo and Zhu	0.16 (0.10, 0.24)	1.97
Wang et al	0.38 (0.35, 0.42)	2.21
Zhang et al	0.12 (0.11, 0.14)	2.25
Zhou et al	0.28 (0.21, 0.35)	2.05
Cong et al	0.55 (0.47, 0.63)	2.05
Chen et al	0.14 (0.12, 0.16)	2.23
Wu et al	0.09 (0.06, 0.12)	2.16
Li et al	0.09 (0.07, 0.10)	2.22
Subtotal (I^2 = 96.08%, p = 0.00)	0.16 (0.13, 0.19)	49.55
female		
Yao et al	0.05 (0.04, 0.07)	2.19
Feng et al	0.06 (0.05, 0.08)	2.21
Chen and Fan	0.02 (0.01, 0.04)	2.15
Gao et al	0.05 (0.04, 0.07)	2.21
Zhang et al	0.03 (0.01, 0.05)	2.17
Liu et al	0.02 (0.01, 0.05)	2.10
Gao and Ma	0.08 (0.05, 0.11)	2.16
Ju-Yu Yen et al	0.10 (0.08, 0.11)	2.23
Zhou et al	0.07 (0.05, 0.10)	2.19
Zhang et al	0.09 (0.07, 0.11)	2.20
Zhao et al	0.09 (0.07, 0.11)	2.22
Chen et al	0.04 (0.02, 0.07)	2.13
Zhang et al	0.03 (0.02, 0.05)	2.19
Luo et al	0.02 (0.01, 0.04)	2.20
Zhou et al	0.10 (0.09, 0.12)	2.25
Luo and Zhu	0.05 (0.03, 0.07)	2.17
Wang et al	0.31 (0.28, 0.33)	2.23
Zhang et al	0.10 (0.09, 0.12)	2.23
Zhou et al	0.16 (0.13, 0.20)	2.17
Cong et al	0.39 (0.34, 0.44)	2.16
Chen et al	0.06 (0.05, 0.07)	2.23
Wu et al	0.06 (0.04, 0.07)	2.22
Li et al	0.04 (0.03, 0.05)	2.24
Subtotal (I^2 = 97.93%, p = 0.00)	0.08 (0.05, 0.10)	50.45
Heterogeneity between groups: p = 0.000		
Overall (I^2 = 97.68%, p = 0.00);	0.11 (0.09, 0.14)	100.00

-.2 -.1 0 .1 .2

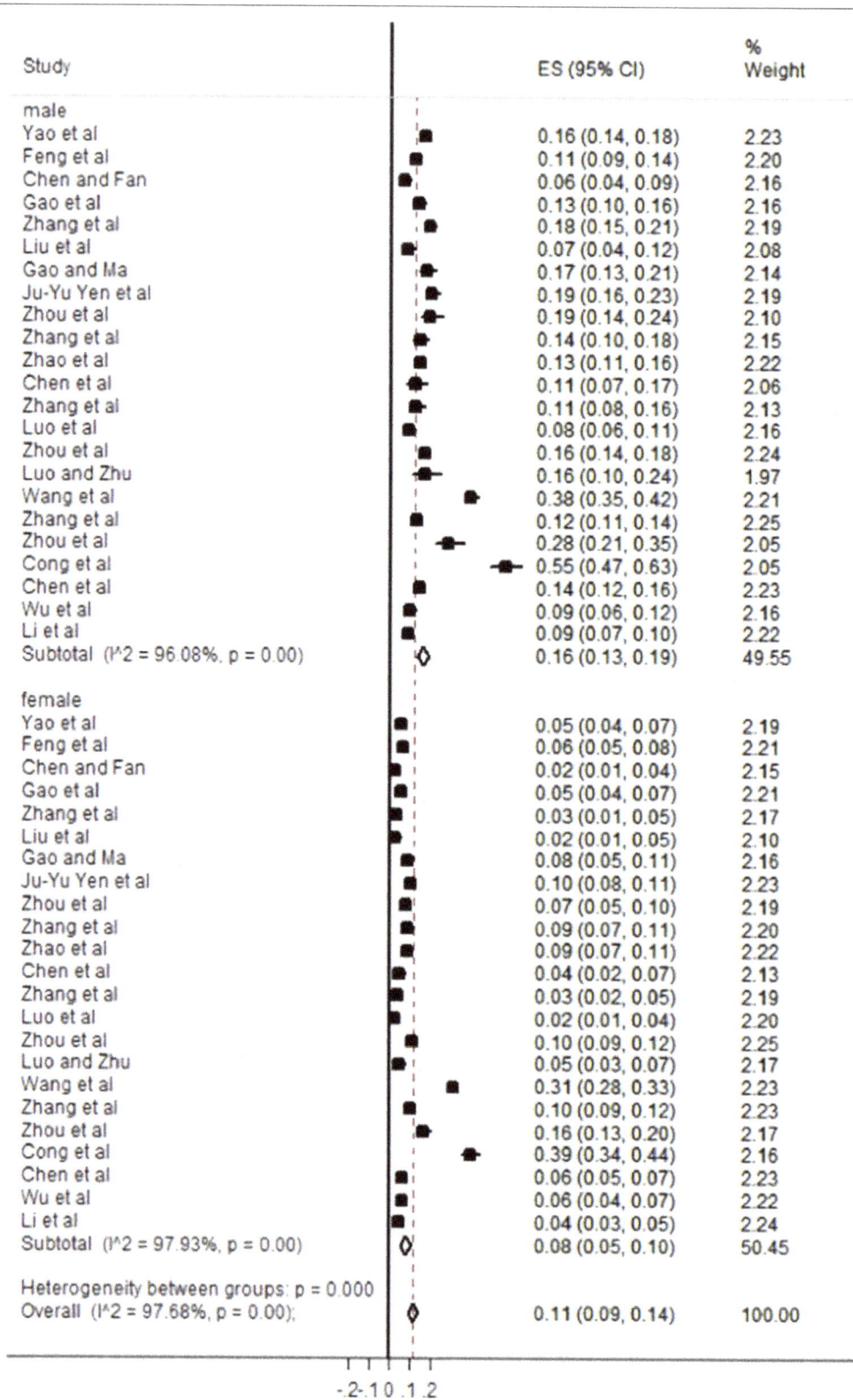

Fig. 3 Forest plot of subgroup analysis based on gender

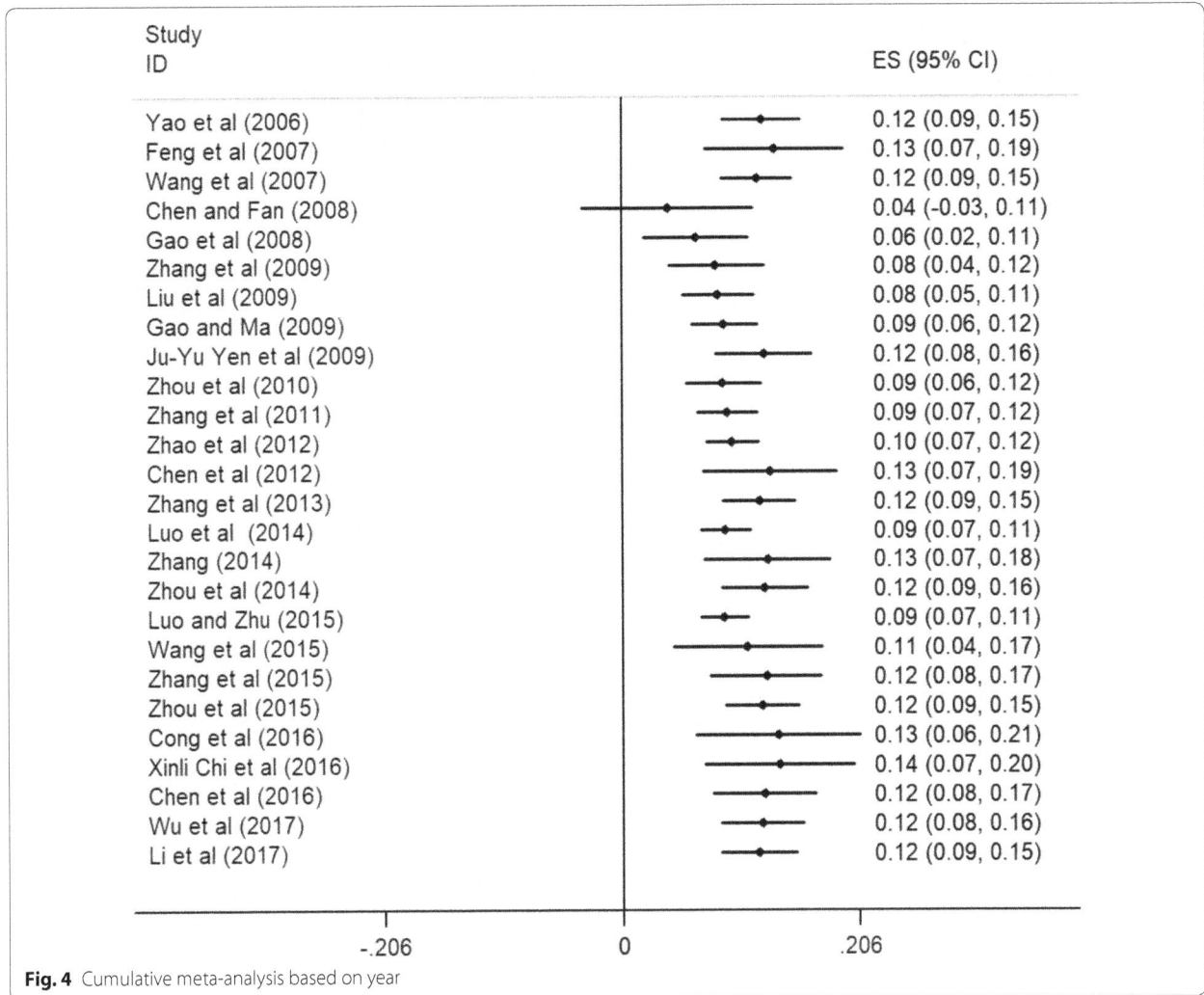

Fig. 4 Cumulative meta-analysis based on year

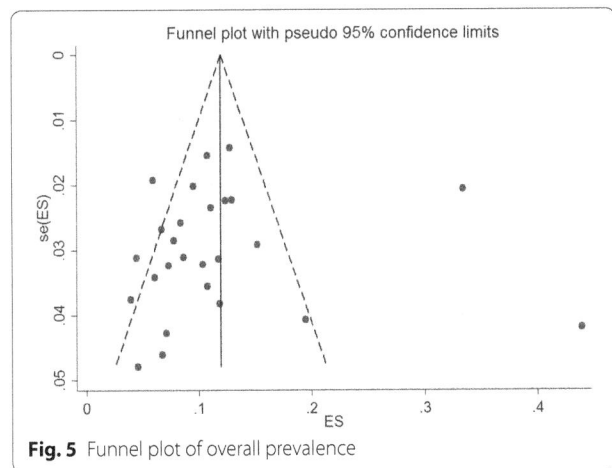

Fig. 5 Funnel plot of overall prevalence

more social activities and athletic sports [28]. In addition, parents should increase communication with their kids and spend more time relieving their inner troubles as well as understanding their needs [29–31]. In my opinion, it is also important to take measures to educate society about the dangers of Internet addiction. First of all, some measures need to be taken in communities and schools where more lectures on Internet addiction can be carried out [32, 33]. Schools and communities must guide students to use the Internet when they enter school and build a good way to communicate with their parents. Secondly, parents need to set up an Internet usage plan for children to make them know the seriousness of the Internet addiction [30]. Finally, the mass media can also organize more social activities such as Internet knowledge competition and make a documentary about Internet addiction so that people learn more about the dangers of Internet addiction. The most important factor is to help people form a reasonable understanding of Internet addiction and change unhealthy lifestyles. It is very necessary for us to pay more attention to the social education of Internet addiction in future studies. Only in this way, Internet addiction will lessen and young people will have a healthy environment to grow up.

Abbreviations

CI: confidence interval; CIAS: Chen Internet Addiction Scale; Young: Young Internet Addiction Scale; CDC: Chinese Center for Disease Control and Prevention; IA: Internet addiction; VI: VIP Database for Chinese Technical Periodicals; DSM-IV: Diagnostic and Statistical Manual of Mental Disorders-Fourth Edition; AHR: Agency for Healthcare Research and Quality; YDQ: Young's Internet Addiction Diagnostic Questionnaire.

Authors' contributions

As for authorship, Y-jS and TZ conceived and designed the study, Y-qW analyzed the data, LL was a major contributor in writing the manuscript. All authors contribute sufficiently to this work. All authors read and approved the final manuscript.

Acknowledgements

Not applicable.

Competing interests

The authors declare that they have no competing interests.

Funding

Study on prevention and cure strategies of college students' psychological and behavioral health in the perspective of preventive medicine (SK2016A0947).

References

1. Beard KW, Wolf EM. Modification in the proposed diagnostic criteria for Internet addiction. Cyberpsychol Behav Impact Internet Multimedia Virtual Reality Behav Soc. 2001;4(3):377.
2. Craparo G, Messina R, Severino S, Fasciano S, Cannella V, Gori A, et al. The relationships between self-efficacy, Internet addiction and shame. Indian J Psychol Med. 2014;36(3):304–7. https://doi.org/10.4103/0253-7176.135386.
3. Jelenchick LA, Becker T, Moreno MA. Assessing the psychometric properties of the Internet Addiction Test (IAT) in US college students. Psychiatry Res. 2012;196(2–3):296.
4. Ghamari F, Mohammadbeigi A, Mohammadsalehi N, et al. Internet Addiction and modeling its risk factors in medical students, Iran. Indian J Psychol Med. 2012;33(2):158–62.
5. Ac-Nikolić E, Zarić D, Nićiforović-Šurković O. Prevalence of Internet Addiction among schoolchildren in Novi Sad. Srp Arh Celok Lek. 2015;143(11–12):719.
6. Ekenze SO, Okafor CI, Ekenze OS, et al. The value of Internet tools in undergraduate surgical education: perspective of medical students in a developing country. World J Surg. 2017;41(3):672–80.
7. Price A. Benefits of the Internet. Br J Gen Pract J R Coll Gen Practit. 1997;47(423):664.
8. Levy JA, Strombeck R. Health benefits and risks of the Internet. J Med Syst. 2002;26(6):495–510.
9. Chou WJ, Huang MF, Chang YP, et al. Social skills deficits and their association with Internet addiction and activities in adolescents with attention-deficit/hyperactivity disorder. J Behav Addict. 2017;6(1):42.
10. Lim J, Gwak AR, Su MP, et al. Are adolescents with Internet addiction prone to aggressive behavior? The mediating effect of clinical comorbidities on the predictability of aggression in adolescents with Internet addiction. Cyberpsychol Behav Soc Netw. 2015;18(5):260.
11. Coniglio MA, Muni V, Giammanco G, et al. Excessive Internet use and Internet addiction: emerging public health issues. Igiene E Sanita Pubblica. 2007;63(2):127.
12. Berner JE, Santander J, Contreras AM, Gómez T. Description of Internet addiction among Chilean medical students: a cross-sectional study. Acad Psychiatry. 2014;38(1):11–4. https://doi.org/10.1007/s40596-013-0022-6 (Epub 2014 Jan 16).
13. Lin MP, Ko HC, Wu JY. Prevalence and psychosocial risk factors associated with Internet addiction in a nationally representative sample of college students in Taiwan. Cyberpsychol Behav Soc Netw. 2011;14(12):741–6. https://doi.org/10.1089/cyber.2010.0574 (Epub 2011 Jun 8).
14. Nestler EJ. Epigenetic mechanisms of drug addiction. Curr Opin Neurobiol. 2013;23(4):521.
15. Mun SY, Lee BS. Effects of an integrated Internet addiction prevention program on elementary students' self-regulation and Internet addiction. J Korean Acad Nurs. 2015;45(2):251–61.
16. Achnio A, Przepiorka A. Dysfunction of self-regulation and self-control in Facebook addiction. Psychiatr Q. 2016;87(3):493–500.
17. Hu J, Dong Y, Chen X, et al. Prevalence of suicide attempts among Chinese adolescents: a meta-analysis of cross-sectional studies. Compr Psychiatry. 2015;61:78–89.
18. Enst WAV, Ochodo E, Scholten RJ, et al. Investigation of publication bias in meta-analyses of diagnostic test accuracy: a meta-epidemiological study. BMC Med Res Methodol. 2014;14(1):70.
19. Wang Z, Zhang YH, Xu QQ. Several methods of published bias assessment. Chin J Health Stat. 2009;26(5):539–41.
20. Bian HY, Li Y, Li N, Liu TW. Meta analysis for Internet addiction rate among adolescents. Chin J School Health. 2016;37(1):67–70.
21. Tateno M, Teo AR, Shirasaka T, Tayama M, Watabe M, Kato TA. Internet addiction and self-evaluated attention-deficit hyperactivity disorder traits among Japanese college students. Psychiatry Clin Neurosci. 2016;70(12):567–72. https://doi.org/10.1111/pcn.12454 (Epub 2016 Oct 24).
22. Khan MA, Shabbir F, Rajput TA. Effect of gender and physical activity on Internet addiction in medical students. Pak J Med Sci. 2017;33(1):191–4. https://doi.org/10.12669/pjms.331.11222.
23. Canan F, Ataoglu A, Ozcetin A, Icmeli C. The association between Internet addiction and dissociation among Turkish college students. Compr Psychiatry. 2012;53(5):422–6. https://doi.org/10.1016/j.comppsych.2011.08.006 (Epub 2011 Oct 13).
24. Zhou XY, Xu F, Wei XL, Zhao L, Pang BH, Chang JB. Internet addiction disorder and mental health in the University Students in Yan'an City. China J Health Psychol. 2015;23(10):1506–9.
25. Luo S, Guo JZ, Hu SJ, Zhuang LH, Wang HJ. Internet addicts' behavior and influencing factors among college students. Chin J Health Stat. 2014;31(3):434–6.
26. Joiner R, Gavin J, Brosnan M, et al. Gender, Internet experience, Internet identification, and Internet anxiety: a ten-year followup. Cyberpsychol Behav Soc Netw. 2012;15(7):370.
27. Guosong S. China's regulations on Internet cafés. China Media Res. 2010;6(3):26–30.
28. Echeburua E, De CP. Addiction to new technologies and to online social networking in young people: a new challenge. Adicciones. 2010;22(2):91–5.
29. Ko CH, Yen JY, Yen CF, et al. Factors predictive for incidence and remission of Internet addiction in young adolescents: a prospective study. Cyberpsychol Behav Impact Internet Multimedia Virtual Real Behav Soc. 2007;10(4):545.
30. Lam LT. Parental mental health and Internet addiction in adolescents. Addict Behav. 2015;42:20.

31. Lin YH, Gau SS. Association between morningness–eveningness and the severity of compulsive Internet use: the moderating role of gender and parenting style. Sleep Med. 2013;14(12):1398–404.

32. Mei S, Yau YHC, Chai J, et al. Problematic Internet use, well-being, self-esteem and self-control: data from a high-school survey in China. Addict Behav. 2016;61:74–9.

33. Christakis DA, Moreno MM, Jelenchick L, et al. Problematic Internet usage in US college students: a pilot study. BMC Med. 2011;9(1):77.

34. Yao YS, Gao C, Zhou FH, Jin YL, Wang EM, Ye DQ. Epidemiological study on Internet use and Internet addiction disorder among college students. Chin J School Health. 2006;27(10):844–6.

35. Feng CY, Xiong M, Huang LY, Luo H, Deng B. Prevalence of Internet addiction disorder and anxiety and depression Among 1497 University Students in Guizhou. Chin J School Health. 2007;28(9):801–2.

36. Wang XZ, Zhao L. The relationship between college students' Internet addiction and personality TRAITS. Chin J School Health. 2007;28(2):164–5.

37. Chen J, Fan JL. A cross-sectional investigation of College Students' Internet addiction and the analysis of its influencing factors. Acta Universitatis Medicinalis Anhui. 2008;43(3):350–3.

38. Gao Y, Li ZL, Wan BH, Li YL, Xu ZG. Investigation on Internet addiction disorder in college students. Chin J School Health. 2008;24(11):1368–9.

39. Zhang LN, Shen QJ, Yang YJ, Zhang T, Cui J, Li H. Psychological and Personality characteristics of college students with Internet addiction disorder in Ningbo. Chin Mental Health J. 2009;23(9):674–6.

40. Liu JA, Feng DX, Wang Q, Liang Y, Meng H, Jin JQ, et al. Study on status and influencing factors of Internet addiction disorder among medical college students. Chin J Soc Med. 2009;26(3):150–2.

41. Gao B, Ma HY. Research on the Internet activities and Internet addiction disorder of college students in Zhejiang Province. Chin J Health Educ. 2009;25(1):11–3.

42. Yen JY, Ko CH, Yen CF, Chen CS, Chen CC. The association between harmful alcohol use and Internet addiction among college students: comparison of personality. Psychiatry Clin Neurosci. 2009;63(2):218–24. https://doi.org/10.1111/j.1440-1819.2009.01943.x.

43. Zhou YQ, Cao JQ, Wang XL, Zhang H, Yang JW. Status of Internet addiction among undergraduates and its influencing factors. Chin Gen Pract. 2010;13(31):3528–30.

44. Zhang T, Yang YX, Bao LQ, Shen YY. An investigation of college students' Internet addiction and analysis of related factors. Strait J Prevent Med. 2011;17(6):24–5.

45. Zhao XY, Hu XB, Zhang MH, Sun YM, Zhao QG, Yang WL. Relationship of Internet addiction and depression among college students in Lanzhou. Chin J School Health. 2012;33(10):1179–81.

46. Chen SY, Zhang XF, Yang CS, Xu P, Chen JL. Study on college students with Internet addiction disorder and their personality characteristics in Wuhan City. Chin J Dis Control Prevent. 2012;16(6):544–6.

47. Zhang BH, Hu S, Sheng J. Relationship between TCM college students'IAD cases and the five-state personality theory. J Shandong Univ. 2013;51(9):105–8.

48. Zhang M. The relationship between Internet addiction and mental health of Uygur College Students. Chin J School Health. 2014;35(10):1559–60.

49. Zhou XQ, Xi XL, Cheng ZH, Shen LY, Li P. Prevalence of Internet addiction disorder and mental health status among college students. Chin J Clin Psychol. 2014;22(4):619–22.

50. Luo R, Zhu DL. A study of personality traits of undergraduates with IAD. J Jiangxi Normal Univ. 2015;48(6):133–6.

51. Wang XD, Gao YS, Lin FF, Chen YC. Analysis of college students' Internet addiction status and its influencing factors in Hainan Province. Chin J Health Educ. 2015;31(12):1152–5.

52. Zhang M, Tang DW, Jiang Q, Deng SP, Zhu XY. Prevalence of Internet addiction and influencing factors among college students in Nantong. Chin J School Health. 2015;36(3):378–80.

53. Cong JN, Huang XM, Zhao YJ. An analysis and prediction of college students' Internet addiction among college students in a medical college. Chin Prim Health Care. 2016;30(8):72–3.

54. Chi X, Lin L, Zhang P. Internet addiction among college students in China: prevalence and psychosocial correlates. Cyberpsychol Behav Soc Netw. 2016;19(9):567–73.

55. Chen YJ, Li L, Hu YH, Guo XP. Relationship between parent–child communication and Internet addiction among college students. Chin J School Health. 2016;37(2):221–3.

56. Wu XS, Dong ZP, Zhu K, Li JD, Wang Q, Liu Y, et al. Analysis of Internet addiction status and influencing factors of college students. J Taishan Med Coll. 2017;38(3):263–5.

57. Li FJ, Sun J, He J, Yang BS, Wang X. Survey on the current situation of Internet addiction among college students, Henan Province, 2013. Prev Med Tribune. 2017;23(7):499–501.

Incidence of depressive symptoms among sexually abused children in Kenya

Teresia Mutavi[1]* ⓘ, Anne Obondo[1], Donald Kokonya[2], Lincoln Khasakhala[1], Anne Mbwayo[1], Francis Njiri[1] and Muthoni Mathai[1]

Abstract

Background: Children who experience sexual abuse undergo various negative psychosocial outcomes such as depressive symptoms. Unfortunately, not many studies have been conducted on the incidence of depressive symptoms among sexually abused children in Kenya. This study sought to ascertain the incidence of depressive symptoms among children who have experienced sexual abuse in Kenya.

Methods: This was a longitudinal study design. It was conducted at Kenyatta National Teaching and Referral Hospital and Nairobi Women's Hospitals in Kenya. One hundred and ninety-one children who had experienced sexual abuse and their parents/legal guardians were invited to participate in the study. The study administered the Becks Depression Inventory and the Child Depression Inventory to the children.

Results: The incidence of depressive symptoms after 1 month of sexual abuse revealed that amongst children who were below 16 years old, 14.6% had minimal-mild depressive symptoms while 85.4% had moderate-severe depressive symptoms. In comparison, children who were 16 years or older, 6.4% had minimal-mild depressive symptoms while 93.6% had moderate-severe depressive symptoms. Children below 16 years old whose parents were separated were found to have depressive symptoms (p < 0.001) as well as those who were presented early for medical care (p < 0.004), while children aged 16 years and above who were abused by strangers were more likely to have depressive symptoms (p < 0.024) and those who were not attending school (p < 0.002).

Conclusion: Sexual abuse of children is world-wide and the Kenyan situation is comparable. Being the victim of sexual abuse as a child has major psychological and emotional sequlae which need to be addressed in Kenya. Children who experience sexual abuse have very high incidence of developing depressive symptoms. All the sexually abused children studied suffered from depressive symptoms and a large majority suffered from major depressive symptoms that should be promptly and effectively addressed to ameliorate psychological suffering among children.

Keywords: Children, Depressive symptoms, Sexual abuse, Kenya

Background

Violence against children is a widespread global problem, causing detrimental health and social outcomes to the child, the family and society [1]. The global estimated prevalence of sexual abuse among girls ranged from 7 to 36% and 5 to 10% among boys [2]. Globally, an estimated one billion children were exposed to violence during the year 2014 compared to two billion children in 2013 who experienced either physical, emotional or sexual violence [3]. Children were found to be affected by sexual abuse across different age groups globally [4]. Sexual abuse had been common among girls than boys and girls were at a higher risk of re-exposure than boys [5].

Accordingly, the odds of having been exposed to sexual abuse had been shown to be greater among girls than boys (OR 1.29; 95% CI 1.2–1.48; p < 0.001) [6]. In Ethiopia, among 267 children who were treated at two hospitals after experiencing sexual abuse, 75.7% were girls and 24.3% were boys [7]. A review paper of African

*Correspondence: terrymutavi@yahoo.com; mutavi.teresia@uonbi.ac.ke
[1] Department of Psychiatry, School of Medicine, College of Health Sciences, University of Nairobi, P.O. Box 74-00519, Mlolongo, Nairobi, Kenya
Full list of author information is available at the end of the article

countries in 2014 reported that the odds for girls experiencing sexual abuse was higher than boys (OR 1.85–3.85 and p < 0.01) [8]. In the year 2011, a Tanzanian study on children aged 13–17 years old found out that nearly two-thirds (63.9%) of the girls and slightly over a third (38.7%) of the boys had experienced sexual abuse [9]. In a Ugandan study of 2014, more girls than boys experienced sexual abuse [$X^2(1407) = 12.44$; $p < 0.0005$] [10]. The prevalence of sexual abuse among children under 18 years of age in Kenya over a period of 5 years (2007–2013) reported that 11.8% of the girls and 3.6% of the boys had been exposed to sexual abuse [11]. An earlier study during the period 2006–2009 found out that 28.3% of the sexual abuse cases among children assessed and treated at Kenyatta National Hospital (KNH), Nairobi Kenya were young and below 18 years of age [12]. Psychosocial outcomes associated with sexual abuse included depression [13], post traumatic-stress disorder (PTSD) and declining school grades among many other negative outcomes [14]. The Ugandan study of 2013 found out that among 1587 children who had experienced childhood traumas had a higher risk of developing depressive symptoms [15]. In the Ethiopian study of 2009, students who reported experiencing different forms of sexual abuse were nearly twice as likely to be classified as having moderate depressive symptoms compared to those who had not been sexually abused [16]. Similarly, in the study of 2015 among 1456 boys in Kenya aged 13–24 years who had experienced sexual abuse, it was found out that 90% of them had depressive symptoms and 14.8% had experienced sexual abuse before the age of 18 years [11]. Another study of 2015 on adolescents aged 13–18 years in Kenya found out that 80% of those who had experienced sexual abuse and other traumatic events had varying degrees of depressive symptoms and 89.2% of them had experienced difficulties in academic performance [17]. This study sought to determine the incidence of depressive symptoms among Kenyan children who had been sexually abused. The children were followed up for a period of 1 year in order to highlight the importance of psychosocial support and to improve the mental health of these children.

Methods

This paper was part of a Kenyan longitudinal study on the psychosocial outcomes associated with sexual abuse among children aged 7–17 years who were treated at the Kenyatta National Hospital (KNH), the National Teaching and Referral Hospital. The study was also conducted at a specialised private Gender-Based Violence (GBV) hospital, the Nairobi Women's Hospital in Nairobi, Kenya [18]. The two are the leading and specialized hospitals in (GBV) in Kenya, based in Nairobi City. Sexually abused

children are medically cared for at the two hospitals with 24-h service at the Gender Based Violence Recovery Centres (GBVRC) or at the Accident & Emergency (A&E) departments [19]. Physical and mental state assessments are conducted by trained medical officers and psychiatrists respectively and data secured confidentially [20]. post exposure prophylactic, emergency contraception, treatment for sexually transmitted infections (STI) and human immunodeficiency virus (HIV) are routinely offered to the survivors who fill in locator forms [21]. The KNH, GBV service centre treats and supports an average of 6 survivors per day while the GBV service centre at the Nairobi Women's Hospital's (NWH) treats and supports an average of 10 survivors. Both centres provide a one stop patient management. This includes provision of emergency post rape medical care, collection and preservation of forensic evidence, Legal Aid, medical intervention, creation of awareness about GBV, trauma counselling, outreach programmes and establishment of support groups for survivors of GBV [22].

This study was approved by the Ethical and Research Committee (ERC) of the KNH/University of Nairobi [23]. The study population comprised of GBV survivors aged 7–17 years. A minimum sample size was set [N = 191] at baseline including an assumed attrition rate of 20% [24, 25]. Four months later, at the first follow up, the attrition rate was 6%, 8 months later it was 6 and 4% at the end of the study period. The cumulative attrition rate was 14% well within the 20% anticipated attrition rate. The attrition was attributed to relocation of the family to the rural areas while others did not return for follow up despite several telephone reminders. The study participants were recruited into the study when they were presented by their care takers for medical and psychosocial care at the two study sites. They were recruited using systematic and purposive (by gender) sampling techniques. After a child had been randomly selected to participate in this study after 1-month exposure to the sexual abuse incidence, the parents/legal guardians were approached to give informed consent to participate in this study and assent from the children. The children were put on the standard prophylactic and therapeutic treatments regimes, usually provided at the GBVR centres in both hospitals [18]. This included Post exposure Prophylaxis (PeP) against HIV and contraceptive prophylaxis (CP), treatment of physical injuries and psychosocial care in the hospitals and or referred to legal services providers. The study participants who were found to be in need of medical care were referred to physicians at the two centres.

A locally designed questionnaire on socio-demographic and sexual abuse profile was administered to the GBV survivors aged 7–17 years. The Beck Depression Inventory (BDI) was used for screening depressive symptoms among children aged 16–17 years because adolescents were considered as mature youth in the study and the Children's Depression Inventory (CDI) was used for screening depressive symptoms in the children aged 7–15.5 years [18]. On the CDI tool, minimal and mild depressive symptoms were regarded as insignificant and moderate and severe depressive symptoms were regarded as pathological [26]. The CDI used was a downward extension of the BDI. Higher scores on the BDI denoted greater severe depressive symptoms. The CDI had high correlational reliability for depressive symptoms with a Cronbach's alpha value of 0.86 for a psychiatric sample and 0.82 for a paediatric medical sample. The total score was the sum of all the separate item scores. Reliability and validity had been established over many years of empirical research. The CDI had been successfully used in the Kenyan children's population [27]. It had also been validated in the Sub Saharan African countries in Rwanda [28], Tanzania [29] and in Malawi [30]. The BDI had been adequately adapted to the Kenyan population [31]. The BDI and the CDI had been translated into Kiswahili versions, a *lingua franca* widely spoken in Kenya, Eastern and Central Africa [29, 30].

Data was collected over a 1-year period at follow up intervals of 4 months. Completed questionnaires were safely and securely stored prior to entry into computer excel sheets. Descriptive statistics were analysed, interpreted and displayed while inferential statistics were statistically analysed using SPSS Version 21. The level of statistical significance was set at 0.05 ($p < 0.05$) with a 95% confidence interval (CI). Bivariate logistic regression analysis and analysis of variance were used to determine associations among variables.

Results
Socio-demographics
One hundred ninety-one (N = 191) sexually abused children were recruited into this study, of whom 12.0% were males and 88.0% were females, giving a male: female ratio of 1:7. The mean and median age were equal at 13 years. The youngest study participant was 7 and oldest the was 17 years of age. The majority (35.1%) of the study participants were young in their mid-adolescence at (13–15 years) of age. Almost a quarter (24.6%) were in their older (16–17 years) childhood ages while slightly less than a quarter (23%) were aged (10–12 years) early adolescence and 17.3% were below adolescence (7–9 years). A statistically significant proportion (96.8%) of the study participants attended school and only 3.2% did not attend school. The parents of over three quarter (75.4%) of the participants were alive while 17.3% of the children had living mothers but no fathers. Less than five percent (4.2%) had fathers only and 3.1% were parentless

(orphaned). Slightly less than three quarters (72.2%) of the parents were married, 19.4% were separated or divorced and 8.4% were of single parentage. Nearly a third (30.4%) of the parents/legal guardians earned less than US$1/day but the majority (37.2%) earned US$1/day, leaving only 29.3% living above the poverty line with a monthly income of more than US$1/day and 3.1% earned more than US$2 a day.

Sexual abuse
Slightly over a half 97 (50.7%) were abused by acquaintances, 80 (41.8%) by a stranger, 3 (1.7%) by a care giver, 9 (4.8%) by biological parent and 2 (1%) by foster parent. Majority 170 (89%) of the participants experienced vaginal anal penetration, 11 (5.8%) experienced touching of the genital, 10 (5.2%) experienced non-genital contact. Majority 172 (90.1%) were made to touch the genitals of the perpetrator, 15 (7.8%) were not made to perform any act and 4 (2.1%) were made to do oral copulation. Ninety two (48.1%) of the abuse incidence happened once, 38 (19.9%) of the abuse happened twice, 30 (15.7%) of the abuse incidence happened three times, 16 (8.4%) of the abuse incidence happened four times and lastly 15 (6.7%) of the abuse incidence happened more than four times. Most 129 (67.9%) the abuse had taken place over a month ago, 42 (22.1%) took place over the past few days, 5 (2.1%) took place over a week ago and 15 (7.9%) had taken place over years ago.

Incidence of depressive symptoms
Depressive symptoms were assessed using CDI at baseline for children below 16 years old and Becks Depression Inventory for children over 16 years. Almost three quarters (3/4) of the study participants (74.3%) experienced moderate depressive symptoms and 11.1% experienced severe depressive symptoms. It was therefore, noted that approximately 85.4% of the sexually abused children in Kenya experienced major depressive symptoms. This meant that sexually abused children in Kenya, suffered major depressive symptoms (T score > 60, equivalent of > 84th percentile) that warranted special mention and attention. Only 14.6% of the children did not experience major depressive symptoms and 3.5% of them suffered from minimal depressive symptoms while 11.1% experienced mild depressive symptoms. During the first follow up, 16% of the study participants had minimal depressive symptoms 81.9% had mild depressive symptoms, 2.1% had moderate depressive symptoms while none had severe depressive symptoms. By extension, during the second follow, up 92% of the children had minimal depressive symptoms and there were no major depressive symptoms after the first follow up (Table 1).

Table 1 Incidence of depressive symptoms (N = 166)

| | Baseline | | Follow ups | | | | | |
| | | | 1 | | 2 | | 3 | |
	N	%	N	%	n	%	n	%
CDI								
Minimal < 10	5	3.5	23	16.0	127	92.0	132	100.0
Mild, 11–16	16	11.1	118	81.9	11	8.0	0	0.0
Moderate, 17–27	107	74.3	3	2.1	0	0.0	0	0.0
Severe > 28	16	11.1	0	0.0	0	0.0	0	0.0
Totals	144	100	144	100	138	100	132	100
BDI								
Minimal, 0–9	0	0.0	0	0.0	26	74.3	27	79.4
Mild, 10–16	3	6.4	14	38.9	9	25.7	7	20.6
Moderate, 17–29	27	57.4	22	61.1	0	0.0	0	0.0
Severe, 30–63	17	36.2	0	0.0	0	0.0	0	0.0
Totals	47	100	36	100	35	100	34	100

This findings study showed that there was a direct relationship between sexual abuse and depressive symptoms. The therapeutic interventions at the GBVRCs in Kenya were rapid and effective as shown by the absence of depressive symptoms, 4 months after the first follow up session and all the children had achieved remission (Table 1).

Children below 16 years of age whose parents were separated were found to be vulnerable to depressive symptoms ($p < 0.001$) as well as those under the of care givers ($p < 0.0001$). The older children aged 16 years and above who were not attending school were found to be more likely to have depressive symptoms ($p < 0.002$), as were children who lived with their fathers ($p < 0.0018$) or were under the care of good Samaritans ($p < 0.0001$) (Table 2).

The female children aged 16–17 years experienced moderate depressive symptoms (mean score = 27.7) while the male experienced severe depressive symptoms (mean score = 29.0) on the BDI II scale. The out of school children experienced severe depressive symptoms (mean score = 43) while those in school experienced moderate depressive symptoms (mean score = 27.1) but those in secondary schools experienced severe depressive symptoms (mean score = 29) compared to those in primary school who experienced moderate depressive symptoms (mean score 26.2). Being raised by the father alone (mean score = 49) or having no parent (mean score = 31) were risk factors for severe depressive symptoms but having both parents (mean score = 26.7) or a mother only (mean score 27.8) led to moderate depressive symptoms.

Table 2 Depressive symptoms in relation to socio demographic characteristics (N191)

| | CDI score | | BDI score | |
	Mean	p-value	Mean	p-value
Gender				
Male	22.3	0.624	29.0	0.867
Female	21.5		27.7	
Attending school				
Yes	21.5	0.667	27.1	0.002
No	19.5		43.0	
School level				
Primary	21.7	0.579	26.2	0.190
Secondary	20.2		29.2	
Have parents				
Both mother and father	22.0	0.575	26.7	0.018
Only mother	20.3		27.8	
Only father	20.1		49.0	
None	26.0		31.0	
Parents marital status				
Married	20.7	0.001	26.3	0.141
Separated	25.9		29.8	
Divorced	18.5		31.0	
Others	19.1		33.1	
Who do you live with				
Good samaritan	20.0	< 0.0001	49.0	< 0.0001
Care giver	20.8		25.6	
Guardian	27.7		32.7	
Others	.		41.0	

Children whose parents were marriage experienced moderate depressive symptoms (mean score = 26.3) compared to divorced (mean score = 31.0, separated (mean score = .29.8 and others (mean score = 33.1) all of whom experienced severe depressive symptoms. Children under the care of good Samaritans (mean score = 49), guardian (mean score. = 27.7) and others (mean score = 41.0) were risk factors for severe depressive symptoms while children under care givers (mean score 25.6) experienced moderate depressive symptoms.

Though statistically insignificant (p < 0.624), both male and female younger children aged 7–15.5 years experienced severe depressive symptoms (mean score 22.3 and 21.5 respectively). On the CDI I depressive symptoms scale, the children out of school experienced mild depressive symptoms (mean score = 19.5) compared to moderate depressive symptoms experienced by those in school (man score = 21.5). Both primary and secondary school children aged 7–15.5 years experienced moderate depressive symptoms (mean score—21.7 and 20.2 respectively). Whether the parents of the children were alive or not, all the children experienced moderate depressive symptoms with high mean scores (both = 22.0), mother only (mean score = 20.3), father only (mean score = 20.1) and none (mean score = 26.0). Whereas the children of divorced and other status of parenthood experienced mild depressive symptoms (mean score = 18.5 and 19.1 respectively), the children of the married parents experienced moderate depressive symptoms (mean score = 20.7) and so to the separated (mean score = 25.9). Living with a good Samaritan (mean score = 20.0), care givers (mean score = 20.8) and guardians (mean score = 27.7) were risk factors for moderate and severe depressive symptoms respectively (Table 2).

Sexually abused young children below 16 years of age, in spite of receiving comprehensive and specialized medical care early were more likely to be depressed (*p* < 0.004), while those above 16 years of age who were abused by strangers were more likely to be depressed (*p* < 0.024). Furthermore, children who were forced to touch the perpetrators' genitals (*p* < 0.011) and those who were taken to the police stations (*p* < 0.032) were more likely to have depressive symptoms (Table 3).

The 7–15.5-year-old children experienced severe depressive symptoms perpetrated by their biological parents (mean score = 26.1), moderate depressive symptoms (mean scores = 21.4 and 21.3) perpetrated by strangers and acquaintances respectively. However, non-parental care givers caused mild depressive symptoms (mean score = 18.0) on the CDI I scale. On the BDI II scale among the 16–17 year old children, biological parents and strangers perpetrated severe depressive symptoms (mean score = 41 and 29.1 respectively),

Table 3 Depressive symptoms in relation to sexual abuse profile (N = 191)

	CDI score		BDI score	
	Mean	p value	Mean	p value
Relationship to perpetrator				
Stranger	21.4	0.199	29.1	0.024
Acquaintance	21.3		26.1	
Non-parental care giver	18.0		15.0	
Biological parent	26.1		41.0	
Perpetrator acts				
Vagina anal penetration	21.3	0.109	27.4	0.230
Touching the genitals	26.5		40.0	
Non-genital contact	18.0		–	
What perpetrator made victim do				
Nothing	19.1	0.458	25.7	0.011
Touching genitals	21.8		49.0	
Oral copulation	20.0		–	
Others	–		27.5	
Frequency of abuse				
Once	20.4	0.129	27.6	0.229
Twice	22.7		27.4	
Three times	22.7		31.0	
Four times	24.9		20.0	
More than four times	20.9		40.0	
How long the abuse taken place				
Days	20.6	0.748	28.0	0.875
Weeks	21.7		22.0	
Months	21.8		27.2	
Years	23.1		27.5	
First place to be taken				
Hospital	21.9	0.469	26.9	0.032
Chief's camp	–		21.0	
Police station	20.4		33.2	
Other	18.0		41.0	
How long before receiving medical care				
Within 1 h	21.9	0.004	26.9	0.223
Within 2 h	25.7		31.0	
Within 12 h	22.7		25.0	
Within 48 h	12.0		24.0	
Within 72 h	21.7		–	
After 72 h	17.6		35.0	

acquaintances caused moderate depressive symptoms (mean score = 26.1) while non-parental care giver was associated with mild depressive symptoms (mean score = 15.0). There was strong association between sexual abuse and depressive symptoms among the older 16–17 years (*p* < 0.024) but this was not the case with the younger children aged 7–15.5 years (*p* < 0.199). As to whether there was a relationship between depressive symptoms and the acts of the perpetrator, there was no statistical significance in both the younger and the older age groups ($p < 0.109$ and 0.230 respectively). Touching the minors' genitals 7–15.5 years (mean score $= 26.5$) evoked severe depressive symptoms to the highest level as well as the 16–17 years old (mean score $= 40.0$) on the BDI II scale. Between the 7–15.5 and the 16–17 year old, the victims experienced severe depressive symptoms (mean score $= 26.5$ and 49.0 respectively) when compelled to touch the perpetrators' genitals compared to the rest, oral copulation (mean score $= 20.0$) for the younger children and none (mean score $= 19.1$) and others (mean score $= 27.5$) and none (mean score $= 25.7$) for the older children. The modal frequency of sexual abuse was four ($\times 4$) times among the younger children aged 7–15.5 years old (mean score $= 24.9$) causing moderate depressive symptoms, though it was not statistically significant ($p < 0.129$). Among the older children (16–17 years), the modal frequency of sexual abuse was $>$four ($\times 4$) times, causing severe depressive symptoms (mean score $= 40$), also not statistically significant ($p < 0.229$). There was moderate depressive symptoms in relation to the severity of sexual abuse with regard to the duration of abuse, ranging from days to years (mean score $= 20.6$–23.1) which produced a pattern showing that the longer the younger children were abused, the severer the depressive symptoms they experienced. In the case of the older children (16–17 years), all of them experienced moderate depressive symptoms (mean score $= 28$–22) and the abuse taking place for days was the highest (mean score $= 28$) which caused the upper end of moderate depressive symptoms. The findings in both categories of children were statistically insignificant ($p < 0.748$ and 0.875 respectively). Following the sexual abuse, the young children were mostly taken to hospitals (mean score $= 21.9$) followed by police stations (mean score $= 20.4$) and other places (mean score $= 18.0$). The older children were largely taken to unknown places (mean score $= 41.0$) followed by police stations (mean score $= 33.2$), then hospitals (mean score $= 26.9$) and Chiefs' camps (mean score $= 21.0$). Within a range of 1–72 h and above, the young victims accessed healthcare within significant short periods ($p < 0.004$), particularly 2 h (mean score $= 25$) while it took longer than 72 h for the older children (p < 0.223) to be taken for healthcare (mean score $= 35$) (Table 3).

Discussion

Sexual abuse in Kenya was widespread and it caused depressive symptoms among children producing similar trends to international findings (1, 3). The mean age in this study was consistent with those of other studies conducted in Kenya [32, 33]. Female children were seven

times ($\times 7$) at risk of sexual abuse in Kenya compared to the males in the mid adolescence age bracket and sexual abuse started in their early ages, just like elsewhere worldwide [1, 2, 5, 6, 10, 32, 33]. These Kenyan findings supported those of previous studies on sexual abuse among children [32, 33] as well as International studies [3, 5, 34]. Almost all cases of sexual abuse were in school, implying that either literacy rate was high and or schooling was a predisposing factor and a large majority were under both parental care in marriage [9, 11]. Most of the victims hailed from families which lived below poverty line and over four-fifths (4/5) of the children experienced severe depressive symptoms beyond the third percentile, quite comparable to studies in the USA [35, 36]. Timely and professional intervention showed that the children could recover fast to full remission within 4 months of the traumatic experience [7, 27]. The findings in this study showed that there was a temporal relationship between sexual abuse and depressive symptoms [11, 13, 16, 17, 37, 38]. These findings were comparable to those in Ethiopia where findings showed that the sexually abused adolescents were twice more likely to experience depressive symptoms than non-abused adolescents [11, 13, 16]. There was vulnerability to sexual abuse among children when parents were divorced or separated and when the children were left in the hands of care givers [38]. The high prevalence [2, 11, 13] and incidence of depressive symptoms particularly among the older children were associated with single parenthood and schooling (almost all the children were in school) but the out of school children experienced severe depressive symptoms that was comparable to other findings [11, 13, 16, 17, 32, 33]. It did not matter whether the parents of the children were alive or not, they all had similar experiences which were comparable with other studies done in Kenya [32]. The younger the children who were sexually abused and those abused by strangers, the severe the depressive symptoms among them [25, 26]. Biological parents who sexually abused their children were found to experience severe depressive symptoms compared to those abused by strangers and there was association between acts of sexual abuse and depressive symptoms [32, 33]. This study also showed that sexual abuse including repeated sexual abuse was common amongst children in Kenya, with associated depressive symptoms which was similar to other studies [5]. Children who were first taken to the hospital within 3 days experienced less depressive symptoms than those who were taken to police stations or elsewhere, a finding similar to that in another study in Kenya [27]. Based on this finding, given that children promptly taken to hospital have less depressive symptoms, it suggests that prompt interventions may have a role in ameliorating depressive symptoms. There appears to be an association between sexual abuse and depressive symptoms, and that therapeutic interventions at the GBVRCs in Kenya are temporally associated with reduction in depressive symptoms, with more rapid intervention associated with less depressive symptoms.

Conclusion

Sexual abuse of children is world-wide and the Kenyan situation is comparable. The act has major psychological and emotional outcomes that need to be addressed in Kenya. Children who experienced sexual abuse had high likelihood of developing depressive symptoms. All children in this study suffered from depressive symptoms 1 month after sexual abuse and that should be urgently addressed to reduce psychological suffering among children in Kenya. Screening and immediate provision of treatment after sexual abuse among children is important to prevent mental health problems among children for the improvement of their psychosocial functioning. Parents whose children have experienced sexual abuse need psychosocial support to enable their children cope with the trauma, thereby quickly facilitating their recovery process.

Abbreviations
SVAC: sexual abuse against children; OR: odds ratio; GBVRC: Gender Based Violence Recovery Centres; BDI: Becks Depression Inventory; CDI: Children's Depression Inventory; ERC: Ethical and Research Committee.

Authors' contributions
TM, AO, MM, conceived, designed the study, FN performed the analysis, DK, LK and AM edited the manuscript. All authors read and approved the final manuscript.

Author details
[1] Department of Psychiatry, School of Medicine, College of Health Sciences, University of Nairobi, P.O. Box 74-00519, Mlolongo, Nairobi, Kenya. [2] Department of Behavioural Sciences & Community Health, School of Medicine, Masinde Muliro University of Science and Technology, Kakamega, Kenya.

Acknowledgements
This study was carried out and funded within the "Mental Health Research for Better Outcomes," a project funded from the National Institute of Mental Health (NIMH) through Grant Award No 4R34MH09913. The content is solely the responsibility of the authors and does not necessarily represent the official views of the National Institute of Mental Health. The University of Washington, provided oversight and resources around child mental health and quantitative research.

Competing interests
The authors declare that they have no competing interests.

References
1. Stoltenborgh M, van IJzendoorn MH, Euser EM, Bakermans-Kranenburg MJ. A global perspective on child sexual abuse: meta-analysis of prevalence around the world. Child maltreat. 2011;16(2):79–101.
2. Pereda N, Guilera G, Forns M, Gomez- Benito J. The prevalence of child sexual abuse in community and student samples: a meta-analysis. Clin Psychol Rev. 2009;29(4):328–38. https://doi.org/10.1016/j.cpr.2009.02.007.
3. Hillis S, Mercy J, Amobi A, Kress H. Global prevalence of past-year violence against children: a systematic review and minimum estimates. Pediatrics. 2016;137(3):1–3.
4. Veenema TG, Thornton CP, Corley A. The public health crisis of child sexual abuse in low and middle income countries: an integrative review of the literature. Int J Nurs Stud. 2015;52(4):864–81.
5. Finkelhor D, Turner HA, Shattuck A, Hamby SL. Violence, crime, and abuse exposure in a national sample of children and youth: an update. JAMA Pediatr. 2013;167(7):614–21.
6. Brown D, Riley L, Butchart A, Meddings D, Kann L, Harvey P. Exposure to physical and sexual abuse and adverse health behaviors in African children: results from the Global school based student health survey. Bull World Health Org. 2009;87:447–55.
7. Girgira T, Tilahun B, Bacha T. Time to presentation, pattern and immediate health effects of alleged child sexual abuse at two tertiary hospitals in Addis Ababa, Ethiopia. BMC Public Health. 2014;14(1):92.
8. Meinck F, Cluver LD, Boyes ME, Mhlongo EL. Risk and protective factors for physical and sexual abuse of children and adolescents in Africa: a review and implications for practice. Trauma Violence Abuse. 2015;16(1):81–107.
9. United Republic of Tanzania. Violence against Children in Tanzania. Dar es Salaam: UNICEF Tanzania; 2011.
10. Mandrup L, Elklit A. Victimization and PTSD in Ugandan youth. Open J Epidemiol. 2014;4(3):141–56.
11. Sumner SA, Mercy AA, Saul J, Motsa-Nzuza N, Kwesigabo G, Buluma R, Marcelin LH, Lina H, Shawa M, Moloney-Kitts M, Kilbane T. Prevalence of sexual abuse against children and use of social services-seven countries, 2007–2013. MMWR Morb Mortal Wkly Rep. 2015;64(21):565–9.
12. Kuria MW, Omondi L, Olando Y, Makenyengo M, Bukusi D. Is sexual abuse a part of war? A 4-year retrospective study on cases of sexual abuse at the Kenyatta National Hospital, Kenya. J Public Health Africa. 2013;4(1):5.
13. Maniglio R. Severe mental illness and criminal victimization: a systematic review. Acta Psychiatr Scand. 2009;119(3):180–91.
14. Khasakhala LI, Ndetei DM, Mathai M, Harder V. Major depressive disorder in a Kenyan youth sample: relationship with parenting behavior and parental psychiatric disorders. Ann Gen Psychiatry. 2013;12(1):15.
15. Kinyanda E, Kizza R, Abbo C, Ndyanabangi S, Levin J. Prevalence and risk factors of depressive symptoms in childhood and adolescence as seen in 4 districts of north-eastern Uganda. BMC Int Health Human Rights. 2013;13(1):19.
16. Gelaye B, Arnold D, Williams MA, Goshu M, Berhane Y. Depression among female college students experiencing gender-based violence in Awassa, Ethiopia. J Interpersonal Violence. 2009;24(3):464–81.
17. Mugambi P, Gitonga C. Adolescent awareness of the psychosocial risk factors for depression in selected secondary schools in Nairobi-Kenya. J Educ Soc Res. 2015;5(3):191.
18. Mutavi T, Mathai M, Obondo A. Post-traumatic stress disorder (PTSD) in sexually abused children and educational status in Kenya: a longitudinal study. J Child Adolesc Behav. 2017. https://doi.org/10.4172/2375-4494.1000357.
19. Mutavi T, Obondo A, Mathai M, Kokonya D, Dako-Gyeke M. Incidence of self-esteem among children exposed to sexual abuse in Kenya. Global Soc Welfare. 2018;5(1):39–47.
20. Bickley L, Szilagyi PG. Bates' guide to physical examination and history-taking. Philadelphia: Lippincott Williams & Wilkins; 2012.
21. Njuki R, Okal J, Warren CE, Obare F, Abuya T, Kanya L, Undie CC, Bellows B, Askew I. Exploring the effectiveness of the output-based aid voucher program to increase uptake of gender-based violence recovery services in Kenya: a qualitative evaluation. BMC Public Health. 2012;12(1):426.
22. Wielding S, Scott A. What women want: social characteristics, gender-based violence and social support preferences in a cohort of women living with HIV. Int J STD AIDS. 2017;28(5):486–90.

23. Beecher MD, Henry K. Ethics and clinical research. In: Ethics and medical decision-making. Abingdon: Routledge; 2017. pp. 3–9.

24. Lemeshow S, Hosmer D, Klar J, Lwanga S. Adequacy of sample size in health studies. Hoboken: WHO, John wiley & Sons; 1990.

25. Heo M. Impact of subject attrition on sample size determinations for longitudinal cluster randomized clinical trials. J Biopharm Stat. 2014;24(3):507–22.

26. Shore L, Toumbourou JW, Lewis AJ, Kremer P. Longitudinal trajectories of child and adolescent depressive symptoms and their predictors—a systematic review and meta-analysis. Child Adolesc Mental Health. 2018;23(2):107–20.

27. Ndetei D, Khasakhala L, Mutiso V, Mbwayo A. Recognition of depression in children in general hospital-based pediatric units in Kenya: practice and policy implications. Ann Gen Psychiatry. 2009;8(1):25.

28. Binagwaho A, Fawzi M, Agbonyitor M, Nsanzimana S, Karema C, Mutabazi V, Kayiteshoga Y. Validating the Children's Depression Inventory in the context of Rwanda. BMC Pediatr. 2016;16:29.

29. Traube D, Dukay V, Kaaya S, Reyes H, Mellins C. Cross- cultural adaptation of Child Depression Inventory for use in Tanzania with children affected by HIV. Vulnerable Child Youth Study. 2010;5(2):174–87.

30. Kim M, Mazenga A, Devandra A, Ahmed S, Kazembe P, Yu X, Nguyen C, Sharp C. Prevalence of depressive symptoms and validation of Becks Depression Inventory-II and the Child Inventory-short among HIV positive adolescent in Malawi. J Int Aids Soc. 2014;17(1):18965.

31. Abubakar A, Kalu RB, Katana K, Kabunda B, Hassan AS, Newton CR, Van de Vijver F. Adaptation and latent structure of the swahili version of beck depression inventory-II in a low literacy population in thecontext of HIV. PloS one. 2016;11(6):e0151030.

32. Ombok CA, Obondo A, Kangethe R, Atwoli L. The prevalence of post-traumatic stress disorder among sexually abused children at kenyatta national hospital in Nairobi, Kenya. East Afr Med J. 2013;90(10):332–7.

33. Syengo M, Kathuku M, Ndetei M. Psychiatric morbidity among sexually abused children and adolescents. East Afr Med J. 2008;85(2):85–91.

34. Brown WD, Riley L, Butchart A, Meddings RD, Kann L, Harvey AP. Exposure to physical and sexual violence and adverse health behaviors in African children: results from the Global school based student health survey. Bull World Health Org. 2009;87(6):447–55.

35. Cancian M, Slack KS, Yang MY. The effect of family income on risk of child maltreatment. Madison: Institute for Research on Poverty, University of Wisconsin-Madison; 2010.

36. Sedlak AJ, Mettenburg J, Basena M, Peta I, McPherson K, Greene A. Fourth national incidence study of child abuse and neglect (NIS-4). Washington, DC: US Department of Health and Human Services; 2010.

37. Shapero BG, Black SK, Liu RT, Klugman J, Bender RE, Abramson LY, Alloy LB. Stressful life events and depression: the effect of childhood emotional abuse on stress reactivity. J Clin Psychol. 2014;70(3):209–30.

38. Münzer A, Fegert JM, Goldbeck L. Psychological symptoms of sexually victimized children and adolescents compared with other maltreatment subtypes. J Child Sexual Abuse. 2016;25(3):326–46.

24

Somatic symptom and related disorders in children and adolescents: evaluation of a naturalistic inpatient multidisciplinary treatment

Pola Heimann[1], Beate Herpertz-Dahlmann[1], Jonas Buning[1], Norbert Wagner[2], Claudia Stollbrink-Peschgens[2], Astrid Dempfle[3] and Georg G. von Polier[1*]

Abstract

Background: This naturalistic study assesses the effectiveness of inpatient multidisciplinary treatment of children and adolescents with somatic symptom disorders (SSD) and investigates the role of pain coping strategies and psychiatric comorbidity (anxiety, depression).

Methods: Sixty children and adolescents (mean age 14.4 years) with SSD who underwent inpatient multidisciplinary treatment were assessed regarding their school attendance, levels of discomfort, coping strategies and psychiatric comorbidity (depression, anxiety) at pretreatment, discharge and 6 months following treatment.

Results: At discharge, the children and adolescents reported improvements in their level of discomfort, psychiatric comorbidities (anxiety, depression) and pain coping strategies, with medium to large effect sizes. Six months following treatment, the improvements remained stable, including significantly higher school attendance rates ($d = 1.6$; $p < 0.01$). Improvement in pain coping was associated with increased school attendance.

Conclusion: Inpatient multidisciplinary treatment is effective in reducing levels of discomfort, psychiatric comorbidity (anxiety, depression), and school absence and in improving coping strategies.

Keywords: Somatic symptom disorder, Multidisciplinary treatment, School attendance, Pain coping strategies, Comorbidity

Background

Somatic symptom disorders (SSD) describe a heterogeneous entity, though the terminology has changed over the years [1, 2]. In the present article they include somatoform disorders, dissociative (or conversion) disorders and somatic disorders with psychiatric comorbidity. Somatic symptom disorders lead to significant functional and emotional impairments e.g., school absence, high socioeconomic costs and frequent use of healthcare services [3, 4]. Recently, increased numbers of children and adolescents suffering from somatic symptom complaints with functional impairments have been reported by van Geelen and colleagues [5]: between 1988 and 2011 the percentage of boys with psychosomatic problems larger than 90th percentile increased from 5.0 to 9.1% and in girls from 16.7 to 24.5% (2619 adolescents included). In particular, factors related to treatment outcomes are poorly understood, and there is a need for further research in this field [3].

In the fifth edition of the Diagnostic and Statistical Manual of Mental Disorders (DSM-5), a new category was introduced known as "somatic symptom and related disorders". The DSM-5 emphasizes a significant functional impairment, as well as excessive thoughts, feelings and behaviors related to somatic symptoms, while the

*Correspondence: gvonpolier@ukaachen.de
[1] Department of Child and Adolescent Psychiatry, Psychosomatics and Psychotherapy, RWTH Aachen University, Aachen, Germany
Full list of author information is available at the end of the article

absence of a medical explanation for the symptoms is no longer necessary [6].

In contrast to the DSM-5, the International Statistical Classification of Diseases and Related Health Problems ICD-10 defines SSD in different categories e.g., somatoform disorder (F45.x) and dissociative and conversion disorder (F44.x) [7].

The most common symptoms reported by children and adolescents with SSD include pain, fatigue, faintness and nausea [8–10]. Specifically, chronic somatic pain (headache, recurrent abdominal and musculoskeletal pain) appears to be very frequent, with up to 25% of children and adolescents being affected in general population samples, including the "German Health Interview and Examination Survey for Children and Adolescents" (KiGGS) [8, 11–13]. Conversion disorders are less frequent, with a prevalence varying between 1–4% and up to 10%, as measured in a pediatric neurological unit [14, 15]. Moreover, data from the KiGGS-survey showed that up to 10.8% of children and adolescents suffer from a chronic somatic disorder and show a threefold increased risk of developing psychiatric comorbidities compared to healthy controls [13]. Likewise, children and adolescents with an SSD show an increased risk of developing psychiatric comorbidity, especially anxious or depressive symptoms [11, 16]. Moreover, adolescents with affective, anxiety and behavior disorders are at risk of developing somatic symptoms such as chronic pain; on the other hand depression and anxiety disorders can be a consequence of chronic pain [17, 18]. Up to 50% of children and adolescents with SSD suffer from psychiatric comorbidity [2]. In addition, affected children and adolescents often face functional long-term impairments resulting in poor academic achievements, an increased risk for later medical treatment and vocational impairment [8, 16, 19]. The emotional burden seems to have an important influence on the long-term treatment outcome [20]. This highlights the importance of consideration and treatment of psychiatric comorbidities during the inpatient multidisciplinary treatment.

Treatment often appears to be unsatisfactory to patients, families and healthcare professionals due to a low acceptance of the concepts of, and interventions for, somatic symptom disorders [1, 8, 11]. For subjects with severe impairments, inpatient multidisciplinary treatment in specialized healthcare units based on a cognitive behavioral approach has been recommended [11, 21]. Notably, a close cooperation among multiple disciplines is warranted, as biological and environmental/social aspects have to be considered [4, 22]. However, a systematic evaluation of treatment approaches is lacking, and specialized healthcare units are rare in Germany and many other developed countries [20].

More specialized multidisciplinary units are needed as unimodal treatment appears to be insufficient for the complexity of the SSD [20]. Compared to sole pediatric and psychiatric treatment, a multidisciplinary treatment approach facilitates a highly specialized treatment and ensures a close collaboration between pediatricians and psychiatrists. Previous studies predominantly focused on chronic somatic pain, while studies investigating SSD, including dissociative (or conversion) disorders and somatic disorders with psychological factors, are scarce [21].

Research of chronic somatic pain in children and adolescents has demonstrated that inpatient multidisciplinary treatment is effective for improving pain intensity, school absence and further pain-related disabilities (e.g., social activities, sports, sleep) [23]. Improvement of pain coping appears to have a strong effect on pain-related treatment outcomes e.g., pain intensity [24–26]. A recently published meta-analysis by Bonvanie and colleagues [21] demonstrated the effectiveness of psychological treatment in improving symptom severity, disability and school attendance at posttreatment and follow-up in children and adolescents with functional somatic symptoms. The type of symptoms did not seem to influence the outcomes [21]. Despite these promising results, research on multidisciplinary treatment of children and adolescents with SSD is scarce, and the mediators of these treatment processes are still not well understood. In addition, an interpretation of the existing studies is limited due to the heterogeneity of the measures used and a lack of data concerning the long-term treatment effects regarding psychosocial functioning (e.g., school attendance) and psychiatric comorbidity [4, 12, 21, 27].

Thus, our study focused on the evaluation of inpatient multidisciplinary treatment of SSD covering all disorders enumerated in DSM-5, with a particular evaluation of distress and impairment (i.e., school absence). In detail, the aims of our study were twofold: first, we aimed to evaluate the effectiveness of an inpatient interdisciplinary treatment for children and adolescents with somatic symptom disorders. The multidisciplinary team consisted of child & adolescent psychiatrists, pediatricians, clinical psychologists, physiotherapists, occupational therapists and nurses. The outcome parameters were a reduction in somatic complaints and psychiatric comorbidity (anxiety, depression) at discharge and upon a 6-month follow-up after treatment completion. At this assessment, school attendance was also evaluated. Second, we aimed to assess the impact of coping strategies and comorbid psychiatric symptoms (depression, anxiety) on changes in functional impairment (i.e., school attendance) and the level of discomfort.

Methods

Patients aged 8–18 years with somatoform disorders, dissociative disorders or chronic somatic disorders with psychiatric comorbidity who were referred to our somatic symptom unit were eligible for inclusion. The requirements for admission included a complete pediatric diagnostic evaluation and an appointment with a member of the treatment team to discuss the indication of inpatient treatment and treatment goals. The exclusion criteria included insufficient knowledge of the German language, duration of treatment of less than 14 days and severe psychiatric comorbidity, such as acute suicidal ideation or psychosis. Regular treatment attendance at individual and group therapies was a precondition for admission and continued participation in the treatment program. Patient assessments were conducted upon admission (T1), discharge (T2) and 6 months following treatment (T3). The local ethics committee approved the study in accordance with the Declaration of Helsinki.

Sample

Seventy-three individuals were screened over a 16-month period, and 60 patients were eligible for inclusion. Eight patients cancelled treatment prematurely, and five patients had to be transferred to the child and adolescent psychiatric unit due to severe psychiatric disorders. Forty-five (75%) of all included patients participated in the follow-up assessment. Study completers did not differ from non-completers in terms of age, sex, distribution of disorders or missed school days upon admission (T1). The details are presented in Table 1.

Measures

School attendance

School attendance was assessed in accordance with a scheme proposed by Hechler et al. (2014) over the 4 weeks prior to admission and over the 4 weeks prior to the 6-month follow-up [37]. School absence was categorized by the amount of missed school days: none (0–1 days), moderate (2–5 days) and high (6–20 days). School attendance was assessed via self-and parental reports.

PPCI

The German version of the revised Pediatric Pain Coping Inventory (PPCI-R), a validated self-report questionnaire, was used to assess pain coping strategies in the children and adolescents [25, 28]. The PPCI-R considers the following subscales: cognitive self-instruction, seeking of social support and passive coping strategies. Passive coping strategies and seeking of social support are defined as behavior-related strategies, while positive self-instruction

Table 1 Demographic and clinical data

	Mean [SD]
Sample size (n)	60
Female (%)	56.7
Age	14.43 [2.0]
Duration of treatment (days)	48.15 [19.7]
Diagnostic distribution	*N [%]*
A primary diagnosis	
Somatoform disorder (F45.x)	47 [78.3]
Dissociative (conversion) disorder (F44.x)	4 [6.7]
Other pediatric diagnosis[a]	9 [15]
B comorbidities	
Depressive episode (F32.x)	27 [45]
Phobic/other anxiety disorder (F40.x/F41.x)	24 [40]
Attention deficit hyperactivity disorder (F90.x)	22 [36.7]
Other F[b]—diagnoses	23 [38.3]

[a] Rheumatic diseases (n = 2), migraine (n = 1), obesity (n = 5), chronic inflammatory bowel syndrome (n = 1)

[b] Obsessive–compulsive disorder (F42.x, n = 2), reaction to severe stress and adjustment disorder (F43.x, n = 6), specific developmental disorders of scholastic skills (F81.x, n = 4), mixed disorders of conduct and emotions (F92.x, n = 1), emotional disorders with onsets specific to childhood (F93.x, n = 1), tic disorders (F95.x, n = 1), somatoform disorder (F45.x, n = 1)

is defined as a cognitive strategy. The summed scores were used for statistical analyses. Lower numbers indicated more adaptive coping strategies [25].

Level of discomfort

The German "Giessen physical complaints inventory for children and adolescents" (GBB-SB) is a self-report questionnaire designed to assess subjective somatic complaints [29]. The GBB-SB includes fatigue, gastric and cardiovascular complaints, rheumatic pain, and cold symptoms that altogether provide a total score of the complaints [30]. The subjective perception of somatic complaints often differs from the clinical findings, especially in somatoform disorders. *T* levels, in accordance with the German norms referred to in the manual, were used for statistical analyses.

Anxiety

The German version of the Spence Children's Anxiety Scale (SCAS), a self-report questionnaire, was used to measure overall anxiety and includes the following six subscales: generalized anxiety, panic/agoraphobia, social phobia, separation anxiety, obsessive–compulsive disorder and physical injury fears [31, 32]. The total SCAS sum scores were used for statistical analyses.

Depression

The German Children's Depression Inventory (DIKJ), a self-assessment questionnaire, was used to measure the severity of depressive symptoms [33]. *T* levels, in accordance to the norms reported in the manual, were used for statistical analyses.

Treatment

For highly affected children and adolescents with SSD, an interdisciplinary inpatient treatment (Monday until Friday) based on cognitive behavioral treatment strategies was recommended [21, 34]. The primary goal of the treatment was to develop adaptive pain coping strategies and to facilitate a return to everyday adolescent life (e.g., regular school attendance, sports, and social activities). The treatment comprised psychotherapy and complimentary therapies such as physiotherapy and social competence training, as well as parental psychoeducation. One important strategy was the supervised gradual exposition to situations in which somatic symptoms frequently occur with the goal to help patients reappraise associated thoughts and feelings increasing somatic symptoms. The parents were invited to participate in the coaching sessions to learn about the individual pathogenesis of SSD and to understand how to reduce overprotective or perpetuate behavior. At the beginning of the treatment, all patients attended a special school at the hospital, with most returning to their classes at their original schools at the end of the treatment. Pharmacological treatment was recommended as an auxiliary intervention in some cases. Of all the patients, 50% (n=30) received no medication, and 21.7% (n=13) were treated with a selective serotonin reuptake inhibitor (SSRI) because of comorbid depression (n=9) and/or anxiety (n=6). Of all the patients 21.7% (n=13) were treated with extended-release methylphenidate, and 1.7% (n=1) were treated with atomoxetine due to comorbid attention deficit hyperactivity disorder. In 5% (n=3) of all patients, a combination of SSRIs and extended-release methylphenidate because of comorbid depression (n=2) or anxiety (n=1) and attention deficit hyperactivity disorder was administered. All patients were drug-naïve at pretreatment. The treatment included regular team meetings to discuss the individual progress of the patients, as well as regular supervisions. The treatment team had prior experience in the therapy of patients with somatic symptom disorders. Before discharge, caregivers were supported in setting up continued care including psychotherapy and child- and adolescent care including medication in some patients. At discharge, all patients had first appointments set for continued ambulant care.

The interdisciplinary inpatient unit in Aachen provides nine treatment units for highly affected children and adolescents. In Germany, inpatient treatment is more widespread compared to similar health care systems in other Western countries with over 6000 psychiatric inpatient treatment units [35]. However, units for children with SSD are scarce in Germany and mostly cared by only one discipline, either child and adolescent psychiatry or pediatrics. The interdisciplinary model presented here is one of the very few in Germany.

Statistical analyses

IBM SPSS version 23 was used to perform all statistical analyses (IBM Corp., Armonk, N.Y.). Sample characteristics were summarized using descriptive statistics. Descriptive statistics were employed for the categorical variables and also for the means and standard deviations (SDs) for the continuous variables. Three time-points were assessed: admission, discharge and the follow-up (6 months after discharge). A test of the distribution of normality revealed that the values of the DIKJ, SCAS and the number of missing school days were not normally distributed. Wilcoxon signed-rank tests (DIKJ, SCAS, and missing school days) and paired *T*-tests (GBB; PPCI) were conducted to assess changes from pre- to posttreatment (T1–T2) and from pretreatment to 6 months after discharge (T1–T3). Due to the use of multiple tests of the same dataset, we adjusted the alpha level using the Bonferroni–Holm procedure [36], which specified a *p* value of 0.0033 for a test to be considered significant. The resulting output of the group comparisons was used to calculate the effect sizes (Cohen's d). Additionally, exploratory post hoc analyses were conducted to investigate the influence of (a) age and sex, or (b) baseline levels of depression or discomfort on the changes in coping strategies, levels of discomfort, depression and anxiety. A repeated measures model with sex as between subject factor and time (T1, T3) as within subject factor was used for (a), while linear regression models were used for (b). Finally, using Pearson correlations, we investigated whether changes in school attendance (T1 to T3) were related to changes (T1 to T3) in pain coping (PPCI), discomfort or comorbidity.

Results

Sample

The demographic and clinical characteristics of the study sample are presented in Table 1. The ages ranged from 9 to 17 years, with a mean age of 14 years ($SD=2.0$). Average school absence during the 4 weeks prior to admission was 11.7 days ($SD=7.9$), and the mean duration of the inpatient treatment was 48 days ($SD=19.7$). Patients who received medication had more severe symptoms, e.g., days of school absence than those without medication ($p < 0.05$).

Treatment effects at discharge

Measures at admission (T1), discharge (T2) and 6 months following treatment (T3) are given in Table 2. Compared

Table 2 Discomfort, pain coping and comorbidity

Measures	Admission	Discharge	Six months after discharge
DIKJ[a]	55.67 [10.08]	49.22 [11.42]*	45.05 [13.73]**
SCAS[b]	26.44 [15.07]	20.08 [17.47]*	15.38 [15.47]**
GBB-SB[b]	59.15 [11.03]	48.96 [14.38]**	48.38 [13.63]**
PPCI[b]	22.86 [8.67]	18.68 [7.14]*	14.21 [7.87]**
PAS[c]	10.20 [4.42]	6.42 [3.78]**	6.11 [3.80]**
SS[c]	4.76 [3.97]	3.33 [2.61]*	1.86 [2.40]**
POS[c]	8.47 [3.29]	9.16 [3.70]	6.31 [4.19]
School absence[d] [in days]	11.92 [7.05]		2.41 [4.28]**
None	5 (10.2%)		29 (64.4%)
Moderate	6 (12.2%)		10 (22.2%)
High	38 (77.6%)		6 (13.3%)

Means and standard-deviations in brackets

* Significant at $p_a < 0.0033$ compared with pretreatment data; ** $p < 0.001$

[a] T-value

[b] Raw-value

[c] *PAS* passive strategies, *ss* seeking for social support, *POS* positive self-instruction

[d] School absence in days for the prior 4 weeks; none = 0–1 days, moderate = 2–5 days, high = > 5 days (%); these subgroups were not included in the comparison tests

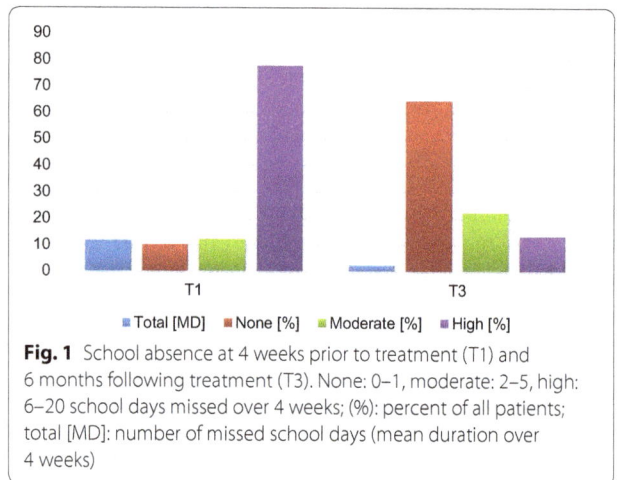

Fig. 1 School absence at 4 weeks prior to treatment (T1) and 6 months following treatment (T3). None: 0–1, moderate: 2–5, high: 6–20 school days missed over 4 weeks; (%): percent of all patients; total [MD]: number of missed school days (mean duration over 4 weeks)

with pretreatment, the effects of the treatment at discharge were noted regarding reduced levels of comorbidity with small to medium effect sizes (anxiety: $d = 0.4$; depression: $d = 0.6$). The level of discomfort was reduced with a large effect size ($d = 0.8$).

Treatment effects 6 months post treatment

Compared with the pretreatment status (admission), treatment effects remained stable 6 months post treatment indicated by significantly reduced levels of discomfort, depression and anxiety and improved coping strategies (Table 2). Moreover, school attendance improved with large effect sizes ($d = 1.6$; Table 2, Fig. 1). Notably, 20 (52%) of the subjects in the high school absence group (>5 days/4 weeks) were rated as having no school absences (0–1 days/4 weeks) at 6 months posttreatment.

When treatment effects 6 months post treatment were compared with the status upon discharge, within subjects' comparisons indicate no changes in depression ($t = 1.16$; $p = 0.26$), anxiety ($t = 0.96$; $p = 0.34$) and levels of discomfort ($t = -0.51$; $p = 0.61$) and further improved coping strategies (PPCI; $t = 3.46$; $p = 0.001$), mainly attributable to reductions in self instructions (POS; $t = 3.47$; $p = 0.001$).

Exploratory post hoc analyses regarding correlates of treatment outcome (i.e., level of discomfort 6 months posttreatment and school attendance), age and gender indicated the following:

a. Age was not associated with treatment outcome. Boys and girls showed comparable levels of discomfort at baseline (GBB raw sum score; boys mean 61.1, sd 11.3; girls mean 58.5, sd 11.1), however, boys showed larger reductions in levels of discomfort at T3 (boys mean 47.8, sd 13.5; girls: mean 49.6, sd 15.3). This was indicated by a significant repeated measures model with GBB T1/T3 as dependent variable and gender as between subjects factor: GBB was reduced over time ($p < 0.001$), and significantly different between sexes ($p = 0.02$ for the time by sex interaction, overall sex effect $p = 0.7$).

b. In a linear regression model, lower levels of discomfort 6 months posttreatment (T3, self-assessment) were predicted by lower depression scores upon admission (T1; $\beta = 0.36$; $t = 2.3$; $p = 0.03$) but not levels of discomfort upon admission ($p = 0.14$). Since depression scores and levels of discomfort were correlated at T1 ($r = 0.28$; $p = 0.04$), a second model only including depression scores at T1 was calculated and results were largely similar ($\beta = 0.41$; $t = 2.7$; $p = 0.01$).

c. Improved school attendance (i.e., delta school absence: T1–T3) was associated with improved pain coping (T1–T3; $r = 0.38$, $p = 0.037$) but not with decreased levels of discomfort or with depressive or anxious symptoms scores.

Discussion

The key finding of this study was that, in children and adolescents with SSD, an inpatient interdisciplinary treatment program is highly effective in reducing somatic complaints, increasing school attendance, developing adaptive coping strategies and improving psychiatric comorbidity (depression, anxiety). Furthermore, our findings highlighted the importance of developing adaptive coping strategies that are associated with improved school attendance.

Our findings were consistent with those of previous studies, which demonstrated that children who were highly affected by chronic pain improved in response to inpatient treatment in regard to functional impairment, pain intensity and quality of life [4, 11, 37, 38]. Although there exists strong evidence for the short-term effectiveness of inpatient treatment, research concerning the long-term outcome is rare, and tools for measuring treatment outcomes need to be standardized for better comparability [38]. A meta-analysis by Hechler and colleagues demonstrated that intensive interdisciplinary pain treatment has positive treatment effects on pain intensity, disability and depressive symptoms, though school functioning and anxiety were excluded due to the heterogeneity in the treatment outcome measures [4]. A recent meta-analysis [21] demonstrated the effectiveness of psychological treatment on functional somatic symptoms. Notably, the *type of symptom* was not associated with the effectiveness of treatment. This may be interpreted in support of the findings of this study that included all somatic symptom disorders and pediatric disorders being complicated by psychological factors.

Second, our results support previous findings that inpatient interdisciplinary treatment can substantially reduce school absence [23]. In accordance with prior research showing that 80–90% of patients with chronic pain show a significant improvement in school attendance, our findings suggest similar results, with only 13.3% maintaining high levels of school absence at 6 months after discharge (i.e., 6–20 school days missed over 4 weeks) [23, 39]. As school attendance is highly important for the development of children and adolescents, factors explaining the persistent school absence rates must urgently be identified [23].

Moreover, previous studies have suggested that adaptive coping strategies play an important role in the treatment of recurrent and chronic pain [40, 41]. While associations of pain coping and improvement in affective symptoms have been inconsistent [42, 43], improvements in functional disability and quality of life have been previously reported [43]. Further, our findings regarding the changes in coping are consistent with former research conducted by Hechler and colleagues [41], who reported identical findings, i.e., reduced passive pain coping and seeking of social support after a multimodal inpatient treatment, with positive self-instruction being maintained. Thus, associations of improved behavioral coping

strategies (more active coping, less seeking of social support) with improved school attendance implies that one promising treatment approach could involve focusing on helping patients become more active in reducing passive coping. One element of our multidisciplinary treatment that helped patients become active were the several treatments of physiotherapy per week, in both group and individual settings. Moreover, this treatment fostered positive social experiences and skills within the patient group, both due to the inpatient setting and specifically in social competence trainings and in supervised group activities. Future research should further investigate which specific treatment strategies are most beneficial in improving behavioral coping. While the importance of coping has been demonstrated in adolescents with chronic somatic pain, our results suggested that improvements in coping strategies are an important treatment target in children and adolescents with SSD as well.

Concerning associations of gender and pain coping, one study demonstrated that reduced seeking of social support was associated with reduced pain intensity in girls but not in boys [41]. In our study, boys showed larger improvements in pain coping strategies compared to girls; however, due to the sample size, we did not explore gender-specific associations of pain coping and the level of discomfort. More research is needed to investigate the role of gender in pain coping, as gender-specific coping strategies may improve the treatment outcomes [32].

Lastly, concerning comorbid affective disorders, our findings support previous data showing that over the course of the inpatient treatment, anxiety and depression improved significantly [4, 11, 37]. However, previous research has been heterogeneous and has not always included specific psychiatric treatments of comorbidities, as conducted in this study. In some cases, treatment of psychiatric comorbidity involved the use of medication that was not previously administered to the patients. This must be considered when interpreting the results of our study. Of note, the improvements in psychiatric comorbidity were not significantly related to changes in school attendance or the level of discomfort. While this finding has been reported previously [44], it should be interpreted with caution due to the sample size this non-finding is based on.

The strengths of this study include the use of the standardized assessment of treatment effects and the inclusion of a 6-month follow up. The limitations apply to the study design, as it evaluates a "natural" clinical treatment program lacking randomization, a control group, a standardized therapeutic manual and structured measures of treatment adherence. Future studies with larger sample sizes are needed to assess which specific treatment strategies add to the effectiveness of an inpatient interdisciplinary treatment and also to investigate the role of coping strategies in more detail.

Conclusion

Inpatient interdisciplinary treatment combining pediatric and psychiatric knowledge and skills is highly effective for SSD in children and adolescents regarding the reduction in somatic complaints, emotional distress, and school absence and the improvement of coping strategies. Untreated somatic symptom and related disorders often result in long-term impairment in affected children and adolescents, including poor academic achievements, an increased risk for later medical treatment and vocational impairments. Thus, it is mandatory to overcome potential barriers to treatment in order to take advantage of multidisciplinary treatment approaches. In this regard, the education of health professionals, teachers and parents regarding recognition and treatment opportunities of SSD is necessary to avoid unnecessary and costly physical examinations, to shorten the duration of illness and to facilitate access to professional treatment.

Abbreviations

SSD: somatic symptom and related disorders; DSM-5: fifth edition of the Diagnostic and Statistical Manual of Mental Disorders; ICD-10: tenth edition International Statistical Classification of Diseases and Related Health Problems; ICD-11: eleventh edition International Statistical Classification of Diseases and Related Health Problems; KiGGS: German Health Interview and Examination Survey for Children and Adolescents; PPCI-R: Revised Pediatric Pain Coping Inventory; GBB-SB: Giessen physical complaints inventory for children and adolescents; SCAS: Spence Children's Anxiety Scale; DIKJ: Children's Depression Inventory; SSRI: selective serotonin reuptake inhibitor; SDs: standard deviations; PAS: passive strategies; SS: seeking for social support; POS: positive self-instruction; MD: mean raw sum difference.

Authors' contributions

BH and JB conceptualised the study. JB supervised data collection, PH, AD and GGP analysed and interpreted the data and drafted the manuscript. BH, NW, and CS revised the manuscript critically. All authors read and approved the final manuscript.

Author details

[1] Department of Child and Adolescent Psychiatry, Psychosomatics and Psychotherapy, RWTH Aachen University, Aachen, Germany. [2] Department of Pediatrics, RWTH Aachen University, Aachen, Germany. [3] Department of Medical Informatics and Statistic, University Schleswig-Holstein, Kiel, Germany.

Competing interests

The authors declare that they have no competing interests.

Funding

All costs for conducting the research were covered by in-house funds.

References

1. Witthöft M, Hiller W. Psychological approaches to origins and treatments of somatoform disorders. Annu Rev Clin Psychol. 2010;6:257–83.
2. Husain H, Browne T, Chalder T. A review of psychological models and interventions for medically unexplained somatic symptoms in children. Child Adolesc Ment Health. 2007;12:2–7.
3. Malas N, Ortiz-Aguayo R, Giles L, Ibeziako P. Pediatric somatic symptom disorders. Curr Psychiatry Rep. 2017;19(2):11.
4. Hechler T, Kanstrup M, Lewandowski A, Simons LE, Wicksell R, Hirschfeld G, et al. Systematic review on intensive interdisciplinary pain treatment of children with chronic pain. Pediatrics. 2015;136:115–27.
5. van Geelen SM, Hagquist C. Are the time trends in adolescent psychosomatic problems related to functional impairment in daily life? A 23-year study among 20,000 15–16 year olds in Sweden. J Psychosom Res. 2016;87:50–6.
6. APA. Diagnostic and statistical manual of mental disorders. Arlington, VA: American Psychiatric Publishing, Inc; 2013.
7. Gureje O, Reed GM. Bodily distress disorder in ICD-11: problems and prospects. World Psychiatry. 2016;15:291–2.
8. Hinton H, Kirk S. Families and healthcare professionals' perceptions of healthcare services for children and young people with medically unexplained symptoms: a narrative review of literature. Health Soc Care Community. 2016. https://doi.org/10.1111/hsc.12184.
9. Garralda M. Somatisation in children. J Child Psychol Psychiatry. 1996;1:13–33.
10. Grattan-Smith P, Dale R. Pediatric functional neurologic symptoms. In: Hallett M, Stone J, Carson A, editors. Handbook of clinical disorders. New York: Elsevier; 2016. p. 489–98.
11. Eccleston C, Malleson PN, Clinch J, Conell H, Sourbut C. Chronic pain in adolescents: evaluation of a programme of interdisciplinary cognitive behaviour therapy. Arch Dis Child. 2003;88:881–5.
12. Eccleston C, Palermo TM, Williames A, Lewandowski A, Morley S. Psychological therapies for the management of chronic and recurrent pain in children and adolescents. Cochrane Database Syst Rev. 2009. https://doi.org/10.1002/14651858.CD003968.
13. Erhart M, Weimann A, Bullinger M. Psychological comorbidity in children and adolescents with chronic somatic diseases. Bundesgesundheitsblatt. 2011;54:66–74.
14. Leary PM. Conversion disorder in childhood-diagnosed too late, investigated too much ? J R Soc Med. 2003;96:436–8.
15. Fegert JM, Kölch M. Klinikmanual. Kinder-und Jugendpsychiatrie und -psychotherapie: Springer; 2013.
16. Ani C, Reading R, Lynn R, Forlee S, Garralda E. Incidence and 12-month outcome of non-transient childhood conversion disorder in the UK and Ireland. Br J Psychiatry. 2012;202:413–8.
17. Tegethoff M, Belardi A, Stalujanis E, Meinlschmidt G. Comorbidity of mental disorders and chronic pain: chronology of onset in adolescents of a national representative cohort. J Pain. 2015;16:1054–64. https://doi.org/10.1016/j.jpain.2015.06.009.
18. Shanahan L, Zucker N, Copeland WE, Bondy CL, Egger HL, Costello EJ. Childhood somatic complaints predict generalized anxiety and depressive disorders during young adulthood in a community sample. Psychol Med. 2015;45:1721–30. https://doi.org/10.1017/s0033291714002840.
19. Thompson R, Delaney P, Flores I, Szigethy E. Cognitive-behavioral therapy for children with comorbid physical illness. Child Adolesc Psychiatr Clin N Am. 2011;20:329–48.
20. Zernikow B, Hermann C. Chronische Schmerzen bei Kindern und Jugendlichen. Schmerz. 2015. https://doi.org/10.1007/s0048 2-015-0036-y.
21. Bonvanie IJ, Kallesoe KH, Janssens KAM, Schröder A, Rosmalen JGM, Rask CU. Psychological interventions for children with functional somatic symptoms: a systematic review and meta-analysis. J Pediatr. 2017;187:272–81.
22. Malas N, Ortiz-Aguayo R, Giles L, Ibeziako P. Pediatric somatic symptom disorders. Curr Psychiatry Rep. 2017;19:11. https://doi.org/10.1007/s1192 0-017-0760-3.
23. Hechler T, Wager J, Zernikow B. Chronic pain treatment in children and adolescents: less is good, more is sometimes better. BMC Pediatr. 2014;14:262.

24. Schneider J, Rief W. Selbstwirksamkeitserwartungen und Therapieerfolge bei Patienten mit anhaltender somatoformer Schmerzstörung (ICD-10: F45.4). Z Klin Psychol Psychother. 2007;36:46–56.

25. Hechler T, Kosfelder J, Denecke H, Dobe M, Hübner B, Martin A. Schmerzbezogene Copingstrategien von Kindern und Jugendlichen mit chronischen Schmerzen—Überprüfung einer deutschen Fassung der Paediatric Pain Coping Inventory (PPCI). Schmerz. 2008;22:442–57.

26. Schulte IE, Petermann F, Noeker M. Functional abdominal pain in childhood: from etiology to maladaptation. Psychother Psychosom. 2010;79:73–86.

27. Palermo T, Eccleston C, Lewandowski A, Wiiliams A, Morley S. Randomized controlled trial of psychological therapies for management of chronic pain in children and adolescents: an updated meta-analytic review. Pain. 2010;148:387–97.

28. Varni JW, Waldron SA, Gragg RA, Rapoff MA, Bernstein BH, Lindsley CB, Newcomb MD. Development of the Waldron/Varni pediatric pain coping inventory. Pain. 1996;67:141–50.

29. Barkmann C, Mack B, Brähler E, Schulte-Markwort M. Der Gießener Beschwerdebogen für Kinder und Jugendliche (GBB-KJ): Faktorielle Validität, Reliabilität und gesamtdeutsche Normierung für 4-bis 18-Jährige im Eltern- und Selbsturteil. Diagnostica. 2008;54:99–111.

30. Barkmann M, Brähler E. GBB-KJ Gießener Beschwerdefragebogen für Kinder und Jugendliche. Bern: Huber; 2009.

31. Spence SH. A measure of anxiety symptoms among children. Behav Res Ther. 1998;36:545–66.

32. Essau CA, Muris P, Ederer EM. Reliability and validity of the "Spence Children's Anxiety Scale" and the "Screen for Children Anxiety Related Emotional Disorders" in German children. J Behav Ther Exp Psychiatry. 2002;33:1–18.

33. Stiensmeier-Pelster J, Schürmann M, Duda K. Depressionsinventar für Kinder und Jugendliche (DIKJ). Handanweisung (3., überarb. und neunormierte Auflage). Göttingen: Hogrefe; 2000.

34. van Dessel N, den Boeft M, van der Wouden JC, Kleinstäuber M, Leone SS, Terluin B, et al. Non-pharmacological interventions for somatoform disorders and medically unexplained physical symptoms (MUPS) in adults. Cochrane Database Syst Rev. 2014. https://doi.org/10.1002/14651 858.CD011142.pub2

35. Statistisches Bundesamt. Krankenhäuser nach Fachabteilungen; Einrichtungen, Betten und Patientenbewegung. Bonn. 2016.

36. Holm S. A simple sequentially rejective multiple test procedure. Scand J Stat. 1979;6:65–70.

37. Hechler T, Ruhe A, Schmidt P, Hirsch J, Wager J, Dobe M, et al. Inpatient-based intensive interdisciplinary pain treatment for highly impaired children with severe chronic pain: randomized controlled trial of efficacy and economic effects. Pain. 2014;155:118–28.

38. Stahlschmidt L, Zernikow B, Wager J. Specialized rehabilitation programs for children and adolescents with severe disabling chronic pain: indications, treatment and outcomes. Children. 2016;12:1–13.

39. Hirschfeld G, Hechler T, Dobe M, Wager J, von Lützau P, Blankenburg M, et al. Maintaining lasting improvements: one-year follow-up of children with severe chronic pain undergoing multimodal inpatient treatment. J Pediatr Psychol. 2013;38:224–36.

40. Eccleston M, Morley S, Williams A. Sytematic review of randomised controlled trials of psychological therapy for chronic pain in children and adolescents, with a subset of meta-analysis of pain relief. Pain. 2002;99:157–65.

41. Hechler T, Kosfelder J, Vocks S, Mönninger T, Blankenburg M, Dobe M, et al. Changes in pain-related coping strategies and their importance for treatment outcome following multimodal inpatient treatment: does sex matter? Pain. 2009;11:472–83.

42. Kashir-Zuck S, Sil S, Lynch-Jordan AM, Ting AV, Peugh J, Schikler KN, et al. Changes in pain coping, catastrophizing and coping efficacy after cognitive-behavioral therapy in children and adolescents with juvenile fibromyalgia. J Pain. 2013;14:492–501.

43. van der Veek SM, De Haan E, Benninga MA, Boer F. Psychological factors addressed in cognitive behaviour therapy for paediatric functional abdominal pain: which are most important to target? J Health Psychol. 2017. https://doi.org/10.1177/1359105317694488.

44. Benore E, D'Auria A, Banez G, Worley S, Tang A. The influence of anxiety reduction on clinical response to pediatric chronic paon rehabilitation. Clin J Pain. 2015;31:375–83.

25

Psychopathology and impairment of quality of life in offspring of psychiatric inpatients in southern Brazil: a preliminary study

Ana Luiza Ache[1*], Paula Fernandes Moretti[2], Gibsi Possapp Rocha[1], Rogéria Recondo[2], Marco Antônio Pacheco[1,2] and Lucas Spanemberg[1,2]

Abstract

Objective: To evaluate the quality of life and risk of psychopathology in the infant and adolescent offspring of psychiatric inpatients from a general hospital unit.

Methods: Offspring (4–17 years old) of psychiatric inpatients were interviewed face-to-face and assessed with the Strengths and Difficulties Questionnaire (SDQ). Interviews with caregivers and the hospitalized parents were also performed. The quality of life of the offspring, psychopathology of their hospitalized parents, and their current caregivers were investigated in order to evaluate any associations between these aspects and psychopathology in the offspring.

Results: Thirty-four children of 25 patients were evaluated, 38.2% of which presented high risk for some type of psychopathology including hyperactivity or attention deficit disorder (38.2%), behavioral disorders (20.6%), and emotional disorders (17.6%). While only the minority of these children (17.6%) were already receiving mental health treatment, another 41.2% of them exhibited some degree of symptoms and were only referred for specialized assessment. Additionally, 61.8% of the children were reported to be suffering from some impairment in their quality of life.

Conclusion: This preliminary study found a high rate of psychopathology in children of psychiatric inpatients. These results corroborate previous evidence that children and adolescents with parents with severe psychopathology are at high risk for developing mental disorders. Public policies and standard protocols of action directed to this population are urgently needed, especially for offspring of parents that are hospitalized in psychiatric in-patient units of general hospitals.

Keywords: Child development, Quality of life, Children psychiatric inpatients, Parent–child relations, Psychopathology

Background

Mental disorders represent a group of pathologies that have the greatest impact on global health burden. Recent findings have demonstrated that the global burden of mental illness accounts for 32.4% of years lived with disability (YLDs) and 13.0% of disability-adjusted life-years (DALYs) [1]. Most mental disorders begin in childhood. Moreover, it is reported that around 50% of mental disorders start before the age of 14 and 75% start before the age of 24 [2]. Thus, prevention and early identification of vulnerable children with psychopathology has been reported as the most effective strategy for reducing the implications and burdens of mental illness [3].

The prevalence of mental disorders in childhood has been increasing, ranging from around 13.4%, in community surveys around the world [4], up to 49% in clinical populations [5]. The US prevalence of youths with serious emotional disturbance with global impairment is about 6.36% [6]. In Brazil, studies have reported a prevalence of 30% of common mental disorders in adolescents [7] with 50% of adult mental disorders

*Correspondence: analuiza90@hotmail.com
[1] Núcleo de Formação em Neurociências da Escola de Medicina da Pontifícia, Universidade Católica do Rio Grande do Sul, Av. Ipiranga 6690, Porto Alegre CEP 90619-900, Brazil
Full list of author information is available at the end of the article

beginning before the age of 18 years [8]. In younger children, a prevalence of 13% of psychiatric disorders was found among 6-year-old children in a birth cohort in southern Brazil [9].

The children of patients with psychiatric disorders are a particularly vulnerable population for the development of psychopathology. Several studies have reported that the offspring of parents with mental problems are up to 13 times more likely to develop the same psychopathology [10–12] and are up to five times more likely to use professional mental health services [13, 14]. In addition, they have a higher risk of criminal convictions [15], self-harm [16], and violence and suicide [17, 18]. Data from the World Health Organization (WHO) World Mental Health Survey estimate that the population-attributable risk proportion for parent disorders is 12.4% across all offspring disorders [19]. Furthermore, it is estimated that about 15.6% of children in Canada are exposed to parents or guardians with psychopathology [20]. In Australia, 14.4% to 23.3% of children have a parent with some non-substance related mental disorder [21, 22]. In the US, the US National Survey of Drug Use and Health (2008–2014) reported that 2.7 million parents (3.8%) and 12.8 million parents (18.2%) had presented a serious mental illness or any mental illness in the past year, respectively [23]. Moreover, data appointed that up to 58% of children with serious emotional disorders have a history of family mental illness and 40% have a history of parent psychiatric hospitalization [24].

Despite the prevalence and the incredibly increased risk for negative outcomes in children of people with mental disorders, this population is often under-detected as well as poorly monitored and treated. A UK community study found that only 37% of children with any psychopathology and children of parents with depression had some recent contact (previous 3 months) with some assistance, of which only 15.2% had contact with a mental health service [25]. Estimates in Brazil are not clear, but a recent survey found that only a small proportion of children or adolescents with any psychiatric disorder (19.8%) were seen by a mental health specialist in the previous 12 months [26]. In addition, children of psychiatric patients, particularly those with severe mental disorders and a history of hospitalizations, present a higher risk of mortality, especially in early childhood and late adolescence [27]. Mothers with mental disorders lose custody or contact with their children more frequently [28]. Moreover, there is no routinization or systematization of mental health evaluations for the children of hospitalized patients. The training of professionals, adequacy of physical area and environments, and psychoeducation aimed at the promotion of children's mental health and prevention of mental disorders are rare and frequently absent in the routines of hospitals, training programs, [29–31], and government policies [24].

Although more than 90% of the world's children and adolescents live in low- and middle-income countries (LMICs), studies on high risk children are rare in these countries. Despite some population surveys, there are few, if any, studies in Brazil that have evaluated high-risk children of hospitalized psychiatric patients. The aim of this study was to investigate the prevalence of mental disorders and the impact on the quality of life in children of inpatients from a psychiatric unit of a general hospital in southern Brazil.

Methods

Sample and design

This was a cross-sectional observational study in which children were sampled over a period of 20 months (from April 2016 to November 2017). The study was carried out at the Psychiatric Inpatient Unit of the São Lucas Hospital, Pontifícia Universidade Católica do Rio Grande do Sul (HSL/PUCRS), a nonprofit university general hospital with 21 psychiatric beds. During the period, were admitted 399 inpatients (420 admissions). The average length of stay is about 30 days, and the average occupancy rate was 85% in the period. Many patients with extreme age (83 elderly and 33 adolescents), did not have children in the study's age group, as well as others 204 adults (an indefinite number of these with dubious or unavailable data). A total of 79 patients had children in the study's age group, although we only had information about the children in 66 cases (97 children). The cases that remained less than 7 days (7 patients, with 10 children) were not interviewed. The final eligible sample was 59 parents of 87 children. We were unable to contact or could not include 53 children (34 parents) for many reasons (such as lack of financial conditions to come to the hospital, the caregiver did not agree with the participation of the children, adopted children, etc.).

Instruments

Clinical and Sociodemographic Questionnaire (CSQ)

This questionnaire was part of the research protocol and contained data about clinical records and interviews with patients, their children, and families. It included questions about parents, caregivers, and their children, such as age, sex, marital status, occupational status, family income, number of people in the house, who the caregiver is during parent hospitalization, and characteristics of the hospitalized parent. In addition, data was collected from routine evaluations of the inpatients selected for the research, such as the psychiatric diagnosis as codified by International Classification of Diseases (ICD-10) after clinical interview.

Strengths and Difficulties Questionnaire (SDQ)

This was a short questionnaire to screen for changes in the behavior of children aged 4–17 with both parent and educator versions. SDQ has become the most widely used research tool for the detection of mental health problems [32] and is currently available in more than 40 languages, including Portuguese. It had 25 items, from which 10 were related to capacities, 14 were about difficulties, and one was neutral item. These items were divided into five subscales for which each one was represented by five statements, namely emotional symptoms, behavioral problems, hyperactivity, relationship problems with colleagues, and pro-social behavior. The instrument was presented in three versions, and was intended to be answered by the children themselves (above 11 years), their parents or guardians, and teachers. There were several answer options: false (zero point for this type of response), plus or less true (one point), and true (two points). Only one option could be selected per item. For each of the five subscales, the score could range from 0 to 10. We proposed that the SDQ would be a promising alternative within the Brazilian scenario where standardized instruments for the evaluation of children's mental health were scarce [32]. For this article, the SDQ individual scores were calculated in the official online website of the questionnaire [33]. This procedure was used to calculate all the dimensions of the instrument, as well as to internalize and externalize symptoms scores and the diagnostic predictors for psychopathology.

Patient Health Questionnaire for Depression and Anxiety (PHQ-4)

The PHQ-4 is an ultra-brief screener for depression and anxiety. Health care staff can administer it or it can be self-administered [34]. A recent study found that higher PHQ-4 scores were strongly associated with functional impairment, disability days, and health care [35]. Total score was determined by adding together the scores for each of the four items. Scores are rated as normal (0–2), mild (3–5), moderate (6–8), and severe (9–12). The PHQ-4 is only a screening tool and does not diagnose depression.

Mood Disorder Questionnaire (MDQ)

The MDQ is a short, single-page, paper and pencil self-report screening instrument for bipolar spectrum disorders for adults. It was divided into three sessions. The first session included 13 Yes/No questions derived from the DSM-IV criteria and clinical experience. The second asked whether several symptoms have been experienced in the same period of time. The third part examined psychosocial impairment, classified as absent, minor, moderate or serious. In the original validation study [36], MDQ positive screening for BDs required that seven or more positive symptoms be reported, with clustering within the same time period and causing moderate to severe problems. The Brazilian version of MDQ was previously demonstrated to be a valid instrument for the screening of bipolar disorders [37].

Quality of Life Evaluation Scale (AUQEI)

This is a quality of life scale developed by Manificat el al [38] and was translated and validated for Brazilian language and culture in children aged from four to 12 years old. This instrument aimed to assess the subjective feeling of well-being by assuming that the developing individual is, and always has been, able to express himself or herself with respect to his or her own subjectivity. The questionnaire was based on the point of view of the child's satisfaction. It had 26 questions covering the domains autonomy, leisure, functions, and family. To facilitate the application and comprehension, the questionnaire used images of four faces that expressed different emotional states. It allowed each child to understand the situations and present their own experience. The scale thus allowed us to obtain a profile of their satisfaction in different situations. It was validated in Brazil with children between 4 and 12 years and exhibited a cutoff point of 48 points for characterizing impairment in quality of life [38]. In order to calculate Z and T scores, we used Brazilian study averages as normative values (50.5 ($\pm$3.5) and 53.5 ($\pm$8.0) for boys and girls, respectively).

The World Health Organization Quality of Life—short version (WHOQOL-BREF)

This instrument evaluates a patient's quality of life and consists of 26 questions, with answers that use a Likert scale (from 1 to 5, the higher the score the better the quality of life). Apart from the first two questions, the instrument has 24 facets that comprise four domains: physical, psychological, social relations, and environment. Psychometric properties were analyzed using cross-sectional data obtained from a survey of adults carried out in 23 countries [39]. The WHOQOL-BREF Portuguese version was validated with high internal consistency (Cronbach's alpha from .71 to .84 for the four domains), high test retest reliability, satisfactory features of discriminant, as well as criterion and concurrent validity [40]. In order to calculate Z and T scores, we used the averages of the validation study as normative values by age groups in each domain [39].

The Clinical Global Impression Scale-Severity (CGI-S)

This is a widely-used assessment tool in psychiatry, is easy to apply and interpret, and is available in the public domain [41]. The CGI-s assesses the degree of patient severity in relation to its psychopathology. Scores range from 1 (normal, not ill) to 7 (among the most severely ill patients). It was routinely used for inpatient assessment and its scores were recorded in the medical records.

Procedures

We collected information from each study group with the following procedures:

- *Inpatients with children* The data about admission and medical and psychiatric history were collected from clinical records. The severity of psychopathology of the inpatients was measured by the clinical staff in the routine evaluation by the CGI-S scale. The patient's psychiatric diagnosis was made by the patient's physician, using International Classification of Diseases (ICD-10) after a clinical interview.
- *Main caregivers* All caregivers answered the CSQ with general information, as well as questions about the clinical aspects of the parent (e.g., number of previous hospitalizations, previous psychiatric treatment and initial psychiatric diagnosis) and questions about the children (e.g., years of study, difficulties before and during the parental hospitalization). Additionally, the caregivers answered the SDQ to screen for changes in the behavior of children; and the PHQ-4 and the MDQ scales, to identify symptoms of anxiety, depression, and bipolar disorder.
- *Offspring of psychiatric inpatients* All children were interviewed clinically for the first researcher (A.L.A.) in order to identify psychopathology in risk factors which could indicate the need for emergency intervention. The quality of life questionnaires were answered according to the child age; children 4–11 years old only answered questions from the AUQUEI and children older than 12 years old answered the WHOQOL-BREF. The SDQ (adolescent version) was answered by the children aged 11–17 years.

Ethical considerations

The research protocol was submitted and approved by the Research Ethics Committee of the São Lucas Hospital of PUCRS (protocol number: 1.438.973) prior to the start of data collection. The participants received a consent term for the caregiver, the term of the consent for minors which was signed by the legal responsible for the children, and the term of assent, which was signed by the minors. All data was kept confidential, except when they constituted risk situations. Cases of children identified with psychopathology were referred for treatment. One case was identified as an emergency situation (suicidal ideation) and referred for assistance in an appropriate setting.

Statistics

Descriptive statistics were used to assess the sample, which was analyzed using absolute numbers, percentages, averages and standard deviations. In order to calculate differences between the averages of the two groups, the Student's t test for independent samples was used. The relationship among the SDQ total and factor scores of the quality of life (WHOQOL-BREF and AUQUEI), clinical impression of the inpatients, and psychopathology of the caregivers was assessed using the Pearson correlation coefficient (r). We considered the following magnitudes of correlation: very low (.00 to .19), weak (.20 to .39), moderate (.40 to .59), strong (from .60 to .79), and very strong (from .80 to 1.00) [42]. To calculate T scores for the quality of live (QOL) questionnaires, we first calculated the Z scores and used the normative scores by sex for the age group according to the normative values. The T scores were obtained by the following formula: $T = 50 + 10Z$, where the value 50 represents the normative average and 10 represents the standard deviation (SD). The QOL impairment was determined as being any value less than a standard deviation below the mean normative scores of the respective QOL scales (for both WHOQOL-BREF and AUQUEI). The significance threshold was considered at $p < .05$. All analyses were conducted using the SPSS program version 23.

Results

The final sample consisted of 34 children from 25 patients. The age ranged from 4 for 17 years old (average was 10.8 ± 4.19). The majority (58.8%) of children was less than 12 years old and of female gender (52.9%). Most children and adolescents were children of hospitalized mothers and lived with their mothers (82.4%), siblings (58.8%), and fathers (47.1%) before hospitalization. Some of these children (17%) had been previously subjected to some previous mental health treatment. Their parents were mainly diagnosed with mood disorders (unipolar depression and bipolar disorder), and most of them were cared for by their mothers before the hospitalization. During the hospitalization, care was provided mainly by other relatives (41.2%) or by fathers (29.4%). The clinical and sociodemographic data are summarized in the Table 1.

Table 2 shows the average scores of SDQ, WHOQOL, AUQEI, the percentage of children with high risk of psychopathology, as well as the clinical features of caregivers and inpatient parents. According to the data from the SDQ, 38.3% of the children were at high risk for

Table 1 Sociodemographic and clinical data of the sample (n = 34) and their hospitalized parents

Variable	M ± SD or percentage
Female sex (%)	52.9
Age (M ± SD)	10.8 ± 4.19 [range from 4 to 17]
Age (%)	
< 12 years	58.8
≥ 12 years	41.1
Number of parents hospitalized (n)	25
Which parent hospitalized (%)	
Mother	85.3
Father	14.7
Age of the hospitalized parent (M ± SD)	38.9 ± 6.8
Age of the mother	38.2 ± 6.8
Age of the father	41.5 ± 9.1
Family income[a]—U$ (M ± SD)	1953 (2341)
Family income[a] (%)	
Up to U$ 1.000,00	48
From U$ 1.000,00 to U$ 2.000,00	28
More than U$ 2.000,00	24
Lives with whom (%)	
Mother	82.4
Father	47.1
Siblings	58.8
Grandparents	14.7
Others	23.5
Number of people in the house (M ± SD)	3.93 ± 1.14
Years of study (Child)	9.41 ± 3.77
Previous treatment (Child %)	17.6
Parenteral psychiatric diagnosis[a] (%)	
Unipolar depression	52
Bipolar disorder	24
Substance use/misuse	16
Personality disorder	4
Organic mental disorders	4
Caregiver before/during hospitalization (%)	
Mother	79.4/8.8
Father	11.8/29.4
Sibling	5.9/17.6
Another relative	11.8/41.2
Non-family caregiver	8.8/23.5

Family income calculated by basic salaries in Reais (R$ 937 or U$ 383; U$ 1.00 ≅ R$ 3.30)

[a] Variables with missing values

Table 2 Clinical findings of inpatients offspring (n = 34), inpatient parents (n = 25) and caregivers (n = 25)

Variables children (n = 34)	M ± SD or percentage
SDQ—informant (M ± SD)	
Overall stress	14.0 ± 7.3
Emotional distress	4.1 ± 2.7
Behavioural difficulties	2.7 ± 2.7
Hyperactivity and concentration difficulties	4.4 ± 3.1
Difficulties getting along with other young people	2.6 ± 1.8
Kind and helpful behaviour	8.3 ± 2.1
Impact of any difficulties on the young person's life	1.0 ± 1.3
Internalizing symptoms (M ± SD)	6.8 ± 3.7
Externalizing symptoms (M ± SD)	7.2 ± 5.1
SDQ—diagnostic predictions (% high risk)	
Any disorder	38.3
Emotional disorder	17.6
Behavioral disorder	20.6
Hyperactivity or concentration disorder	38.2
WHOQOL[a] (M ± SD)	
Physical	15.4 ± 2.4
Psychological	13.4 ± 2.5
Social	14.1 ± 4.4
Environmental	14.1 ± 2.4
Overall	15.0 ± 2.9
AUQEI[b] (M ± SD)	44.9 ± 6.0
QOL—impairment (%)	61.8
Children referred for psychiatric evaluation (%)	
Already in treatment	17.6
Referred for psychiatric evaluation	41.2
Variables caregivers (n = 25)	
PHQ depression caregivers (M ± SD)	2.3 ± 1.7
PHQ anxiety—caregivers (M ± SD)	2.9 ± 2.0
PHQ-4 total—caregivers (M ± SD)	5.2 ± 3.4
PHQ-4 categories—symptoms in caregivers (%)	
None	20.8
Mild	33.3
Moderate	29.2
Severe	16.7
Variables inpatient parents (n = 25)	
Clinical Global Impression-Severity (CGI-S)—parent impatient (M ± SD)	5.2 ± 1.0
Primary caregiver is the inpatient (%)	70.6

SDQ Strengths and Difficulties Questionnaire total, WHOQOL World Health Organization Quality of Life questionnaire; AUQUEI Quality of Life Evaluation Scale, PHQ Patient Health Questionnaire

[a] Used only for adolescents (> 12 and < 18 years; n = 13)

[b] Used only by children (from 4 to 12 years; n = 20)

developing a psychiatric illness, including attention deficit hyperactivity disorder (38.2%), behavioral disorders (20.6%), and emotional disorders (17.6%). Of the offspring assessed in the present study, 41.2% were determined to be in situations of suffering or vulnerability and were

recommended for psychiatric monitoring. These children were referred for outpatient psychiatric care when necessary. One child presented suicide ideation and was referred to an emergency department. Moreover, 61.8%

Table 3 Correlations among Strengths and Difficulties Questionnaire (SDQ) total and factors scores, internalizing and externalizing problems, and clinical variables of child and adolescents and their parents

	SDQt	EMO	CON	HYPer	PEER	PROs	IMP	EXT	INT
QOLphy[a]	− .619*	− .510	− .500	− .293	− .458	.493	− .743**	− .419	− .595*
QOLpsy[a]	− .513	− .466	− .592*	− .233	.014	.670*	− .420	− .405	− .418
QOLsoc[a]	− .630*	− .619*	− .635*	− .207	− .273	.371	− .709**	− .400	− .640*
QOLenv[a]	− .247	− .429	− .316	.214	− .459	.074	− .455	.053	− .523
AUQUEI[b]	.075	− .085	.052	.158	.109	.460*	− .196	.115	− .006
PHQdep	.244	.201	.233	.022	.281	− .045	.136	.138	.292
PHQans	.399*	.336	.395*	.115	.297	− .212	.176	.283	.401*
PHQtotal	.394*	.352*	.372*	.088	.329	− .124	.221	.243	.394*
CGIpar	.213	.132	.125	.102	.284	− .204	.223	.130	.242

SDQt Strengths and Difficulties Questionnaire (SDQ) total score, *EMO* SDQ Emotional problems scale, *CON* SDQ Conduct problems Scale, *HYPer* SDQ Hyperactivity scale, *PEER* SDQ Peer problems scale, *PROs* SDQ Prosocial scale, *IMP* SDQ impact scale, *EXT* externalizing problems, *INT* Internalizing problems, *QOLfhy* WHOQOL physical domain, *QOLpsy* WHOQOL psychological domain, *QOLsoc* WHOQOL social domain, *QOLanv* WHOQOL environmental domain, *AUQUEI* Quality of Life Evaluation Scale, *PHQdep* Patient Health Questionnaire-depression, *PHQans* Patient Health Questionnaire-anxiety, *PHQtotal* Patient Health Questionnaire total score, *CGIpar* Clinical Global Impression inpatient parent

[a] Used only for adolescents (> 12 and < 18 years; n = 13)

[b] Used only by children (from 4 to 12 years; n = 20)

* p < .05

of them presented impairment in their quality of life. In 70.6% of cases, the primary caregiver before admission was the inpatient, and they presented an average CGI of 5.2 (markedly ill). The average score of psychopathology of caregivers during parental hospitalization (as measure by PHQ) was 5.2 (mild to moderate distress) with high scores for anxiety.

The correlations between SDQ total and factors scores, internalizing and externalizing problems, and clinical variables of child and adolescents and their parents are presented in Table 3. SDQ total scores and some SDQ dimensions reached strong negative correlations between mental hospitalization of parents with domains of quality of life in adolescents, mainly in physical and social domains. In children, prosocial scores achieved a moderate positive correlation with quality of life. Scores of psychopathology in caregivers, particularly for anxiety, reached a weak to moderate positive correlation with several domains of SDQ, mainly with emotional problems, conduct problems, and internalizing symptoms.

Discussion

Parental mental disorders have a dramatic impact on the next generation. In particular, offspring of parents with major mental disorders have an elevated risk of developing a mental disorder. Based on that assumption, the aim of this study was to evaluate the impact of parental mental illness on children of psychiatric inpatients. The children were evaluated through the perception of the caregiver during the hospitalization and their own perception and these evaluations were then correlated with

clinical data of the hospitalized parent. We found that the offspring of inpatients presented high risk for psychopathology as well as impairment in the quality of life. A large proportion of the children was referred for specialized evaluation, especially those whose inpatient parent and/or caregiver during admission presented severe symptoms of psychopathology. As far as we could verify, this was the first study in Brazil evaluating the offspring of psychiatric inpatients.

Studies on children and adolescent psychopathology are relatively rare in low- and middle-income countries [3]. A large part of the research addressing the influence of parental psychopathology in offspring study adults [43–45]. Most of the studies to date have examined community samples. In a worldwide meta-analytic study, Polanczyk et al. determined that there was a 8.3% (in Africa) and 14.2% (in South America and Caribbean) prevalence of mental disorders in children and adolescents in the community [4]. In non-clinical samples of Brazilian children and adolescents, the prevalence of mental disorders range from 13% (in younger children) [9] to 30% (for common mental disorders in adolescents) [7]. In a high-risk cohort, Salum et al. reported mental disorder prevalence to be 19.9% of mental disorders from a random sample and 29.7% in the high-risk strata [46]. As such, the prevalence of 38.3% of mental disorders in our sample is higher than community non-clinical and high-risk samples. This result was higher than the 32% of psychopathology found in children of German parents with severe mental disorders [47]. This rate is also higher than the 23.7% prevalence of any psychopathology in children of patients with depression in the UK [25].

In our study, the hospitalized parent of 70.6% of the 34 children was their primary caregiver prior to psychiatric hospitalization. This may indicate that they were in the custody of parents that were potentially compromised in their care skills. Data from the UK show that at least a quarter of adults admitted to hospital settings (acute settings) have dependent children and between 50 and 66% of people with severe mental illness live with children under 18 years of age [48]. The intense relationship between children and seriously ill caregivers with psychiatric disorders often produces disorganized families and may lead to the development of pathologies in these children. The literature is extensive on the subject of growing with a mentally ill parent and the increased risk of persistent emotional and behavioral disorders in these children [25, 49–51]. Emotional and behavioral problems are related to low social competence [52]. In addition, the relationship with the child may be compromised, as studies report that parents with mental illness have problems with parenting in daily life, including difficulties in talking to children about their mental illness, maintaining discipline, and giving limits. Parental behavior can change due to disease symptoms or side effects of medications. Moreover, feelings of guilt, shame, and fear regarding adverse effects can also affect the parent's relationship with the children [53]. Furthermore, when the primary caregiver is hospitalized, there may be an abrupt change in the dynamics of care of these children and the substitute caregiver does not always has a close link with them.

In addition to the mentally ill parent, we found that almost half of the children caregivers during the parent's hospitalization had moderate (29.2%) to severe (16.7%) distress symptoms. Furthermore, the distress symptoms of caregivers were significantly associated with scores of emotional and conduct problems and internalizing symptoms. Thus, even when separated from their more psychiatric-diseased parent, half of these children were still exposed to caregivers (the other parent or other family member) with significant psychiatric symptoms. Studies have shown that when both parents are affected by psychopathology, the offspring have at least a double risk of psychopathology, behavior problems, or suicide [11, 17].

The quality of life (QOL) was impaired in 61.8% of our sample of children from psychiatric inpatients. Additionally, we found a significant negative association of high magnitude among several WHOQOL domains and emotional, conduct and internalizing problems in adolescents. Furthermore, was found a significant positive association of moderate magnitude between the Prosocial Scale and QOF in children. These results corroborate

previous findings that parents with more serious illnesses are expected to have children with impaired quality of life, emotional distress, and behavior problems [47]. Although there are many questions about the term quality of life, and this term is considered by many authors to be difficult to evaluate [38], studies have shown that mentally ill children have a lower health-related quality of life (HRQL) than healthy or somatically ill children [47]. The effect of having a mentally ill parent on QOL may be related to mental distress and may evolve into more serious problems in the future.

The well-being of children of inpatients with mental disorders is a aspect that is not systematically collected by institutions, since the focus of the intervention remains centered on the inpatient. When the relative is hospitalized, it is an opportunity for the health service to protect and potentially strengthen the bond between the children their parents and promote the detection of mental problems and well-being of the children [54]. The results of our study indicate that there is a major need to evaluate and refer to the treatment of the children of inpatients who are often neglected due to the serious health situation of their main caregiver. Of the children evaluated in the present study, 17.8% were already in treatment, which may be considered a low rate for a population at risk. In addition, we found that another 41% of the children had some mental health problem that needed specialized evaluation, so they were referred to specialized professionals. Early intervention and prevention offer the possibility to avoid mental health problems in adults and improve personal well-being and productivity [3].

It was determined that in relation to parental diagnoses, unipolar depression was prevalent in 52% of hospitalized relatives. This is often an incapacitating psychiatric illness that leads to difficulties in self-care and self-management. These difficulties can have repercussions on family relationships and impact the lives of the children. Descendants of parents with major depression disorders have higher rates of psychiatric disorder than children of parents who are not affected. Children with unipolar depression are more likely to have a parent with unipolar depression than other parental diseases [55]. Common parenting styles among parents with depression, such as low levels of child monitoring, may also play a role in the development of childhood mental health problems [13]. Hammen [56] found that the patterns of parenting established by depressed mothers can be learned by their children, who later parent the same way and maintain negative patterns of interaction over generations. Most studies examining parental mental illness have assessed adults with depressive symptoms and have found a 3–4 fold increase in symptomatology in children compared to controls [12]. The type of psychiatric illness, severity, associated impairments, as well as the degree of support from other family members seems to influence this risk. Compared with children of healthy parents, those living with serious mental illness may also be exposed to greater material deprivation, increased adult responsibilities and self-care, and increased risk of maltreatment and neglect [47].

The adequate identification of children at risk allows a quick referral for care. The possibility of intervention and follow-up of these children could reduce the suffering and psychiatric symptoms in children and adolescents, as shown by international strategies and studies like Preventive Basic Care Management (PBCM) [55], and Let's Talk in Australia [57], which are programs that aim to identify if the children of patients with mental disorders situations need intervention and to promote well-being and quality of life. Screening and early intervention in children from high-risk psychopathology groups is a challenge that needs to be addressed. In tertiary environments, the first step is to identify patients with children, which is often difficult because they are not questioned and such information is not recorded in medical records. This is a subject that is rarely touched upon in medical practice and is still stigmatized because it is very difficult for parents to talk about these problems with their doctors [29]. There is evidence that both children and parents benefit from adequate identification, as this may influence the treatment and recovery of psychiatric illness. Thus, identifying and supporting an individual's parenting role can provide hope, a sense of action, self-determination, and meaning, all aligned with a recovery approach. For those parents with a mental illness, parental support can provide a sense of competence, belonging, identity, hope and meaning that is well aligned with the concept of personal recovery [57]. In addition to the arguments of how societal costs can be reduced by early intervention, there is also ethical responsibility to the most vulnerable young people, who can have their full developmental potential thwarted [3]. We still have a lot to do for these children and adolescents in order to identify risk situations, try to alleviate suffering and prevent new diseases.

This study has several limitations. First, our sample size is very small, which excluded the ability to use several analytical strategies. Our sample size suffered a lot of losses due to logistical difficulties (i.e., location of caregivers, difficulties of accessing them to the hospital, and refusal of many parents to allow the evaluation of their children) and the non-routinization of this type of assessment in the unit. However, we believe that the data presented is significant and may still be underestimate the effect of having a parent with mental illness on the well-being of a child. Nevertheless, we are implementing an evaluation routine for children of inpatients

based this study. Second, the sample consisted of patients and their children from only one psychiatric unit, which decreases its external validity. However, since screening programs are not usually used in our environment, we believe that our data is indicative of a much larger problem, and replications will be required. In addition, short hospitalizations, with less than a week, also made some evaluations unviable. Finally, the data on psychopathology in children were collected from their caregivers, which may have influenced the evaluation, since many of them also exhibited psychiatric symptoms. However, quality of life assessments were conducted directly with children and adolescents, allowing a more direct measure of the impact of parental symptoms in their lives.

This work reinforces the importance of the routine screening of psychopathology in children of hospitalized psychiatric patients. Several barriers related to economic factors, integration of the health system, inadequate insurance coverage and unavailability, and overloading of the teams make it difficult for children and adolescents to access health services [58]. The development of assistance is also hampered by lack of government policy, inadequate funding, and a dearth of trained professionals [3]. Thus, we believe that the insertion of the evaluation routine of children of patients can be an important step for the identification of vulnerable children and adolescents stresses the need for institutions and governments to construct public policies that prioritize this issue.

Authors' contributions

ALA and LS conceptualized the study. LS performed the statistical analyses. All authors drafted the first version of the manuscript. All authors had substantial contributions to the interpretation of data for the work, revised it critically for important intellectual content and approved the final version submitted to the journal. All authors agreed with all aspects of the work in ensuring that questions related to the accuracy or integrity of any part of the work are appropriately investigated and resolved. All authors read and approved the final manuscript.

Author details

[1] Núcleo de Formação em Neurociências da Escola de Medicina da Pontifícia, Universidade Católica do Rio Grande do Sul, Av. Ipiranga 6690, Porto Alegre CEP 90619-900, Brazil. [2] Hospital São Lucas da Pontifícia Universidade Católica do Rio Grande do Sul, Av. Ipiranga 6690, 6º andar sul, Porto Alegre CEP 90619-900, Brazil.

Competing interests

The authors declare that they have no competing interests.

References

1. Vigo D, Thornicroft G, Atun R. Estimating the true global burden of mental illness. Lancet Psychiatry. 2016;3(2):171–8.
2. Kessler RC, et al. Lifetime prevalence and age-of-onset distributions of DSM-IV disorders in the National Comorbidity Survey Replication. Arch Gen Psychiatry. 2005;62(6):593–602.
3. Kieling C, et al. Child and adolescent mental health worldwide: evidence for action. Lancet. 2011;378(9801):1515–25.
4. Polanczyk GV, et al. Annual research review: a meta-analysis of the worldwide prevalence of mental disorders in children and adolescents. J Child Psychol Psychiatry. 2015;56(3):345–65.
5. Bronsard G, et al. The prevalence of mental disorders among children and adolescents in the child welfare system: a systematic review and meta-analysis. Medicine. 2016;95(7):e2622.
6. Williams NJ, Scott L, Aarons GA. Prevalence of serious emotional disturbance among U.S. children: a meta-analysis. Psychiatr Serv. 2017;69(1):32–40.
7. Lopes CS, et al. ERICA: prevalence of common mental disorders in Brazilian adolescents. Rev Saude Publica. 2016;50(Suppl 1):14s.
8. Viana MC, Andrade LH. Lifetime prevalence, age and gender distribution and age-of-onset of psychiatric disorders in the Sao Paulo Metropolitan Area, Brazil: results from the Sao Paulo Megacity Mental Health Survey. Rev Bras Psiquiatr. 2012;34(3):249–60.
9. Petresco S, et al. Prevalence and comorbidity of psychiatric disorders among 6-year-old children: 2004 Pelotas Birth Cohort. Soc Psychiatry Psychiatr Epidemiol. 2014;49(6):975–83.
10. Dean K, et al. Full spectrum of psychiatric outcomes among offspring with parental history of mental disorder. Arch Gen Psychiatry. 2010;67(8):822–9.
11. Gottesman II, et al. Severe mental disorders in offspring with 2 psychiatrically ill parents. Arch Gen Psychiatry. 2010;67(3):252–7.
12. Weissman MM, et al. Remissions in maternal depression and child psychopathology: a STAR*D-child report. JAMA. 2006;295(12):1389–98.
13. Olfson M, et al. Parental depression, child mental health problems, and health care utilization. Med Care. 2003;41(6):716–21.
14. Mowbray CT, et al. Children of mothers diagnosed with serious mental illness: patterns and predictors of service use. Ment Health Serv Res. 2004;6(3):167–83.
15. Dean K, et al. Criminal conviction among offspring with parental history of mental disorder. Psychol Med. 2012;42(3):571–81.
16. Simioni AR, Pan PM, Gadelha A, et al. Prevalence, clinical correlates and maternal psychopathology of deliberate self-harm in children and early adolescents: results from a large community study. Rev Bras Psiquiatr. 2018;40(1):48–55.
17. Mok PL, et al. Parental psychiatric disease and risks of attempted suicide and violent criminal offending in offspring: a population-based cohort study. JAMA Psychiatry. 2016;73(10):1015–22.
18. Gureje O, et al. Parental psychopathology and the risk of suicidal behavior in their offspring: results from the World Mental Health surveys. Mol Psychiatry. 2011;16(12):1221–33.
19. McLaughlin KA, et al. Parent psychopathology and offspring mental disorders: results from the WHO World Mental Health Surveys. Br J Psychiatry. 2012;200(4):290–9.
20. Bassani DG, Padoin CV, Veldhuizen S. Counting children at risk: exploring a method to estimate the number of children exposed to parental mental illness using adult health survey data. Soc Psychiatry Psychiatr Epidemiol. 2008;43(11):927–35.
21. Maybery DJ, et al. Prevalence of parental mental illness in Australian families. Psychiatr Bull. 2009;33(1):22–6.
22. Reupert AE, Maybery JD, Kowalenko NM. Children whose parents have a mental illness: prevalence, need and treatment. Med J Aust. 2013;199(3 Suppl):S7–9.
23. Stambaugh LF, et al. Prevalence of serious mental illness among parents in the United States: results from the National Survey of Drug Use and Health, 2008-2014. Ann Epidemiol. 2017;27(3):222–4.
24. Biebel K, et al. The responsiveness of State Mental Health Authorities to parents with mental illness. Adm Policy Ment Health. 2004;32(1):31–48.
25. Potter R, et al. Missed opportunities: mental disorder in children of parents with depression. Br J Gen Pract. 2012;62(600):e487–93.
26. Paula CS, et al. The mental health care gap among children and adolescents: data from an epidemiological survey from four Brazilian regions. PLoS ONE. 2014;9(2):e88241.
27. Webb RT, et al. Mortality risk among offspring of psychiatric inpatients: a population-based follow-up to early adulthood. Am J Psychiatry. 2006;163(12):2170–7.
28. Nicholson J. Parenting and recovery for mothers with mental disorders. In: Levin BL, Becker MA, editors. A public health perspective of women's mental health. New York: Springer; 2010. p. 415.
29. Ramchandani P, Stein A. The impact of parental psychiatric disorder on children. BMJ. 2003;327(7409):242–3.
30. Howard LM, et al. Predictors of parenting outcome in women with psychotic disorders discharged from mother and baby units. Acta Psychiatr Scand. 2004;110(5):347–55.
31. Lauritzen C, et al. Factors that may facilitate or hinder a family-focus in the treatment of parents with a mental illness. J Child Fam Stud. 2015;24(4):864–71.
32. Saur AM, Loureiro SR. Psychometric properties of the Strengths and Difficulties Questionnaire: a literature review. Estudos de Psicologia. 2012;29:609–29.
33. DAWBA. SDQ Information for researchers and professionals about the Strengths & Difficulties Questionnaires. DAWBA family of mental heath measures. 2012. http://www.sdqinfo.com. Accessed 25th Nov 2017.
34. Spitzer R, Williams JBW, Kroenke K. Instruction manual: instructions for patient health questionnaire (PHQ) and GAD-7 measures. 2016. http://www.phqscreeners.com/select-screener. Accessed 13 May 2017.
35. Kroenke K, Spitzer RL, Williams JBW, et al. An ultra-brief screening scale for anxiety and depression: the PHQ-4. Psychosomatics. 2009;50(6):613–21.
36. Hirschfeld RM, Williams JB, Spitzer RL, et al. Development and validation of a screening instrument for bipolar spectrum disorder: the Mood Disorder Questionnaire. Am J Psychiatry. 2000;157(11):1873–5.
37. Castelo MS, Carvalho ER, Gerhard ES, Costa CM, Ferreira ED, Carvalho AF. Validity of the Mood Disorder Questionnaire in a Brazilian psychiatric population. Rev Bras Psiquiatr. 2010;32:424–8.
38. Assumpção FB, Kuczynski E, Sprovieri MH, Aranha EM. Quality of life evaluation scale (AUQEI): validity and reliability of a quality of life scale for children from 4 to 12 years-old. Arq Neuropsiquiatr. 2000;58:119–27.
39. Skevington SM, et al. The World Health Organization's WHOQOL-BREF quality of life assessment: psychometric properties and results of the international field trial. A report from the WHOQOL group. Qual Life Res. 2004;13(2):299–310.
40. Fleck MP, et al. Application of the Portuguese version of the abbreviated instrument of quality life WHOQOL-bref. Rev Saude Publica. 2000;34(2):178–83.
41. Guy W. ECDEU assessment manual for psychopharmacology. Rockville: US Department of Health, Education, and Welfare Public Health Service Alcohol, Drug Abuse, and Mental Health Administration; 1976. p. 603.
42. Evans JD. Straightforward statistics for the behavioral sciences. 12th ed. Pacific Grove: Brooks/Cole Pub. Co; 1996. p. 600.
43. Oladeji BD, Gureje O. Parental mental disorders and suicidal behavior in the Nigerian survey of mental health and well-being. Arch Suicide Res. 2011;15(4):372–83.
44. Santana GL, et al. The influence of parental psychopathology on offspring suicidal behavior across the lifespan. PLoS ONE. 2015;10(7):e0134970.
45. Atwoli L, et al. Association between parental psychopathology and suicidal behavior among adult offspring: results from the cross-sectional South African Stress and Health survey. BMC Psychiatry. 2014;14:65.
46. Salum GA, et al. High risk cohort study for psychiatric disorders in childhood: rationale, design, methods and preliminary results. Int J Methods Psychiatr Res. 2015;24(1):58–73.
47. Silke Wiegand-Grefe SH, Franz Petermann, Angela Plass. Psychopathology and quality of life in children of mentally ill parents, in mental illnesses—evaluation, treatments and implications. In: L'Abate L, editor. InTech; 2012.
48. Bee P, Berzins K, Calam R, et al. Defining quality of life in the children of parents with severe mental illness: a preliminary stakeholder-led model. PLoS One. 2013;8(9):e73739.
49. Rutter M, Quinton D. Parental psychiatric disorder: effects on children. Psychol Med. 1984;14(4):853–80.

50. Biederman J, et al. Patterns of psychopathology and dysfunction in high-risk children of parents with panic disorder and major depression. Am J Psychiatry. 2001;158(1):49–57.

51. Middeldorp CM, et al. Parents of children with psychopathology: psychiatric problems and the association with their child's problems. Eur Child Adolesc Psychiatry. 2016;25(8):919–27.

52. Larson RW. Toward a psychology of positive youth development. Am Psychol. 2000;55(1):170–83.

53. Krumm S, Becker T, Wiegand-Grefe S. Mental health services for parents affected by mental illness. Curr Opin Psychiatry. 2013;26(4):362–8.

54. Ostman M, Hansson L. Children in families with a severely mentally ill member. Prevalence and needs for support. Soc Psychiatry Psychiatr Epidemiol. 2002;37(5):243–8.

55. Wansink HJ, Drost RMWA, Paulus ATG, et al. Cost-effectiveness of preventive case management for parents with a mental illness: a randomized controlled trial from three economic perspectives. BMC Health Serv Res. 2016;16:228.

56. Hammen C. Depression runs in families—the social context of risk and resilience in children of depressed mothers. New York: Springer; 1991. p. 275.

57. Maybery D, Goodyear M, Reupert A, et al. Developing an Australian-first recovery model for parents in Victorian mental health and family services: a study protocol for a randomised controlled trial. BMC Psychiatry. 2017;17(1):198.

58. Patel V, et al. Improving access to care for children with mental disorders: a global perspective. Arch Dis Child. 2013;98(5):323–7.

Permissions

All chapters in this book were first published in CAPMH, by BioMed Central; hereby published with permission under the Creative Commons Attribution License or equivalent. Every chapter published in this book has been scrutinized by our experts. Their significance has been extensively debated. The topics covered herein carry significant findings which will fuel the growth of the discipline. They may even be implemented as practical applications or may be referred to as a beginning point for another development.

The contributors of this book come from diverse backgrounds, making this book a truly international effort. This book will bring forth new frontiers with its revolutionizing research information and detailed analysis of the nascent developments around the world.

We would like to thank all the contributing authors for lending their expertise to make the book truly unique. They have played a crucial role in the development of this book. Without their invaluable contributions this book wouldn't have been possible. They have made vital efforts to compile up to date information on the varied aspects of this subject to make this book a valuable addition to the collection of many professionals and students.

This book was conceptualized with the vision of imparting up-to-date information and advanced data in this field. To ensure the same, a matchless editorial board was set up. Every individual on the board went through rigorous rounds of assessment to prove their worth. After which they invested a large part of their time researching and compiling the most relevant data for our readers.

The editorial board has been involved in producing this book since its inception. They have spent rigorous hours researching and exploring the diverse topics which have resulted in the successful publishing of this book. They have passed on their knowledge of decades through this book. To expedite this challenging task, the publisher supported the team at every step. A small team of assistant editors was also appointed to further simplify the editing procedure and attain best results for the readers.

Apart from the editorial board, the designing team has also invested a significant amount of their time in understanding the subject and creating the most relevant covers. They scrutinized every image to scout for the most suitable representation of the subject and create an appropriate cover for the book.

The publishing team has been an ardent support to the editorial, designing and production team. Their endless efforts to recruit the best for this project, has resulted in the accomplishment of this book. They are a veteran in the field of academics and their pool of knowledge is as vast as their experience in printing. Their expertise and guidance has proved useful at every step. Their uncompromising quality standards have made this book an exceptional effort. Their encouragement from time to time has been an inspiration for everyone.

The publisher and the editorial board hope that this book will prove to be a valuable piece of knowledge for researchers, students, practitioners and scholars across the globe.

List of Contributors

Andreas Witt, Rebecca C. Brown, Paul L. Plener and Jörg M. Fegert
Department of Child and Adolescent Psychiatry/ Psychotherapy, University of Ulm, Steinhövelstr. 5, 89073 Ulm, Germany

Elmar Brähler
Department of Psychosomatic Medicine and Psychotherapy, University Medical Center of Johannes Gutenberg University Mainz, Mainz, Germany
Department of Medical Psychology and Medical Sociology, University of Leipzig, Leipzig, Germany

Mahmood Karimy, Esmaeel Vali and Farzaneh Vali
Social Determinants of Health Research Center, Saveh University of Medical Sciences, Saveh, Iran

Ahmad Fakhri
Department of Psychiatry, Ahvaz Jundishapur University of Medical Sciences, Ahvaz, Iran

Feliciano H. Veiga
Institute of Education, University of Lisbon, Lisbon, Portugal

L. A. R. Stein
Psychology Dept., University of RI, Kingston, RI, USA
Behavioral and Social Sciences Dept., Brown University School of Public Health, Providence, RI, USA
RI Training School, Cranston, RI, USA

Marzieh Araban
Social Determinants of Health Research Center, Department of Health Education and Promotion, Public Health School, Ahvaz Jundishapur University of Medical Sciences Campus, Golestan BLVD, Ahvaz 61375-15751, Iran
Department of Health Education and Promotion, Public Health School, Ahvaz Jundishapur University of Medical Sciences Campus, Golestan BLVD, Ahvaz 61375-15751, Iran

Barbara Fallon, Joanne Filippelli, Tara Black and Nicolette Joh-Carnella
Factor-Inwentash Faculty of Social Work, University of Toronto, 246 Bloor Street West, Toronto, ON M6S 3W6, Canada

Nico Trocmé
McGill University, 3506 University Street, Room#301, Montreal, QC H3A 2A7, Canada

Elisabeth A. W. Janssen-de Ruijter and Chijs van Nieuwenhuizen
GGzE Centre for Child and Adolescent Psychiatry, (DP 8001), 5600 AX Eindhoven, The Netherlands
Scientific Center for Care and Welfare (Tranzo), Tilburg University, Tilburg, The Netherlands

Eva A. Mulder
Leiden University Medical Center, Leiden, The Netherlands
Intermetzo-Pluryn, Nijmegen, The Netherlands

Jeroen K. Vermunt
Department of Methodology and Statistics, Tilburg University, Tilburg, The Netherlands

Ingvild Oxås Henriksen
Regional Centre for Child and Youth Mental Health and Child Welfare, Faculty of Medicine, NTNU, Trondheim, Norway

Ingunn Ranøyen and Marit Sæbø Indredavik
Regional Centre for Child and Youth Mental Health and Child Welfare, Faculty of Medicine, NTNU, Trondheim, Norway
Department of Child and Adolescent Psychiatry, St. Olavs Hospital, Trondheim University Hospital, Trondheim, Norway

Frode Stenseng
Regional Centre for Child and Youth Mental Health and Child Welfare, Faculty of Medicine, NTNU, Trondheim, Norway
Queen Maud University College, Trondheim, Norway

Oraynab Abou Abbas
King Abdullah International Medical Research Center and King Saud Bin Abdulaziz University for Health Sciences, Riyadh, Kingdom of Saudi Arabia

Fadia AlBuhairan
King Abdullah International Medical Research Center and King Saud Bin Abdulaziz University for Health Sciences, Riyadh, Kingdom of Saudi Arabia
Department of Pediatrics, King Abdullah Specialized Children's Hospital, King Abdulaziz Medical City, Riyadh, Kingdom of Saudi Arabia
Bloomberg School of Public Health, Johns Hopkins University, Baltimore, MD, USA

Veronica Kirsch, Ferdinand Keller, Dunja Tutus and Lutz Goldbeck
Department of Child and Adolescent Psychiatry and Psychotherapy, University of Ulm, Steinhoevelstr. 5, 89075 Ulm, Germany

Laura van Duin, Floor Bevaart, Carmen H. Paalman, Marie-Jolette A. Luijks, Josjan Zijlmans, Reshmi Marhe, Theo A. H. Doreleijers and Arne Popma
Department of Child and Adolescent Psychiatry, VU University Medical Center, Meibergdreef 5, 1105 AZ Amsterdam, The Netherlands

Arjan A. J. Blokland
Leiden Law School, Leiden University, Institute of Criminal Law and Criminology, 2300 RA Leiden, The Netherlands

Marie Laure Baranne and Bruno Falissard
CESP, INSERM U1018, Université Paris-Saclay, Université Paris-Sud, UVSQ, APHP, Paris, France

Sanne L. Hillege and Lieke van Domburgh
Department of Child and Adolescent Psychiatry, VU University Medical Center, Duivendrecht, Amsterdam 1115 ZG, The Netherlands
Intermetzo-Pluryn, Nijmegen, The Netherlands

Eddy F. J. M. Brand
Department of Justice, National Agency of Correctional Institutions, The Hague, The Netherlands

Eva A. Mulder
Intermetzo-Pluryn, Nijmegen, The Netherlands
Curium-LUMC, Leiden University Medical Center, Leiden, The Netherlands

Robert R. J. M. Vermeiren
Department of Child and Adolescent Psychiatry, VU University Medical Center, Duivendrecht, P.O. Box 303, Amsterdam 1115 ZG, The Netherlands
Curium-LUMC, Leiden University Medical Center, Leiden, The Netherlands

L. Poulmarc'h, S. Colin, M. Valentin and J. Pradère
Service Universitaire de Psychiatrie de l'Adolescent, Argenteuil Hospital Centre, Argenteuil, France

J. Sibeoni, E. Costa-Drolon and A. Revah-Levy
Service Universitaire de Psychiatrie de l'Adolescent, Argenteuil Hospital Centre, Argenteuil, France
ECSTRA Team, UMR-1153, Inserm, Paris Diderot University, Sorbonne Paris Cite, Paris, France

Judy Wanjiru Mbuthia, Mary Wangari Kuria and Caleb Joseph Othieno
Department of Psychiatry, College of Health Sciences, University of Nairobi, Nairobi 00202, Kenya

Manasi Kumar
Department of Psychiatry, College of Health Sciences, University of Nairobi, P.O.Box 19676, Nairobi 00202, Kenya
Research Department of Clinical Health and Educational Psychology, University College London, Gower Street, London WC1E 6BT, UK

Fredrik Falkenström
Department of Behavioural Sciences and Learning, Linköping University, Linköping, Sweden

Inge Simons and Henk Rigter
Department of Child and Adolescent Psychiatry, Curium-Leiden University Medical Center, 2300 AA Leiden, The Netherlands

Eva Mulder
Department of Child and Adolescent Psychiatry, Curium-Leiden University Medical Center, Post Box 15, 2300 AA Leiden, The Netherlands
Intermetzo-Pluryn, 6500 AB Nijmegen, The Netherlands

René Breuk
Intermetzo-Pluryn, 6500 AB Nijmegen, The Netherlands

Kees Mos
Youth Interventions Foundation, 2300 AA Leiden, The Netherlands

Lieke van Domburgh
Intermetzo-Pluryn, Post Box 53, 6500 AB Nijmegen, The Netherlands
Department of Child and Adolescent Psychiatry, De Bascule-VUmc, Post Box 303, 1115 ZG Duivendrecht, The Netherlands

Robert Vermeiren
Department of Child and Adolescent Psychiatry, Curium-Leiden University Medical Center, Post Box 15, 2300 AA Leiden, The Netherlands
Department of Child and Adolescent Psychiatry, De Bascule-VUmc, Post Box 303, 1115 ZG Duivendrecht, The Netherlands

Minha Hong
Department of Psychiatry, Myongji Hospital, Seonam University, College of Medicine, Goyang, Republic of Korea

Han Nah Cho and Ah Reum Kim
Hallym University Suicide and School Mental Health Institute, Hallym University, Anyang, Republic of Korea

Hyun Ju Hong
Hallym University Suicide and School Mental Health Institute, Hallym University, Anyang, Republic of Korea
Department of Psychiatry, Hallym University Sacred Heart Hospital, College of Medicine, Hallym University of Korea, Anyang, Republic of Korea

Yong-Sil Kweon
Hallym University Suicide and School Mental Health Institute, Hallym University, Anyang, Republic of Korea
Department of Psychiatry, Uijeongbu St. Mary's Hospital, College of Medicine, The Catholic University of Korea, 222 Banpo-daero, Seocho-gu, Seoul 16591, Republic of Korea

Soo Jin Kwon
Nursing Science Research Institute, Chung-Ang University, Seoul, Republic of Korea

Yoonjung Kim and Yeunhee Kwak
Faculty of Red Cross College of Nursing, Chung-Ang University, 84 Heukseok-Ro, Dongjack-Gu, Seoul 156-756, Republic of Korea

Sauharda Rai, Safar Bikram Adhikari and Nanda Raj Acharya
Transcultural Psychosocial Organization Nepal (TPO Nepal), Anek Marga, Baluwatar, Kathmandu, Nepal

Bonnie N. Kaiser
Duke Global Health Institute, Duke University, Durham, NC, USA

Brandon A. Kohrt
Transcultural Psychosocial Organization Nepal (TPO Nepal), Anek Marga, Baluwatar, Kathmandu, Nepal
Duke Global Health Institute, Duke University, Durham, NC, USA
Department of Psychiatry and Behavioral Sciences, George Washington University, Washington, DC, USA
Department of Psychiatry, Duke University, Durham, NC, USA

Joanna Lockwood, David Daley and Kapil Sayal
Division of Psychiatry and Applied Psychology, Institute of Mental Health, University of Nottingham, University of Nottingham Innovation Park, Triumph Road, Nottingham NG7 2TU, UK
Centre for ADHD and Neurodevelopmental Disorders Across the Lifespan, Institute of Mental Health, University of Nottingham, Nottingham, UK

Ellen Townsend and Leonie Royes
Self-Harm Research Group, School of Psychology, University of Nottingham, Nottingham, UK

Michelle Siu Min Lauw, Abishek Mathew Abraham and Cheryl Bee Lock Loh
Department of Psychological Medicine, Changi General Hospital, 2 Simei Street 3, Singapore 529889, Singapore

Ole Jakob Storebø
Child and Adolescent Psychiatric Department, Region Zealand, Denmark
Psychiatric Research Unit, Region Zealand, Denmark
Institute of Psychology, University of Southern Denmark, Odense, Denmark

Anders Bo Bojesen and Niels Bilenberg
Child and Adolescent Psychiatric Department and, Psychiatric Research Unit, University of Southern Denmark, Odense, Denmark

Erik Simonsen
Psychiatric Research Unit, Region Zealand, Denmark
Department of Clinical Medicine, University of Copenhagen, Copenhagen, Denmark

Yael Shmueli-Goetz
Anna Freud National Centre for Children and Families, London, UK

Pernille Darling Rasmussen
Child and Adolescent Psychiatric Department, Region Zealand, Denmark
Psychiatric Research Unit, Region Zealand, Denmark
Child and Adolescent Psychiatric Department and, Psychiatric Research Unit, University of Southern Denmark, Odense, Denmark
Ny Østergade 12, 4000 Roskilde, Denmark

Han Byul Lee
Sunflower Center of Southern Gyeonggi for Women and Children Victims of Violence, Suwon, Republic of Korea

Kyoung Min Shin
Hanyang Cyber University, Seoul, Republic of Korea

Young Ki Chung and Hyoung Yoon Chang
Sunflower Center of Southern Gyeonggi for Women and Children Victims of Violence, Suwon, Republic of Korea
Department of Psychiatry and Behavioral Sciences, Ajou University School of Medicine, 164 World Cup-ro, Yeongtong-gu, Suwon, Suwon-si 16409, Republic of Korea
Center for Traumatic Stress, Ajou University Medical Center, Suwon, Republic of Korea

Namhee Kim
Department of Psychiatry and Behavioral Sciences, Ajou University School of Medicine, 164 World Cup-ro, Yeongtong-gu, Suwon, Suwon-si 16409, Republic of Korea
Center for Traumatic Stress, Ajou University Medical Center, Suwon, Republic of Korea

Yee Jin Shin
Yonsei University College of Medicine, Seoul, Republic of Korea

Un-Sun Chung
Kyungpook National University Hospital, Daegu, Republic of Korea

Seung Min Bae
Gil Hospital, Gachon University College of Medicine, Incheon, Republic of Korea

Minha Hong
Myongji Hospital, Seonam University College of Medicine, Goyang, Republic of Korea

Yuko Urao
Research Centre for Child Mental Development, Chiba University Graduate School of Medicine, 1-8-1 Inohana, Chuo-ku, Chiba 260-8670, Japan

Michiko Yoshida
Department of Cognitive Behavioural Physiology, Chiba University Graduate School of Medicine, 1-8-1 Inohana, Chuo-ku, Chiba 260-8670, Japan

Eiji Shimizu
Research Centre for Child Mental Development, Chiba University Graduate School of Medicine, 1-8-1 Inohana, Chuo-ku, Chiba 260-8670, Japan
Department of Cognitive Behavioural Physiology, Chiba University Graduate School of Medicine, 1-8-1 Inohana, Chuo-ku, Chiba 260-8670, Japan

Yasunori Sato
Department of Global Clinical Research, Chiba University Graduate School of Medicine, 1-8-1 Inohana, Chuo-ku, Chiba 260-8670, Japan

Shin-ichi Ishikawa
Department of Psychology, Doshisha University, 1-3 Tatara Miyakodani, Kyotanabe, Kyoto 610-0394, Japan

Takako Koshiba
Department of International Communication, Kanda University of International Studies, 1-4-1 Wakaba Mihama-ku, Chiba 261-0014, Japan

Yao-jun Shao, Tong Zheng, Yan-qiu Wang, Ling Liu, Yan Chen and Ying-shui Yao
Faculty of Epidemiology and Statistics, School of Public Health, Wannan Medical College, 22 Wenchang West Road, Yijiang District, Wuhu 241002, Anhui, People's Republic of China

Teresia Mutavi, Anne Obondo, Lincoln Khasakhala, Anne Mbwayo, Francis Njiri and Muthoni Mathai
Department of Psychiatry, School of Medicine, College of Health Sciences, University of Nairobi, Mlolongo, Nairobi, Kenya

Donald Kokonya
Department of Behavioural Sciences and Community Health, School of Medicine, Masinde Muliro University of Science and Technology, Kakamega, Kenya

Pola Heimann, Beate Herpertz-Dahlmann, Jonas Buning and Georg G. von Polier
Department of Child and Adolescent Psychiatry, Psychosomatics and Psychotherapy, RWTH Aachen University, Aachen, Germany

Norbert Wagner and Claudia Stollbrink-Peschgens
Department of Pediatrics, RWTH Aachen University, Aachen, Germany

Astrid Dempfle
Department of Medical Informatics and Statistic, University Schleswig-Holstein, Kiel, Germany

Ana Luiza Ache and Gibsi Possapp Rocha
Núcleo de Formação em Neurosciências da Escola de Medicina da Pontifícia, Universidade Católica do Rio Grande do Sul, Av. Ipiranga 6690, Porto Alegre CEP 90619-900, Brazil

Paula Fernandes Moretti and Rogéria Recondo
Hospital São Lucas da Pontifícia Universidade Católica do Rio Grande do Sul, Av. Ipiranga 6690, 6º andar sul, Porto Alegre CEP 90619-900, Brazil

Marco Antônio Pacheco and Lucas Spanemberg
Núcleo de Formação em Neurosciências da Escola de Medicina da Pontifícia, Universidade Católica do Rio Grande do Sul, Av. Ipiranga 6690, Porto Alegre CEP 90619-900, Brazil
Hospital São Lucas da Pontifícia Universidade Católica do Rio Grande do Sul, Av. Ipiranga 6690, 6º andar sul, Porto Alegre CEP 90619−900, Brazil

Index

www.ingramcontent.com/pod-product-compliance
Lightning Source LLC
Chambersburg PA
CBHW061303190326
41458CB00011B/3755